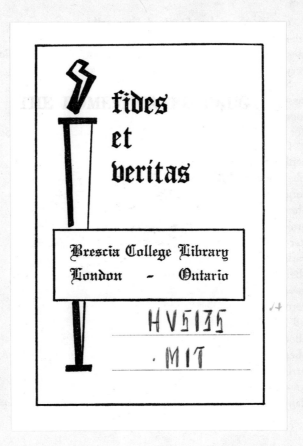

CONTRIBUTORS

C. Norman Alexander, *Stanford University*

Selden D. Bacon, *The State University of New Jersey*

James A. Belasco, *State University of New York at Buffalo*

Henry B. Bruyn, *University of California Medical School, San Francisco*

Ernest Q. Campbell, *Vanderbilt University*

Roderick S. Carman, *University of Colorado*

Peter H. Grossman, *Community Mental Health Service, Santa Clara County, California*

Joseph R. Gusfield, *University of Illinois*

Richard Jessor, *University of Colorado*

George L. Maddox, *Duke University*

Ephraim Harold Mizruchi, *Syracuse University*

Harold A. Mulford, *University of Iowa*

Peter Park, *University of Massachusetts*

Charles Peek, III, *University of Georgia*

Robert Perrucci, *Purdue University*

Lawrence Riggs, *College of Wooster*

Everett M. Rogers, *Michigan State University*

Paul M. Roman, *University of Georgia*

Robert D. Russell, *Southern Illinois University*

Robert Straus, *University of Kentucky College of Medicine*

Harrison M. Trice, *Cornell University*

Harry S. Warner,

Allan F. Williams, *The Medical Foundation, Boston, Massachusetts*

THE
DOMESTICATED DRUG

DRINKING AMONG COLLEGIANS

George L. Maddox, *Editor*

COLLEGE & UNIVERSITY PRESS · *Publishers*
NEW HAVEN, CONN.

"FOR THE MEMBERS OF THE DRINKING
BEHAVIOR COMMITTEE, SOCIETY FOR THE
STUDY OF SOCIAL PROBLEMS."

MANUFACTURED IN THE UNITED STATES OF AMERICA BY
UNITED PRINTING SERVICES, INC.
NEW HAVEN, CONN.

ACKNOWLEDGMENTS

We thank the following publishers and authors for permission to reprint copyrighted material in whole or in part:

Harry S. Warner, "Alcohol Trends in College Life," Board of Temperance, Prohibition and Public Morals of the Methodist Episcopal Church, 1938.

George L. Maddox, "Adolescence and Alcohol," in Raymond G. McCarthy (Ed.), *Alcohol Education for Classroom and Community*. McGraw-Hill, 1964. Abridged from pages 32-47.

George L. Maddox, "Role Making: Negotiations in Emergent Drinking Careers," *Social Science Quarterly*, Vol. 49, pp. 331-349, 1968.

Ernest Q. Campbell, "The Internalization of Moral Norms," *Sociometry*, Vol. 27, 1964, pp. 391-412.

Joseph R. Gusfield, "The Structural Context of College Drinking," *Quarterly Journal of Studies on Alcohol*, Vol. 22, 1961, pp. 428-443.

Richard Jessor, *et al.*, "Expectations of Need Satisfaction and Drinking Patterns of College Students," *Quarterly Journal of Studies on Alcohol*, Vol. 29, 1968, pp. 101-116.

Ephraim H. Mizruchi and Robert Perrucci, "Norm Qualities and Deviant Behavior," revised and extended from *American Sociological Review*, Vol. 27, 1962, pp. 391-399; and in E. H. Mizruchi (Ed.), *The Substance of Sociology*, 1967, Meredith Publishing Company, pp. 259-270, by permission of Appleton-Century-Crofts.

PREFACE

For more than a decade the Society for the Study of Social Problems has sponsored the publication of books which have seemed especially timely and useful to its members in general or to the members of one or another of its special committees. During this time, for example, volumes have appeared on mental health and mental disorder; on work and leisure; on understanding deviance; and on the opportunities and problems of applied sociology. The Society derives royalties from the sale of such books and this income is, in turn, used to further the work of the Society.

In 1962, the Drinking Behavior Committee, one of the special interest groups within the Society for the Study of Social Problems, encouraged David J. Pittman of Washington University and Charles R. Snyder of Southern Illinois University to edit a volume surveying, reviewing, and summarizing the accumulated research on drinking behavior in the social sciences. This volume, published by John Wiley and Sons, Inc., appeared as *Society, Culture, and Drinking Behavior*. In September, 1965, the proposal which culminated in the present volume was made to and accepted by the Committee on Drinking Behavior. Over a decade had passed since Straus and Bacon had published their systematic survey of drinking in college. In the intervening years occasional articles on drinking among older youth appeared in various sources. For those interested in drinking among collegians —educators, research social scientists, college administrators, the informed adult, and perhaps students themselves—access to the available articles was inconvenient. But perhaps of greater significance, the available articles, considered cumulatively, left many relevant issues untouched.

This volume does not raise all the issues worth raising. Readers on more than one occasion will feel that other issues warrant attention and that some of the issues considered warrant more attention than they receive. Nevertheless, it is hoped that this volume will be of interest and prove useful not only for members of the Society for the Study of Social Problems but also for a wide variety of readers. For the teachers and students of courses in sociology and social problems, this volume should prove to be useful supplementary reading in an area of unusual intrinsic interest for students. For college administrators, the research reviewed and the interpretations of drinking behavior among collegians should provide some perspective in the chapters which follow, on one of the more persistently troublesome issues found on many college campuses. They may be especially troubled by the suggestion which is repeatedly made in this volume that the American college campus reflects in its drinking rules much of the confusion endemic in our society historically in regard to drinking. In a sense, many colleges not only have problems involving student drinking; collegiate rules about drinking are also part of and contribute to that problem. For the research social scientist, the empirical studies reported in this volume illustrate the ways in which the study of drinking behavior, while interesting in its own right, can be used to understand in general terms social aspects of human development; role playing, role taking, and role making; the impact of social norms and structure on behavior; and aspects of conformity and deviance. Hopefully, there will be something also for the general reader who wants to get only an impression of what collegians are thinking about and doing with beverage alcohol. Insofar as possible, highly technical research material has been minimized or at least balanced with material and with a style that should interest the general reader.

The work of many people is reflected in a volume such as this. Although they are too numerous to name specifically, special thanks must be given to the contributors whose work made the volume possible. Their only reward will be my thanks and the satisfaction they derive from having made a contribution to the work of the Society for the Study of Social Problems.

GEORGE L. MADDOX

Duke University
August, 1967

CONTENTS

Section C. Drinking Means Many Things

PART ONE
PERSPECTIVE

INTRODUCTORY NOTE

V ISITORS TO OUR SOCIETY frequently get the impression that we are preoccupied with drinking and drink with a certain sadness. This impression stems in part from their observation that, among the estimated 70 per cent of adults who drink more or less regularly, many drinkers appear to be troubled and troublesome. The impression that many Americans drink and contemplate drinking sadly is reinforced even more by what visitors hear Americans say about alcoholic beverages.

Americans seem unable to take drinking for granted, as an aspect of life to be enjoyed graciously or ignored. We talk a lot about drinking. Drinkers frequently feel they must explain why they drink as much or as little as they do. Abstainers seem compelled to justify their behavior, as though it mattered, or to mask their abstinence by the appearance of drinking. Drinking in our society is far from incidental behavior which follows incidentally and naturally when good friends get together; the prospect of having a few drinks is as likely, if not more likely, to be the occasion for getting together. If those who get together to drink are not really friends, no matter. The happy hours in America, whether in homes or in public places, are an institution which provides the appearance of friendship and intimacy without requiring its substance.

Preoccupation with drinking in the United States can be explained, at least in part. Liquor has troubled us for a long time. The American colonists were, as often as not, hard drinkers. Some of them discovered that liquor could be profitable as well as pleasurable when they explored the potentialities of exchanging rum and slaves. But even in Colonial times there were misgivings about drinking. Benjamin Rush, a physician and one of the signers of the Declaration of Independence, was a harbinger of what was to come. Dr. Rush attacked the widespread notion of his time that liquor was good for working folk. By the 1840's a substantial number of Americans were doubting publicly that drinking was good for anyone. Their original notion was to promote temperance (i.e., moderation) through moral suasion. In time some of these doubters organized themselves into po-

13

litical pressure groups dedicated to legal restraint of all drinking and became the forerunners of national prohibition in the twentieth century. These same people coined the idea that made Mr. Welch a rich man; their theologians concluded belatedly that the Bible supported only total abstinence. Grape juice in the communion cup became traditional among many Protestant groups following eighteen centuries during which Christians had used wine gladly in the celebration of the sacraments.

Substantial prohibitionist sentiment and activity in a nation of hard drinkers are not easy to explain and have no simple explanation. But one of the important factors was an idea. For lack of a better label, this idea can be designated the *work ethic*. Its roots were deep in the religious tradition of Protestantism, particularly Calvinism. According to this way of looking at life, work is man's central life task, the great balance wheel of his life. Correspondingly, fun and games are typically suspect; the only kind thing that can be said for non-work activity is that it is re-creative, allowing a man to return to his labor a better worker. And, above all, the work ethic stresses the maintenance of self-control in the interest, presumably, of engaging with religious devotion in conspicuous productivity. An individual with such an orientation to life would, predictably, perceive drinking to be antithetical to the efficient, work-oriented life. If he drank, one would expect him to drink somewhat sadly, perhaps a bit guiltily too, and at considerable cost to his self-esteem. Seen from the perspective of the work ethic, liquor could do something to a drinker; it could do nothing for him that could not or should not be done some other way.

The prohibitionists did their best to save the nation from the inefficiencies which drinkers characteristically seemed to seek, exhibit, and tolerate and the influence of prohibitionists was at its height in the early decades of this century. Most Americans refused to be saved from some measure of inefficiency, however, and by the 1930's national prohibition came legally to an end. Currently, every state recognizes the legal sale of alcoholic beverages. Most people are probably pleased that alcoholic beverages are legally available. Since a substantial majority of adults drink at one time or another, this seems to be a reasonable assumption. But many people, whether they themselves drink or not, apparently still regard drinking as a sad experience. Every state has a statute requiring instruction about alcohol for

youth and the predominant interest of such instruction is to indoctrinate young people about the evils of alcohol. The message
is packaged many different ways but, more often than not, that
message is "Don't drink." Whether this means that drinking is
never justified, not justified until one is legally of age, or not
advisable until one understands the implications of what he is
doing is usually not very clear. Only rarely does anyone seem
to care very much about this ambiguity, at least not enough to
insist on clarification. In almost every state, the legal purchase
of liquor is reserved for those 21 years of age. Even then, a
drinker finds alcoholic beverages burdened with a tax that can
be interpreted only as punitive and finds himself hedged with
restrictions designed to make drinking inconvenient. If the drinker is a collegian, he commonly finds administrative restrictions
on his behavior even more stringent than the state enforces for
citizens generally. In colleges that continue to assume administrators are *in loco parentis*, administrative rules that are no more
stringent than the state requires, e.g., rules that would permit
a 21-year-old student to drink openly and remain in good standing if his behavior were otherwise appropriate, remain uncommon and must be treated as a mark of liberality or moral indifference, depending on who does the evaluating. Studied ambiguity in drinking rules, their application, or both, characterize
the situation on most college campuses in the United States.

Poking fun at the indications of our uneasiness about drinking
is easy enough to do. The morally convinced abstainer can and
surely does sound like a spoilsport at times. He may even
manufacture or perpetuate some demonstrably false information
to support his contention that no drinking is really defensible.
Unfortunately, the shriller and more extreme the denunciations
of liquor, the easier it becomes to overlook the gross inepti-
tude of quite a few Americans in holding their liquor and
to avoid discussing frankly what it means to drink responsibly.
Alcohol-related problems do not need exaggeration; even conservative estimates of overdrinking and drinking abuses in our
society suggest a serious and disturbing situation. The seriousness of some common problems among drinkers surely concerns
all thoughtful people, drinkers and abstainers alike. Consider,
for example, intoxication.

Intoxication is a common type of inefficiency among drinkers.
Exactly how common being high, tight, or drunk is among drink-

ers is not known exactly, but some loss of control while drinking is frequently reported by both high school students and collegians. Among adults, public drunkenness is one of the most frequent occasions for arrest, and drinking while driving is demonstrably a factor associated with a high proportion, perhaps half, of all fatal automobile accidents. Precise, valid statistics are hard to come by in discussions of drunkenness and its consequences. In the great majority of instances, intoxication from drinking alcoholic beverages is probably only mild and its personal and social effects are probably inconsequential. But there is little room for argument that gross inefficiencies in drinking behavior are also common and that, in a substantial number of cases, loss of self-control takes place without adequate provision being made by the drinker for himself or for others with whom he might be in contact. There is a still more dramatic abuse of drinking, alcoholism.

An estimated five million adults, some 6 per cent of those who drink, are in serious trouble. This is nothing more than an educated guess, but most knowledgeable people agree that the incidence of severe drinking problems is high in the United States. While all these people are not in trouble as a result of their drinking for exactly the same reasons or to the same degree, they have one thing in common: They are preoccupied with drinking. Liquor has become the hub around which their lives revolve. Having drunk too much for too long, they have a high probability of being seriously impaired physically, psychologically, and socially. Being mildly out of control is the occasional experience of most drinkers. Even the moderate social drinker may deliberately seek now and then some relief from the usual constraints of the workaday world, especially if his drinking is to be in a safe, protected environment with family or friends. For the alcoholic, however, seeking relief from the experience of himself and the world in which he lives through overdrinking and intoxication is a preoccupation which preempts every other concern. His drinking is frequently out of control even when there is no reasonable expectation of safety for himself or others; and the length of time his drinking is out of control reduces his capacity for personal and social functioning below the level significant people in his environment will accept and finally below the level he can tolerate himself. He eventually hits bottom. Although Americans frequently are amused by the intoxicated person who is gentlemanly, benign, and in control to an appropriate degree, no one is really amused by an alcoholic. As the National Council on Alcoholism tells everyone who will listen, the alcoholic is seriously and, unless helped, often fatally ill. The alcoholic can be helped, the National Council adds, but the intervention that is usually required is extensive. The rehabilitation of ubiquitous alcoholics taxes severely the reserves of compassion and helping resources of any community whose citizens are informed and concerned about the rich men, poor men, beggarmen, thieves, doctors, lawyers, merchants, and chiefs whose drinking is intolerably inefficient.

Americans do not have the highest per capita consumption of alcoholic beverages in the world. They do have one of the highest rates of alcoholism and more than their share of trouble with excessive drinking. The casual observer would have to wonder, along with the prohibitionist, why a nation so preoccupied with the potential problems associated with drinking and so aware of actual drinking abuses continues to find drinking worthwhile. The answer is disarmingly simple: alcoholic beverages presumably do something for drinkers that they want done. And they want that something enough to take their chances with what drinking in the unusual instance might do to them or to others. That sounds irresponsible and there is no question that under some circumstances drinkers are irresponsible. But there is really no convincing evidence that drinkers are generally more irresponsible or less concerned about responsibility than most people. After all, most people including many citizens who certainly appear to be responsible, are drinkers.

What do most drinkers expect drinking to do for them? There is no single, simple answer since drinking means different things to different people. Most people expect drinking to say something about who they are, to identify them with a cultural tradition and a style of life. Some men say something about themselves by standing and gulping their drinks, others by sitting and sipping. In either case, to ignore where, with whom, when, and how a person drinks and concentrate on the fact that the drinker is consuming so many ounces of absolute alcohol is to miss the social aspects of drinking altogether. Drinking can be and is for many what is done when congenial people get together; it is an experience which is integrated and integrating in their lives. More than that, there is a mystic quality to drinking which our ancient ancestors surely recognized when they talked of alcohol as *aqua vitae*. Birth, communion, betrothal, death—all have historically been celebrated with the cup by religious people.

Drinking is also associated with the transformation and transcendence of reality as it is ordinarily perceived by secular and religious folk alike. The use of alcoholic beverages to modify reality may be utilitarian as well as mystical. In an efficiency-oriented society, drinking to inebriety is surely the perpetuation of an ancient and socially recognized form of inefficiency. Alcohol is man's original tranquilizer, one of his means of tuning out the insistent demands of the workaday world; it is one of his ways of making himself and his world seem just a little bit nicer than in fact either is. For youth, no longer children but not yet adults, drinking can be a declaration of independence and more. Their role as children can be dissolved in alcohol and drinking can be an introduction to the world of adults. Alcohol can also have less subtle, more blatant utilitarian functions too.

With drink in hand, an individual may have ideas about making a girl or a sale as well as remaking himself and his world. Our culture, which takes due note of various chemical comforts, has an elaborate mythology about drinking as a facilitator of sex and commerce. Like all mythology, the expectations about what alcohol can do to and for people who have places to go and things to do are a wondrous mixture of fact and fancy. The shared expectation that a drink or two facilitates a deal, sexual or otherwise, may help the drinker to fulfill his wishes. The known inhibition-reducing effects of alcohol on the central nervous system surely make a contribution too.

Drinking as a social integrator or as a means of reality modification usually seems harmless enough and may even seem a happy antidote to some of the personal ills which so many people experience in a segmented, inhibited society. For most, drinking apparently looks just that way. But, the drinking abuses on the part of a persistent, substantial minority cloud the picture. What starts as an expression of conviviality sometimes gets out of hand. Facilitation in remaking one's world with a drink or two can, and does for some, become a habit which looks very much like an attempt to escape from the world and from personal responsibility. For some, alcohol, a domesticated drug, ceases to be a beverage and becomes a chemical means of cooling out.

Why an individual cools out with alcohol is not altogether clear. There are clearly other ways to get the job done. Man's capacity to devise crutches of one sort or another apparently is infinite; the chemical comforts such as alcohol, medically prescribed tranquilizers, heroin, and LSD only hint at his ingenuity. It is sufficient here to note that, among the crutches available to the walking wounded in our society, alcohol continues to have a fatal attraction to a degree not found in most other societies, even those in which heavy drinking is common. While it is conceivable that an individual who is well integrated personally and socially can accidentally and inadvertently drink himself into some serious problems, there is increasing evidence that more commonly the problem lies in the man rather than in the bottle. People who have trouble living when they are sober run high risks when they drink. The relief which drinking offers troubled people is only temporary; and worse, drinking masks their underlying problems, increases the risk of social punishment, and dissipates whatever competence they have for problem solving. Even the awareness of the extremely high cost of drinking as an escape from reality does not and will not deter a persistent minority of escapist drinkers in our society. As a clinician with long years of experience with escapist drinkers once astutely observed, if you think an alcoholic is miserable when he is drinking, you ought to know him when he is sober.

The drinking behavior of Americans has not demonstrably taken a turn for the worse over the last three decades and there are a few hopeful signs. There are some indications, for example, that while the number of abstainers may be shrinking a bit, there is no convincing evidence of mass defection and there are some indications that voluntarily abstinent individuals are a bit more relaxed and comfortable with their abstinence. Drinking excesses, which are admittedly too common, are not demonstrably becoming more prevalent. There is perhaps only a little comfort in the observation that the situation is not as bad as it might be, given the peculiarities in the American way of drinking. But, if one concedes that drinking is here to stay, a concession which only a small minority will refuse to make, the apparently growing preference for beverage with a low alcoholic content and for drinking at home is a salutary factor. Of potentially greater significance is a fundamental change in attitudes toward drinking in our society.

Historically there has been a tendency for Americans to divide people into wets and drys, bad guys and good guys, even when most people who took sides about drinking knew that real issues are never so simple as that. One of the most unfortunate results of this simple response to a complex question was an undercutting of any basis for significant dialogue between and among those who drank and those who did not. Perhaps even worse, in the interest of self-defense, drinkers tended to minimize the possibilities of drinking abuses as much as abstainers tended to exaggerate them. Neither antagonist found much incentive for the conscious development of a responsible drinking ethic or of a convincing case for voluntary abstinence. Drinkers and abstainers alike have managed to avoid for a very long time an inquiry into whether, as long as a person is going to drink, there are some ways that are preferable to others. They have managed to avoid discussing whether, as long as a person is considering drinking, there are some things he ought to know about drinking. Drinkers and abstainers alike have spent very little time in trying to understand the historical roots of abstinence from alcohol and the complex motivations of abstainers.

We may be witnessing in our time a radical transformation in our thinking about drinking. We talk increasingly in our society as though we can and should distinguish between drinkers and alcoholics; occasionally people even talk as though alcoholics may not drink in the usual sense of that word at all. Drinkers and abstainers occasionally demonstrate a capacity to break through their ambivalence toward the alcoholic at least to the extent necessary to contemplate humane treatment for these refugees from life and to join forces against this extreme form of irresponsible drinking in a highly mechanized society. The alcohol beverage industry, with an enlightened self-interest which Americans should find it easy to understand, has played an increasingly important role in the development of education about the responsible use of alcohol. Some major religious groups, especially those historically committed to abstinence, have apparently decided to recognize that most Americans, including many of their own members, drink. They have understandably had some second thoughts, not about the wisdom and virtue of voluntary abstinence, but about a policy which automatically labels all drinkers as sinners and which provides no adequate basis for dialogue with these members who drink.

Dialogue does not necessarily solve problems. Yet dialogue among drinkers, among abstainers, and between them, is an important first step toward the development of a viable philosophy for America in regard to drinking and abstinence. Dialogue may help drinkers evaluate the motives for their drinking and help motivate them to explore the ways and means to reduce irresponsible drinking to the bare minimum. Dialogue may help abstainers evaluate their motives for abstinence and may help them explore the ways and means of making voluntary abstinence a viable option in a drinking society. The persistent minority for whom drinking does nothing that cannot be done in some other way certainly deserve support and need all the support they can get.

A happy conclusion to the increasing dialogue about the place of drinking and abstinence in the life of responsible men is hardly likely in the near future. But continuing discussion will be better enlightened and to the point as there is more and better information about what various groups of Americans think about and do with alcohol. This book is intended as a description and interpretation of patterns of drinking and abstinence among collegians.

Collegians are particularly good subjects for study. College students constitute a substantial and highly visible minority of older youth in this country. If present trends continue, in the near future a majority of youth between the ages of 18 and 22 will be on one or another college campus. In any case, both Robert Straus (chapter 1) and Harry S. Warner (chapter 2) agree that collegians stand out in the social portrait of our society as a vivid cross-section of prevailing attitudes, customs, and trends. College students are a commentary on the generation that rears them; they are a prophecy about the generation that will inherit the future. This fact contributes to their social visibility and the continual concern which adults exhibit with what students are thinking and doing.

Looking back fifteen years, Straus (chapter 1) notes that the research which he and Selden Bacon published in *Drinking in College* (New Haven: Yale University Press, 1953) refuted the prevalent notion of the college drinker as a distinctive breed. Most collegians, they found, drank moderately and usually began drinking before they entered college anyway. A small minority of college students—an estimated 6 per cent of the men and 1 per cent of the women—did present troublesome problems with drinking. But these troubles did not seem to have any single, simple explanation—Straus speculates that the sources were personal and situational—certainly not that being in college provides an explanation. Straus is particularly interested in the possibility that drinkers who have experienced extremely negative moral sanctions against drinking may be especially vulnerable.

Although Straus's characterization of drinking behavior among college students at mid-century has the authority of survey evidence carefully gathered and analyzed, his conclusions were anticipated by the perceptive review of historical documents and limited survey data by Harry S. Warner (chapter 2). Warner provides a colorful historical account of drinking among collegians in the United States over the past two centuries and of the collegian's faithful reflection of the rise and fall of prohibition in this country in the past century. If there is the slight suggestion of regret that prohibition failed in Warner's account, which was written in 1938 only shortly after the end of national prohibition, it is hardly surprising. Harry Warner has been a forceful proponent for abstinence during all his adult years. And, if he relies on statistics which appear questionable to the modern student of survey research, this is only a reminder that all survey research, past and present, needs careful scrutiny. Warner clearly has a positive feeling for older youth and for college life, which he continually exhibits. And, given his preference for abstinence, his conclusion is all the more striking: "College alcoholic pleasures, customs, and consequences are not different from those elsewhere in influential society." Although as a feature of publicity and public interest drinking among collegians has a place of its own, drinking among them follows social, class, family, and community standards.

The current evidence, such as it is, continues to indicate that exposure to higher education does not produce a distinctive kind of drinker. Harold Mulford, for example, reports in chapter 3 that, while the probability that an individual drinks increases with years of exposure to formal education, the difference between those who have only finished high school and those who have gone on to college is slight. Heavy drinking does appear to be higher among those who have had some exposure to college but this relationship is clearly complex and varies depending on the sex, place of residence, and religious affiliation of the drinker. Moreover, the drinker with some college experience, while he may drink more heavily than others, may well have less trouble with his drinking and may be less preoccupied with it than those with little education. Mulford is appropriately cautious in stating this conclusion. Actually, we have only tentative notions of what exposure to higher education means and how this exposure shapes the drinking behavior of collegians. Some of the chapters in Part II of this volume will provide some suggestions on these points. Moreover, as yet we have no simple procedure for identifying the emerging problem drinker among older youth. Some of the chapters in Part II may also be helpful on this point too.

For the most part, then, college drinkers continue to provide a portrait, though perhaps sometimes a caricature, of drinking behavior in society generally. And, in spite of some indications of increasing tension between the generations, of intensified identity crises among the young, and of increasing affluence which has mechanized more and more young people, drinking behavior among collegians has remained very much the same over several decades. The fluctuations in drinking behavior on the campuses, such as a surge of prohibitionist sentiment in the 1920's, have paralleled changes in the larger society. This is a testimony to the extent to which alcohol is our domesticated drug.

Of all the chemical modifiers available to us for the modification of personal perception and feeling and for the redefinition of social reality, alcohol is among the oldest, is one of the best understood, and hence most reliable, and is clearly the most popular. It is significant that when Bernard Barber in a recent review of man's uses and abuses of varied substances which have been called "drugs" (*Drugs and Society;* Russell Sage, 1967), alcohol received limited and ambiguous treatment. This is partly a reflection of public and professional preoccupation with "dangerous drugs" such as heroin and more recently LSD (for example, Richard Blum and associates, *Utopiates;* Atherton, 1965) or with drugs with especially troublesome legal histories such as marijuana (for example, Richard Goldstein, *One in Seven: Drugs on the Campus;* Walker, 1966).

There is a certain amusing quality to the attention being given to drug use on college campuses today. Straus correctly observes that drugs other than alcohol now receive the attention formerly given alcohol. He also is correct in noting that, while we can only speculate about the incidence of LSD or marijuana use by college students, marijuana and LSD are not effective rivals for alcohol as the contemporary drug of choice. The possibility that the older youth who formerly would have been the excessive drinker is now the most likely to experiment with the less-domesticated drugs is an additional commentary on the domestication of alcohol. Alcohol may, in fact, increasingly be the drug of choice for the "squares."

The domestication of any drug is, of course, a relative matter. Wide use in conventional ways and shared myths about how abuse can be minimized may and surely do mask drug abuse in a society. Alcohol is a case in point. Although the evidence is spotty, it is reasonable to guess that the actual incidence of trouble due to drinking on any college campus is far in excess of trouble due to the use of all other drugs combined.

In sum, this volume is intended to put the drinking behavior of college students in perspective. The domestication of alcohol is documented. So are the indications that this domestication is more complete in our social mythology than in fact. In their drinking as in so many other ways, college students continue to be a fair portrait, occasionally a caricature, of the society which produces them and of what society is becoming.

THE DOMESTICATED DRUG

Chapter 1

DRINKING IN COLLEGE IN THE
PERSPECTIVE OF SOCIAL CHANGE

ROBERT STRAUS

University of Kentucky, College of Medicine

TWENTY YEARS have now passed since planning was initiated for a study of the drinking customs and attitudes of American college students, the report of which was published in 1953 as *Drinking in College*.[1]

This chapter will provide a review of the background against which the study was conceived and conducted, summarize some of the principal findings, and speculate on how applicable these findings may be today in the perspective of changes in the social context of student drinking which have occurred during the past 20 years.

In 1947, few facts about drinking customs in the United States were known. Instead prevailing stereotypes based primarily on conjecture and misinformation provided distorted impressions of the nature of drinking behavior and drinking customs. The survey of college drinking was conceived as part of a larger program of multi-disciplinary study, then under way at the Yale Laboratory of Applied Physiology, concerned with many aspects of drinking behavior and alcohol-related problems.

College students, it was felt, could provide a particularly fruitful source of basic information about drinking customs because they were at an age when the onset of drinking for many people either takes place, or has been so recent that fairly accurate recall of factors associated with early drinking behavior is possible. Similarly, non-drinking college students could pro-

---

[1] Robert Straus and Selden D. Bacon, *Drinking in College* (New Haven: Yale University Press, 1953).

vide recent or contemporary data on their decisions to abstain and recount the pressures for or against drinking which they were experiencing. In the late 1940's, there were still many World War II veterans in college and they afforded an unusual opportunity to explore possible differences in drinking behavior between veterans and non-veterans who were living in a similar social situation.

Young people who attend college have generally been more conspicuous than their non-student peers who have usually joined the labor force and are scattered throughout the community. In some societies, the student population has been able to exert considerable political force.

Contemporary documents from every period since the founding of America's first colleges reveal that adults have been concerned about the behavior of college students. In 1967, this apprehension is focused on the use of cannabis, LSD and on the hippie movement. Although the real objects of concern are by no means limited to college students—in fact the majority may well be college dropouts or college-age hangers-on—such movements and the associated behavior are generally represented as a college problem. Similarly in 1947, drinking and intoxication provided the major focus for society's uneasiness about college youth. References in the contemporary press reflected the assumptions that many students drank, that most of these drank frequently and excessively, and that the result was often intoxication with ensuing embarrassment, disgrace, or serious problems. In *Drinking in College* this tendency was documented both historically and from the then contemporary scene. Even the "news" of the college drinking study was given wide publicity in the mass media, most of it reflecting the distortions of prevailing stereotypes, rather than fact. It was shown that almost any conspicuous untoward behavior involving students was apt to be blamed on drinking, sometimes in spite of contrary evidence.[2] Public attitudes and reactions toward college

[2] The tendency to blame drinking for any untoward incident involving college students was illustrated by a news item (circa 1950) about vandalism which occurred while a group of students were picnicking in a public park. Although the story reported in one paragraph that the vandalism had been positively traced by the police to a group of town troublemakers, another paragraph and the headline assumed that the students were responsible and placed blame on the "liquor problem."

drinking reflected the confusion and anxiety with which society faced broader questions regarding both socialization of youth and moral integration of drinking customs.

Because, in 1947, misconceptions about drinking seemed especially rampant with respect to the drinking behavior of college students, it was hoped that a study aimed at providing some factual knowledge to replace speculation could provide a basis for realistic explanations of behavior as well as suggest more realistic and effective action by persons concerned with the "problem" of student drinking, including educators, college administrators, parents, religious leaders, legislators, employers, judges, physicians, public health authorities and others called on to make policy decisions or provide guidance for young people.

Data for the study were furnished during 1949-51 by nearly 17,000 students from 27 American colleges and universities selected to provide representation of various kinds of schools and located in all major regions of the country, including students with varied sociocultural characteristics. Primary data were provided through questionnaires administered to students in classroom groups by a representative of the survey who provided a standardized explanation of the nature of the study. Supplementary data were gathered from discussions with students, faculty and administrators, a review of official and non-official campus policies toward drinking, and surveillance of the sociocultural context of the campus with respect to drinking.

Findings of the Study

Data from *Drinking in College* revealed wide variations in the incidence and nature of alcohol usage by students depending on such factors as age, sex, type of college, family income, religious affiliation and participation, and the incidence of drinking by parents and close friends.

Among the male students, users[3] of alcohol ranged from 92 per cent in private nonsectarian colleges, to 65 per cent in private colleges governed by a temperance doctrine; from 86 per cent of those with family income over $10,000 to 66 per cent of those with family income under $2,500; from 100 per cent of the

[3] "Users" of alcohol included all students who reported having consumed alcoholic beverages apart from experimental, joking or ceremonial use before age 11 or purely incidental, isolated experiences.

Jewish students who participated in formal religious activity at least weekly (and only 91 per cent of those who were irregular or non-participant in their religion) to only 21 per cent of the Mormon students who participated in their religion at least weekly (but 77 per cent of the Mormon students who were irregular or non-active); from 90 per cent of Catholic to 50 per cent of Protestant students who were regular religious participants; from 69 per cent of the freshmen to 87 per cent of the seniors; from 92 per cent of those whose parents both used alcohol to only 58 per cent of those whose parents both abstained; from 89 per cent of those whose close friends drank to only 16 per cent of those whose close friends abstained.

Women students showed similar but even greater ranges. Users ranged from 89 per cent in private nonsectarian women's colleges (and only 84 per cent in private nonsectarian coeducational schools) to 39 per cent in private temperance-oriented colleges; from 79 per cent of those with family income over $10,000 to only 30 per cent of those with family income below $2,500; from 83 per cent of those who were Jewish and regular religious participants to only 6 per cent of the Mormon regular participants (but 48 per cent of the Mormon irregular or non-participants); from 80 per cent of Catholics to 43 per cent of Protestants who attended church at least weekly; from 46 per cent of the freshmen to 77 per cent of the seniors; from 83 per cent of those whose parents were both users to 23 per cent of those whose parents both abstained; from 79 per cent of those whose close friends were users to 5 per cent of those whose close friends abstained.

Among college users, 79 per cent of the men and 65 per cent of the women reported having started drinking (beyond experimental, joking, ceremonial, or isolated incidents) before entering college.

By themselves, these various percentages must be interpreted with great care for they deal with gross averages, but they do suggest some distinctive patterns and relationships. It was found, for example, that most college students who use alcohol started to drink before entering college. The incidence of parental drinking had a clear relationship to the incidence of student drinking, although nearly three-fifths of the men and over one-fifth of the women whose parents both abstained were themselves users. There was a close relationship between the incidence of drinking among students and their close friends. There were significant religious differences and, especially within religious faiths, there were differences between regular and irregular or non-participants in religious activity. Other data suggested that age, sex, income, ethnicity are also significant factors related to drinking or abstaining. Together these data served to underline that the use or non-use of alcoholic beverages is a form of social behavior significantly affected by characteristics of the social environment. Yet, while social criteria establish ranges of behavior within which most individuals respond, there remains considerable latitude for individual variation and choice.

Most students indicated that they had received "specific advice concerning the use of alcoholic beverages" and over half of these indicated that they had been advised to abstain. Furthermore, 30 per cent of the men and 56 per cent of the women so advised were indeed abstainers compared with only 18 per cent of the men and 35 per cent of the women who reported that they had never been so advised. There were striking differences in the apparent effectiveness of advice against drinking depending on its source. While sanctions against drinking, as compared with no such advice, were moderately effective when they came from parents, advice not to drink which originated with the school or the church appeared actually less effective than no advice. Yet, when abstainers were asked why they refrained from drinking, religious or moral grounds were cited more frequently than the disapproval of parents. As might be expected, religious grounds for abstaining were given the greatest value by the Mormons whose religion resolutely condemns drinking, and no value by the relatively few Jewish abstainers in whose religion drinking has important symbolic meaning.

Of special interest was the relationship between student drinking and the perceived sanctions of their colleges. Colleges were assigned "liberality scores" based on several measures of their relative position in condemning or condoning drinking by students. There were, as might be expected, relatively more student users of alcohol in schools with high-liberality scores and fewer student users in schools with strong formal sanctions against drinking. It should not be interpreted from these findings that college sanctions, per se, influenced students' decisions to drink or not to drink, for as we have already seen most students who drank started doing so before entering college.

On the other hand, there was evidence to suggest that liberal colleges provided more effective controls against excessive drinking. While the non-liberal colleges had relatively fewer drinkers, the male students who did drink at such schools had relatively higher rates of drunkenness and of problems associated with intoxication. It was concluded that students who drink in violation of generally accepted practice are apt to go further in their drinking than students for whom the use of alcoholic beverages is not made an issue. This reaction was illustrated by a student in a school which had strong sanctions against drinking who noted: "When you go to the trouble of driving 50 miles to drink, you don't have just two drinks."

The influence of parental practices and attitudes on the drinking behavior of college students was evident from several kinds of data. About a third of the men and over half of the women reported that their first drinking beyond childhood experiences occurred in their own homes and/or in the company of family members. As already noted, parental example and parental advice appeared to be moderately significant influences especially with daughters, although many more students than parents were using alcohol.

Data on the types of alcoholic beverage used by college students revealed wide variations, influenced by such factors as the context of drinking, companions when drinking, reasons for drinking, and by such practical considerations as the availability and cost of different types of beverage.

Among college men, beer was clearly the beverage of most frequent use and was also slightly preferred over distilled spirits. College women users, on the other hand, used distilled spirits just as frequently as beer and most expressed a preference for spirits. Most male beer users did so in male company, while most who used spirits did so in mixed company. Women, on the other hand, reported that most of their drinking, irrespective of beverage type, took place in mixed company. The beer-drinking fellowship stood out as a pattern common to male students in virtually every college studied.

As noted earlier, popular stereotypes in 1947 were found to depict most college students as engaging in frequent and heavy drinking leading to unfortunate or disgraceful behavior, and they assumed that most inappropriate behavior involving students was caused by excessive drinking. Evidence from the drinking in college study clearly refuted the image conveyed by such stereotypes. Of all the students who drank, only a fifth of the men and a tenth of the women reported frequencies greater than once a week. When the quantity of drinking was computed on the basis of approximate absolute alcohol per average drink, again moderation was the rule. More than 95 per cent of students of both sexes consumed only smaller (less than 1.4 ounces of absolute alcohol) or medium (between 1.5 and 3 ounces of absolute alcohol) amounts of wine on any drinking occasion. More than 90 per cent consumed only smaller or medium amounts of beer. Only 7 per cent of the women and 29 per cent of the men reported consuming larger (3 ounces or more of absolute alcohol) amounts of distilled spirits. Furthermore, the category for "larger" amounts included, at its lower limits, amounts of alcohol which would rarely be accompanied by manifest signs of effect from alcohol and many students who reported taking "larger" amounts, drank very infrequently. When an over-all index of quantity and frequency was constructed, the category of greatest quantity-frequency for men included, at its lower limit, men whose drinking did not exceed three cocktails or four glasses of beer at a time with frequencies no greater than twice a week. Even with these minimal criteria, the highest quantity-frequency scale type included only 17 per cent of the male users or 14 per cent of all male students.

Clearly, the nature of student drinking was influenced much more by a complex configuration of social background and maturation experiences than by factors specific to attendance at college. The various aspects of drinking discussed thus far—who, what, how much, when, where, with whom, and from what age—showed correlations with such factors as ethnic and religious background, parental custom, family income, social activities, and usual companions.

The major problems of drinking are usually associated with the effect of alcohol on behavior. This was measured in the study by the operationally defined terms "high," "tight," "drunk," and "passed out." A significant finding was the small proportion of students experiencing the more advanced degrees of effect from alcohol and the infrequency of such incidents for most students.

Specifically, among users, a fifth of the men and half of the women reported never having experienced even moderate effects from alcohol ("tight") while 38 per cent of the men and

82 per cent of the women had never been "drunk," and two-thirds of the men and 91 per cent of the women had never consumed alcohol to the point of passing out. Furthermore, a majority of those who had experienced the extreme effects of alcohol, had done so only once. Only 10 per cent of the men and less than 0.5 per cent of the women had been drunk more than ten times and only 1 per cent of the men had passed out more than ten times. These findings also were inconsistent with the stereotypes of frequent heavy drinking and intoxication among college students.

A much more significant finding, however, was derived from the fact that experiences of extreme effect from alcohol did not correlate with the sociocultural factors which were found to be associated with other criteria of drinking. While family income was found to be a significant predictor of the probability that a student would drink or not drink, and also a predictor of the quantity and frequency of drinking and the types of beverages used, there were absolutely no significant relationships between family income and the frequency with which drinkers had become tight, drunk, or had passed out.

When religious and ethnic groups were compared according to incidence of various levels of intoxication, the Jewish and Italian groups, which included the highest incidence of alcohol users, reported by far the least frequent intoxication, while the highest rates of intoxication were found among the male Mormon students, whose use of alcohol seemed to involve a reaction against the strong prohibitive pressures of their church.

A clear relationship was found between frequency of intoxication and the relative importance which students attached to the use of alcohol for its intoxicating effects in listing their reasons for drinking. Students whose drinking patterns reflected such prodromal signs of pathology as anticipatory and surreptitious drinking and students who scored high on a scale of social complications associated with drinking were also most apt to have experienced frequent intoxication.

From these findings, it was concluded that although social and cultural forces played a very significant role with respect to the adoption or non-adoption of drinking as a behavior pattern, and although, after adoption, these factors were still important in detecting the mode, frequency, and general intensity with which individuals engaged in drinking; for those students whose drinking involved extreme modes, intensities and frequencies of expression, cultural and social forces played a small role while individual and situational forces were increasingly significant.

Although it was not anticipated that alcoholism would be a significant problem in the college-age population, an effort was made to identify students whose patterns of alcohol consumption and associated behavior included possible prodromal signs of chronic pathological drinking. This required differentiation between incidental problem drinking such as an isolated experience of intoxication and that which was patterned and repetitive. For this purpose a number of factors were used which alcoholics have reported retrospectively as characteristic of their incipient problem drinking. First, a Guttman type scale of social complications associated with drinking was constructed using these items: failure to meet obligations, damage to friendships, accident or injury, and formal punishment or discipline. Two-thirds of the men and 85 per cent of the women who used alcohol scored "0" or no complications on the scale. The higher values of "3" and "4" on the scale included only 6 per cent of the men and less than 0.7 per cent of the women. Social complication scale ratings were found to be very highly correlated with the tendency to place a special stress on drinking (anticipatory and surreptitious drinking) and with such additional warning signs as having experienced a "blackout" (temporary amnesia) when drinking, having become drunk alone, having become aggressive when drinking, and having used alcohol before or instead of breakfast.

Most of the students who reported any of the complications or other warning signs, reported only one or two incidents. However, for those students whose frequency with complications or warning signs was more than incidental, patterns were evident which suggested the possibility of identifying incipient alcoholism even at the early stages manifested in college-age drinkers. It was estimated that perhaps 6 per cent of the male student drinkers and 1 per cent of the women demonstrated positive signs of potential problem drinking.

Because 44 per cent of the men who participated in the study during the years 1949 through 1951 were veterans, there was an excellent opportunity to test speculation regarding the possible impact of experience in the armed forces on their drinking patterns. Would the armed forces have provided greater opportunities or greater incentives for drinking? What impact might be attributed to the abrupt change from a social setting characterized by emphasis on individual initiative and individual needs to one calling for subordination of the individual to the organization? What impact might the discipline, monotony, and rigidity of military life and the sanctions of military peer groups have on the use of alcohol as a way of either enhancing or obliterating the experience of off-duty situations?

Veterans in the study differed from non-veterans in a number of basic characteristics. Particularly, the veterans were older and of lower family income. However, when allowances were made for age differences, remarkable similarities appeared between veterans and non-veterans in terms of patterns of alcohol consumption, frequency of intoxication, measures of complications and special stress on drinking, and even reasons for drinking. Therefore, findings of the study did not support a theory that the stresses, restrictions, or sanctions of military service left any distinctive mark on the drinking patterns of most veterans who went on to college. Furthermore, there was no evidence that drinking practices initiated while in service had led to any particular extensive or intensive drinking patterns in veterans.

In addition to studying patterns of drinking behavior among students, the survey also sought data on students' attitudes toward drinking, drunkenness, abstaining, and related matters. A fairly high degree of consistency was found between the students' own drinking behavior and their opinions regarding the propriety of drinking in others. Drinking attitudes also tended to be in keeping with actual behavior when measured according to such criteria as religion, ethnicity, and family income. There was even fair consistency in the attitude expressed toward drinking by people of college age and drinking by older persons. The male students had more liberal attitudes than women regarding drinking in others and students of both sexes accorded more freedom to men than to women; but most students, male and female, favored drinking in moderation irrespective of sex or age. Despite this, nearly half of the men and a third of the women indicated approval of the "double standard which prescribes greater license in drinking to men than to women."

When comparisons were made according to religion, family income, and the type of college, it was found that attitudes toward drinking in others were remarkably similar to actual practices except that the percentages of abstainers in almost every category exceeded the percentages of those who felt that others should abstain. The proportion of students favoring abstention in others was highest in abstainers and lowest among the users with a high quantity-frequency index. The vast majority of students, irrespective of their own drinking pattern, expressed either respect or indifference toward abstainers who made no point of their abstention, but about half of the students expressed disapproval, scorn, or resentment toward abstainers who tried to influence the behavior of others. The tendency to reject the militant abstainer followed expected lines according to religion, family income, and quantity-frequency index with resentment more frequently expressed by Jewish and Catholic students, those of higher income, and those who were themselves users, and with respect most frequently expressed by Mormons and Protestants, those of lower income, and those who either abstained themselves or were low quantity-frequency users.

Attitudes toward drunkenness in others revealed that relatively few students were indifferent or tolerant and that most expressed disgust or loss of respect. Students of both sexes were less tolerant of drunkenness in women than in men although male students were less intolerant of drunkenness in men than were female students. Jewish, Catholic, and Protestant male students were all about equally distributed between tolerance and intolerance toward drunkenness in other men, while intolerance was the dominant response of Mormon men. Abstainers and moderate users were less tolerant than higher quantity-frequency users. Although students who had experienced drunkenness themselves were more tolerant than those who had never been drunk, still about a third of the former expressed disapproval of drunkenness in others.

In general, most data on attitudes, whether toward drinking, drunkenness, or abstention in others, revealed double standards according to sex. The most vivid evidence of double standards was found in the students' responses to questions regarding the identification of behavior associated with drinking which students considered as "going too far." Most responses from male students pertaining to drinking by men described "going too far" in terms of aggressive, violent, or anti-social activity. Typical responses included "reckless driving," "abusing others," "profanity," "becoming violent," "fighting," and "getting out of hand."

Perhaps one response in five referred to sexual aggression. However, the same male respondents saw "going too far" in women almost exclusively in terms of sexual transgression. Typical responses included "sexual misbehavior," "acting loose in morals," "sex promiscuity," "not knowing what they are doing in affairs with men," "flirting," "petting," "when they get sexy," and "sexual intercourse." Women respondents tended to specify sexual activity as "going too far" for both sexes although many of their responses suggested aggressive sexual behavior for the male ("trying to force one to neck with you," "taking advantage of situations with female companions") while implying seductive sexuality on the part of the female ("arousing sexual behavior," "making passes at men," "promiscuity"). Discussions with students brought out further that the double standard with respect to drinking was obviously intertwined with a double standard regarding sexual activity which generally accorded greater freedom of action to men than to women. With respect to the aggression-sexuality contrast revealed in male attitudes toward "going too far" by men and by women, it must be remembered that most drinking by women was in mixed company, while much male drinking and especially heavier male drinking took place only in the company of other men.

Quite a different set of questions revealed a further association of drinking with sexuality in the attitudes and perhaps in the behavior of many students. Students were asked whether they felt that drinking generally precipitates feelings of sexual excitement or accompanies or facilitates petting and necking or sexual intercourse. Positive responses were expressed by 51 per cent of both men and women with respect to feelings of sexual excitement, by 63 per cent of the men and 54 per cent of the women with respect to petting and necking, and by 47 per cent of the men and 31 per cent of the women with respect to sexual intercourse. Although these questions were phrased so that responses could be based on opinion (about others) rather than personal experience it was significant that married students, both men and women, provided a higher percentage of positive responses to each question than did single students. In fact, 67 per cent of the married men and 45 per cent of the married women associated drinking with sexual intercourse. Of further significance was the fact that positive responses to all three questions among single male students were most frequent among the abstainers and high quantity-frequency users while among married students, it was the moderate users who were most apt to associate drinking with sexual activity. In the case of some abstainers, an association between moral sanctions governing both illicit drinking and illicit sexual activity seems probable. In the case of married students, most of whom had only recently initiated a marital sexual relationship, it is possible that small amounts of alcohol had proved functional in alleviating anxiety and thus facilitating a more comfortable exploration for sexual compatibility and fulfillment.

The Findings in the Perspective of Social Change

Repeatedly and consistently the data of *Drinking in College* indicated that much of the behavior and many of the attitudes of college students in the United States in the period 1949-51 reflected the customs and norms which prevailed in the larger society. Especially with respect to such questions as who drinks, how much and how frequently, when, where, with whom, and what beverages are used or preferred, drinking by college students reflected the forces of custom deep-rooted in religious symbolism, ethnic traditions, and family practices and values. Patterns discernible at particular colleges reflected to a large degree cultural traditions of the population groups from which that college's students were drawn.

When such factors as excessive consumption of alcohol, frequent intoxication, social complications and the warning signs of problem drinking were studied, however, no such culturally supported patterns were discernible. On the contrary, the very same cultural pressures against drinking which seemed at least partially effective in restricting the number of drinkers on a campus, within a region or among members of a particular religious or ethnic group, were found to be quite ineffective in limiting excesses of drinking among those students who chose to be users of alcohol in the face of strong negative sanctions.

In retrospect, the findings of *Drinking in College* suggested that negative sanctions provided a special symbolic meaning for drinking on the part of those students who found a particular need to reject authority, to assert their adulthood, or to cope with the painful stresses and anxiety which are often associated with late adolescence. This may help explain why no significant differences were found in the drinking patterns of veterans and non-veterans. Veterans were, on the average, older and most had already experienced or bypassed the storm and stress which characterizes many young people of college age during their transition from dependency to adult status. The greater maturity of veterans may well have offset the impact of any veteran-related experiences which might have been expected to contribute to drinking excess.

In the years since the publication of *Drinking in College* many factors have altered the experience of adolescence in our society. Unprecedented and rapidly accelerating rates of change affecting almost every facet of life in society have increased the pressures for advanced education. At the same time they have increased the gap between young people and their parents' generation.

James S. Coleman[4] has documented the increasing influence of age peers and the decreasing role of parents as the persons from whom adolescents tend to acquire many attitudes, values, and responses. Rapid change has tended to weaken the common bonds which many young people and their parents have found in school subject matter. Not only are there the "new math" and new sciences, but new methods of teaching languages, the fine arts, and even ancient history. Numerous activities which parents and their children traditionally shared have been shifting from such basic adult functions as farming, home maintenance, sewing, cooking or housekeeping, to child centered social and recreational activities in which the success of the child is often exploited to meet the parents' status or recreational needs. Parents' own occupational roles are threatened with obsolescence. All of these factors have tended to decrease the significance of parents as role models for their children and to intensify a tendency for adolescents to reject adult authority while they strive for the privileges, rights, and freedom of adult status.

At the same time, traditional symbolic respect for the wisdom and experience of elders has been shattered by the current dilemmas in which the United States finds itself with respect to the Viet Nam war, the cold war generally, and the crises of race relations. Increasingly the older generation is seen as the bungling creator of problems for which the current generation of youth

[4] James S. Coleman, *The Adolescent Society* (New York: Free Press, 1961).

must pay dearly. Uncertainties associated both with these massive problems and with rapid change make it difficult for the college-age population to make long-range career plans or to envision stable family and community living. Without fixed goals in the outer world, many youths are tempted to turn inward for enlightenment and to seek security in a greater awareness of introspective sensations and illusions.

During the period since the publication of *Drinking in College*, the meaning of being a college student has changed in a number of ways. Most colleges have greatly increased their enrollment. Many new colleges have been created to meet the rapidly rising demand for higher education. Without academic traditions, these new schools often resemble a business enterprise more than an educational institution. At older, more prestigeful colleges, pressures on faculty to engage in research, consultation, and service have imposed seriously on the time and interest which professors devote to students and on their commitment to teaching. Massive research institutes and skyscraper dormitories are replacing the "halls of ivy." College athletics are becoming increasingly professional. The colleges no longer represent the termination of preparation for a life career, but are just an interlude in a continuing process of education. College life has been altered by the trend toward earlier marriage which sees on many campuses half of the students married before they graduate. All of these factors have been associated with a decrease in the special significance of college life and in the respect accorded by students to college faculty, deans, and counselors who, like parents, find that their influence on the attitudes, values, and behavior of students is waning. Correspondingly, there has been developing a movement of student self-assertion symbolized by an increasingly militant student government, by student participation in numerous protest movements, and by student experimentation in various efforts to enhance their awareness of themselves.

Since the completion of *Drinking in College,* a number of changes in alcohol use by college students also seem apparent. On the positive side, it is probable that student sophistication about alcohol has increased commensurate with increased opportunities to acquire a sound factual basis for intelligent decisions about alcohol use. Recently, student use of marijuana, LSD, and other pharmacological agents has almost replaced student drinking as the major focus of adult concern. To the extent that drinking is less prominently associated with student misbehavior it will probably be less useful as a means of attracting attention to themselves by students who feel a special need for self-assertion.

On those campuses where the use of marijuana or LSD has been in vogue, it is also probable that many of the users of these materials are students who otherwise would be misusing alcohol. Thus, the hallucinatory and psychedelic drugs have probably been replacing alcohol as a form of escape for some students. It is not possible to estimate how many students are now using these substances. It is clear that the incidence and nature of use varies greatly in different areas and on different campuses. It is also probable that the impressions created by the popular press greatly exaggerate these problems just as they have previously exaggerated the problems of student drinking.

On the other hand, there appears to have been an increase in the acceptance of escapism behavior generally among students, and in the approval of escapism reasons for drinking. Also, it seems reasonable to assume some increase in the use of alcohol by college students as a means of asserting adulthood and rejecting authority, especially in those localities where the formal enforcement of legal restrictions has enhanced this symbolic meaning of drinking. When alcohol is used as an expression of rebellion or self-assertion or as a means of escape, it can be assumed that such use often involves drinking in order to achieve intoxication.

The problem of drinking by young people has been complicated by an increase in the use of automobiles by students while in college and by the greatly increased freedom from college imposed sanctions which the automobile has provided. For many young people, the automobile is a much more significant symbol of independence than is alcohol. The acquisition of a driver's license is an extremely important rite of passage for the adolescent today; the ownership of an automobile is another. These provide both independence from home and college, a means of self-expression, and an opportunity to engage in those activities which are forbidden by the adult world including carefree driving, sex experimentation, and drinking. The rising rate of automobile accidents involving young people (and often alcohol) is a grim testimonial to the lethal combination of poor judgment and inexperience in driving combined with the same qualities in drinking.

The problems of drinking and driving by young people have been particularly conspicuous in areas where there are variations in the laws governing the sale or use of alcoholic beverages. At this writing only New York and Louisiana permit drinking at age 18. All other states define drinking legally as an adult behavior permissible only at age 21. Several states make some exceptions before age 21 with respect to beer or wine, or drinking with the consent of or in the presence of parents. There are two states which exempt married youth and one which exempts members of the armed forces. Kentucky permits voting and entering into a legal contract at age 18, but not drinking. Variations in the legal age of drinking between states, and in local option regarding drinking and enforcement practices within states, have created many situations in which young people use automobiles in order to drive to a place where they can drink. As noted earlier, such practices are not conducive to moderate drinking.

In summary, this chapter has reviewed the background of a survey on college drinking attitudes and customs which was initiated in 1947 and has summarized the findings which were published in 1953. Numerous factors of social change which have characterized the last 20 years were then discussed including changes in the nature of society, the nature and meaning of a college experience, and the relationships between adolescents and older generations. It has been suggested that pressures associated with the rapidity and nature of recent social change have intensified the need which many young people feel to assert their independence, to reject inconsistent and restrictive authority, or to seek ways of coping with the stresses of uncertainty, frustration, disillusionment, and groping for self-identity.

Theoretically, all of these factors might be expected to have led to an increase in the frequency and quantity of alcohol use by college students and in the incidence of social complications and potential problem drinking. There is no evidence to support or refute such a theory. However, in spite of the grim picture of pressures which impinge on today's college youth, there are some reasons for optimism with respect to college drinking per se. It seems clear that on some campuses those students who in the past would have used drinking and intoxication in order to resolve unbearable stress or cope with problems of identity,

are now using other pharmacological agents. The use of marijuana, LSD and related materials is not based on custom nor does
it symbolize adult behavior; it represents primarily a youth centered cultural response which combines protest with escape.

Fortunately, however, the vast majority of today's students
appear to have found satisfactory ways of coping with the problems of social change which have been identified in this chapter.
The findings of *Drinking in College* revealed that most college
students who used alcohol in the period around 1950 did so
moderately. Although many events since 1950 might be expected
to increase the incidence of drinking for intoxication and other
misuses of alcohol, the opposite effect is equally likely. The
same changes in the nature of society, the nature of colleges and
college life, and in intergenerational relationships appear to have
contributed to an earlier transition from dependency and to have
hastened the maturation process of contemporary youth. With
an earlier and greater sense of independence has come an enhanced sense of responsibility. As this is combined with increased knowledge about the nature of alcohol, its traditional
customary uses, its effects on man, and its potential misuse, there
appear to be good reasons for believing that intelligent choice
of action with respect to alcohol can be expected from the majority of college students.

Chapter 2

ALCOHOL TRENDS IN COLLEGE LIFE: HISTORICAL PERSPECTIVES*

HARRY S. WARNER

I. *Early College Traditions*

CONVIVIAL DRINKING TRADITIONS and the variety of culture associated with them have come by a long trail into a considerable part of modern college life. Not different essentially from other customs, practices, and philosophies that for ages have been a part of the quest for alcoholic sensations, college drinking, nevertheless, has age-old characteristics of its own. For the years of life called "student" and the period of growth called "collegiate" are filled with heightened experiences, struggles of freedom and rebellion, vivid, colorful, and spectacular.

Consequently, college customs and capers, desires and rationalizations gain attention and publicity beyond those of other groups. The questioning and attitudes of students and future possibilities in leadership appeal to the imagination of all as do those, also, of instructors and other representatives of higher education. They stand out in the social picture of a people or a period.

College drinking customs may be taken for study, therefore, as a vivid cross-section of the prevailing attitudes, customs, and trends at different periods in the alcoholic liquor controversy and problem of this country. As a Swedish writer says of university

---

* Originally published by The Board of Temperance, Prohibition and Public Morals of the Methodist Episcopal Church and reprinted here by permission of the author and of the Board of Social Concerns, the Methodist Church, successor to the Board of Temperance of that organization.

drinking in his country, "The customs and opinions of student life to a very great degree influence the habits and ways of thinking of the educated classes" of the country.

At the time of the founding of the first colleges in North America, Harvard, Yale, William and Mary, and the others, alcoholic sociability was a regular and assumed part of influential and nearly all other shades of society. Liquor seemed as necessary at social functions, in polite and everyday social intercourse as food, wit, and conversation. Each nationality and shipload of adventure-seeking colonists, even the Puritans, brought with them the drinking traditions and customs of the homeland. The first colleges, taking their standards from Oxford and Cambridge, included the ale, beer, and other customs popular in the English universities. In earlier times, various colleges at Oxford brewed their own varieties. The English universities held festivities known as "college ales," had a great variety of ancient and later drinking occasions, developed famous student taverns, and wrote a mass of literature, poetry, and song in praise of drink. These or their equivalent were accepted as a traditional part of sociability by the colleges established in the Colonial period.

Harvard and Yale each had a "buttery," an annex to the commons at which extras between meals, refreshments, and various articles, including beer, cider, and at times harder liquor could be purchased. In 1748 at Yale the steward in charge was allowed 12 barrels of beer for the year and later, as the college grew, 20 barrels. One purpose of the buttery was to prevent students from having an excuse for frequenting public houses and taverns in town. "Beer was furnished at dinners for many years" at Yale, "then cider took its place and beer was allowed at supper until 1759" (1, p. 253). Harvard had a rule that no resident of the college could use distilled spirits or mixed drinks when entertaining and no undergraduate might "keep by him brandy, rum or any distilled spirituous liquors without leave from the President or a Tutor." Other colleges also had restrictions as to "hard" liquors, but few as to beer and wine. On special occasions in the college hall at Yale "a barrel of wine was elevated on the table and none were expected to leave until 'mid shouts and songs and harangues, the barrel was emptied" (2, p. 651). To the first commencement at Dartmouth, a founder who had secured the charter brought "a roast ox and a barrel of rum." By 1800 a leading club at Harvard had made Washington's birthday a convivial occasion with a procession of students to Porter's tavern and a night of revelry:

> And each one to evince his spunk,
> Vied with his neighbor to get drunk.

Later, toward the end of the past century, the influence and culture of German universities gained wide attention in the universities of the United States. Graduate students in large numbers, returning from Germany with their new Ph.D.'s, brought into the younger faculty and student clubs of some of the colleges the traditional beer drinking customs, assumptions, and philosophies of Mid-Europe. Together with a similar influence from Paris and its universities, this tended to reinforce the prestige of the drinking customs of the Colonial heritage that were losing their hold in the early years of the present century.

Yet during the entire history of college education in the United States, alcoholic practices, whether of English origin made native in the Colonial Period, or of formal French wine origin, the later German variety, or the unrestrained and individualistic types of drinking native to the New World, have all varied greatly in different types of colleges and at different periods. The attitudes and practices in the church-founded and "small-colleges" of whatever origin for a century or more have contrasted greatly with many of those in the older and more conservative colleges. In many of the former alcoholic customs never gained dignified standing; social and personal drinking usually were under disapproval, and were not, as in the European universities, a recognized part of the life of the community.

II. *In the Years of the Saloon*

By 1900 two deeply divergent trends were to be seen side by side in American college communities: one, a strong and increased questioning of the place and value of alcoholic liquors in the community and in personal use, because of their many unfortunate social consequences; and the other, a growing consciousness and attitude of defense of the traditional drinking privileges combined with efforts to retain support for the criticized customs.

This was the period of the open saloon. Liquor was available and cheap to all who sought it, in all except five states and in limited areas in many other states. Large cities, small towns, college towns, and a few exceptions, and country crossroads had their drinking places. Hotels had bars, breweries in foreign sections of the great cities delivered beer to homes of the Mid-European colonies, a few women in these colonies and in "high society" drank hard cider formed in farmers' cellars, and "moonshine" flourished from the stills in the eastern and southern mountains. But these were little more than incidental features. It was the day of the great American saloon where men went to drink, remained to boast, received the news and drink, "set it up" and drank again; the saloon was the place where men met men; it was the "poor man's club," the profligate's club for the habit-developed sons of the middle classes and the well-to-do.

In college communities, also, liquor indulgence tended toward the drinking saloon and hotel bar. In these downtown congregating places and in those on the edge of the campus that equipped their rooms with tables, steins, and decorations for student club use, in the fraternity and other drinking parties, and at occasional big celebrations most of the drinking and trouble occurred. Colleges had discontinued the earlier practice of providing liquors for their students and also the restrictions against going down town. Whereas at Harvard in 1837 "wine was furnished at dinners as well as cider," by 1898 no wine, beer, or other liquor could be used at the student-controlled commons where 1,120 ate daily. Changes in policy occurred frequently and rules varied greatly from college to college, but on the whole the trend of liquor was away from college auspices. Then, during the fifteen years following 1900 in one college or university community after another saloons were pushed back from the campus by local vote or other state law, one mile, two miles, four miles, or from the county, because of their demoralizing effect on student and community life. And for abundant reason.

The use and extent of liquor were serious. An investigator of 1903 after intensive research and observation, talks with students and professors, and examination of records reported that as many as 90 per cent of the students in one eastern university center drank in their freshman year and 95 per cent in their senior year, that 35 per cent drank heavily, and that 15 per cent became drunkards (3, p. 18). He said, "I have been around to the other universities to a considerable extent as manager of two of the university athletic organizations. . . . At Princeton it is beer, beer, beer. . . . the body of students in my mind drink even more than do Harvard men. . . . At Yale drinking is recognized to so great a degree that clubs have their tables at the barrooms . . . and at some of the bars the students carve their names in the tables." The tabletops are preserved as souvenirs of the year on the walls of the saloon and new tops put on the tables for another year of names. "At Cornell the conditions are somewhat the same, although I do not believe Cornell students carry their excesses as far. . . . At Columbia there exists more debauchery on account of the resorts of the city." Answering sensational criticisms of the colleges about 1911, a writer in the *Boston American* said that on "official figures" the proportion of students who drank at the great university mentioned was in 1908, 56 per cent; 1909, 59 per cent; 1910, 45 per cent; 1911, 60 per cent (4).

The big games were a frequent occasion for alcoholic festivities. Following a Georgetown-University of Virginia game, 1913, *The Washington Star* reported that "the police worked overtime gathering up nearly a hundred young drunks, who had to put up $10 or sleep in a cell. . . . In front of one thirst parlor a line of police waited until midnight, when the lights were made dim and about twenty drunks spilled outward toward the curb. . . . In one hotel . . . the riot started early in the evening, the drinking rooms were crowded by eight o'clock, and mobs fought for possession of the tables . . . the ejection of a drunk was a monumental affair, as two policemen had to battle with upward of twenty alleged collegiates. . . . And the boys and girls who stayed seemed to like it" (5).

As late as 1915 a writer in the Harvard *Crimson* stated that 75 per cent of the students joined in the drinking customs of the university community. Liquid refreshments were the rule at class and other functions and the non-drinkers, a minority, through class membership were compelled to help pay for the beer which they declined to drink. One of the militant few protesting in the *Crimson* against this forced wetness wrote, "it is not class meetings alone from which many are excluded through an unwillingness to make themselves conspicuous by their abstinence."

Commenting on the public results of drinking at Wisconsin, a Madison newspaper said, "The drunken student . . . vomiting, uttering foul language . . . open nastiness of vocalization which almost justified recourse to the shotgun. . . . And our eighty-eight or ninety saloons, what part are they playing in this humiliating business?" An observer wrote, "in the saloon at the brewery last night there were not less than a dozen students, several of them carrying away supplies of beer, one having a suitcase filled . . . this they told me is the regular thing" (6).

On the West Coast, college drinking customs of the East were combined with those that had come out of the pioneer days of California and the mining camps of the "gold rush" years. At the University of California "wet" celebrations were held in San Francisco away from the campus. The banquets often ended in smashing dishes, throwing steins, and with the men under the table. An old ferry boat on the Bay became a drinking center for student clubs. "Beer night" around the "Big C" on the hillside above Berkeley was a yearly event, an annual Sophomore "beer-bust" celebrated in defiance of rival university teams before the big games. Kegs of beer were rolled to the top of the hill and the class and its friends spent the night guarding and drinking. Yet the President of the University, in 1912, stated that 70 per cent of the students were abstainers; that the trouble came from the 30 per cent who "run things," control student politics and publications, dazzle the "dubs," and emphasize the drink traditions of the past.

The intercollegiate games were accompanied by much drinking. After a football victory at Stanford, President David Starr Jordan reported that "Two hundred students from the University of California spent the night on the campus. The fraternity houses were open all night. Two hundred rowdies marched through the library. . . . Beer kegs were carried over to the steps of the sorority house. A student went to a saloon downtown, got drunk, got into the wrong house. Someone shot him" (3). After these events Stanford banished liquor from the University and its surroundings.

The following incidents illustrate conditions in many college communities in "the old days" and some of the types of excess that had to be faced in many of the larger and some of the smaller college centers.

1. The openly recognized celebration or consolation drinking bouts after the big games when restraint was removed, training

broken, and large numbers present. The tendency to "break loose" often led to great excesses.

2. The campus-edge saloons with tables for clubs and fraternities in imitation of German customs. This was the period when German culture was most influential in American colleges. The student saloon, with its pictures, tables, and steins expressed imported customs. But at only a few of the larger universities and technical colleges did "beer night" gain standing as a regular feature of class, fraternity, departmental, or other group sociability.

3. At social functions the use of smaller, rather "polite" amounts of wines and liquors prevailed much more widely. In many college towns faculty affairs set the example for this sort of drinking.

4. Ordinary saloon and hotel barroom drinking in groups, often continued late at night, was the greatest source of trouble and the most prevalent form. In university towns, saloons near the campus catered to students, appealing to fraternity, class, and other interests. In the cities, hotels and club barrooms added many other questionable attractions.

The influence of college drinking in forming life habits and the way these habits worked out later received special study at this time. At Dartmouth, a seminar class under Professor Charles F. Emerson, about 1916, studied the personal histories of the members of classes graduated between 1869 and 1879 and the effects of alcohol were traced from college over a period of 35 years. Of the 320 men graduating, 92, or 29 per cent, used liquor while 228 students, 71 per cent, did not. After 35 years, it was found that of the college liquor users 59 per cent were living, of the college non-users, 78 per cent were living; or, stating it another way, 41 per cent of those who drank while in college had died and but 22 per cent of the abstainers had died in 35 years.

In the saloon years the social use of liquors was the accepted tradition in the older and more influential colleges, in polite society, on formal occasions, and at celebrations by students and alumni. Many individuals declined to participate, "radicals" or "fanatics" even attended convivial dinners and parties. On the whole, however, prevailing customs did not make it easy for non-drinkers. It required more than average strength of personality for a student, or faculty member either, to stand out against the assumed or actual attitudes of those who led the drinking in places of influence. Traditions were too strong in the opposite direction.

III. *The Break from Tradition*

The decade 1910-20 was marked by increased questioning and conflict over alcoholic liquor and its social and economic consequences. Students, faculty members, and college communities in many parts of the country and in all but a few of the more conservative colleges had a share in it. The place and significance of the whole tradition of alcoholic beverage in modern life was challenged, made realistic, and given a measure of scientific evaluation. The college no less than the country as a whole, at least that part of it west of the Atlantic seaboard, became "liquor minded" as a result of a century of struggle against the saloon and drunkenness. The social and community implications of alcoholic indulgence became important. The attention of millions turned toward the never-ending crop of degraded manhood and neglected childhood found wherever drink selling and drinking customs prevailed; this new social consciousness refused to regard the question longer as one only of "personal liberty." And students and professors in increasing numbers, as well as others, were interested in doing something about it.

Two trends should be noted: (a) In the more conservative and socially influential college communities old traditions and practices continued popular, although increasingly questioned and reduced in frequency. A process began similar to that in the smaller and denominational institutions. (b) In practically all other colleges and universities, especially those in the Central and Southern states, and also among a minority group of students and faculty members in the conservative schools, an aggressive attitude developed that had its outlet chiefly in local and state efforts to restrict or banish the legalized sale of intoxicants.

In the larger universities and colleges the freedom of individuals to refrain from drinking at social functions and retain standing gradually came to be recognized; the number and variety of gatherings that depended upon alcohol for entertainment decreased. Dinners, banquets, and parties depended less on liquor as an aid to wit. Many fraternities "went dry." The celebrations after the big games continued to have an abundance of liquor enthusiasm or consolation; bootlegging against faculty, student body, and legal restrictions was abundant; and downtown saloons, where they remained, had their full share of student patronage. But on the average in large colleges and smaller, even where old traditions remained strongest, the frequency and popularity of liquor were declining. Academic customs supporting it steadily lost prestige. In their place developed, as in the "freshwater colleges" earlier, a sense of social concern and the conviction that alcoholic drink would soon be out of date and should be eliminated from modern college life. In hundreds of universities and colleges student groups and individual teachers took active service in efforts to reduce the community and state evils of the saloon and the liquor traffic. A poll of Yale seniors, in 1913, as to personal practice revealed 155 abstainers to 128 users in the class (7). By 1915 Professor Irving Fisher, Yale economist, was in a position to write, "So far has the anti-liquor movement in the colleges proceeded that a man who frankly opposes its use is more respected than the man who condones it."

At such universities as Michigan, Ohio State, Indiana, Minnesota, Nebraska, and Kansas the social affairs of the university were largely free from the sentiment that favored the use of intoxicants at banquets and dinners. Regulations against drinking in saloons became more severe. At the University of Missouri, it was reported that drinking was practically eliminated by the removal of saloons from the city. At Illinois, in 1912, the student vote was largely responsible for removing the saloons from Urbana and Champaign.

An early example of united student activity in regard to drinking customs in a large university occurred at Michigan in 1898 when 500 undergraduates, a few professors cooperating, pledged themselves to oppose the saloons in Ann Arbor, some of them next to the campus, and many patronized by students. The effort included attempts to reduce drinking in fraternities, among the drinkers on the faculty, and at the celebrations of athletic victories. Soon after this campaign saloons were closed, but the social drinking customs and wet celebrations continued.

A later University of Michigan student movement in 1916 (8) was more effective. Led by a popular athlete, a left tackle on the varsity eleven, it included the creation of opinion for better college standards, law enforcement in the city, and stricter abstinence among athletes. After the date, the boast of a football captain ten years earlier "that I can drink my whole team under the table" was succeeded by the newer, scientific policy of positive opposition to drinking by athletic coaches and leaders.

A dramatic contest in student opinion against well-established drinking customs occurred at the University of California in a three-year campaign beginning in 1910. For years sophomore night at the "Big C" on the hill above the campus was a noted event. On the night preceding the chief game of the season the sophomores had the responsibility of guarding the letter from encroaching Stanford men, who each year attempted to paint it red. Kegs of beer were regularly provided to keep the guards awake. But the class of 1910, the majority being non-drinkers, attempted to substitute coffee, sandwiches, and doughnuts. Nevertheless after midnight the beer arrived. The next day a reaction occurred, more decisive action was taken, and this form of "beer night" came to an end. During the following two years by persistent organized effort the students opposed to liquor introduced and carried by a vote of 627 to 138 an amendment against the "use of intoxicants at any banquet, dinner, supper, luncheon, rally, smoker, or social event given by any student organization" at the University of California (9).

A similar struggle in student opinion at Cornell University for the removal of the drink tradition from student activities centered on the annual Junior Feed, a popular banquet held usually away from the campus where liquor facilities were more abundant. After a series of efforts for four years the organized student opposition won their campaign. In addition, by circulating petitions, securing speakers, and their personal activities, these students helped carry through the state legislature a bill that removed the saloons from Ithaca.

A student movement of several years that had as much influence outside the University among alumni as it did inside took place at Yale where drink traditions were hoary with age. It was the tradition that Yale men could hold their liquor. Beginning with a group studying the problem, attitudes grew stronger from year to year until many definite anti-liquor steps had been taken. Some of the fraternities voluntarily banished the use of liquor in their houses. In 1915, after three months of discussion, the senior class of Yale College voted, 115 to 101, to discontinue liquor at their graduating party. By another vote of 169 to 51 they dropped liquor from their future class reunions. The graduating class of Sheffield Scientific School took similar steps (10).

These movements were followed by an appeal to Yale alumni to approve what the undergraduates had done by eliminating alcoholic indulgence at their own class celebrations at the University. The appeal to the alumni by the Committee of Seventy-One, which included leading football, crew, newspaper, and senior class men was signed by William Howard Taft, Yale, '78, and mailed to 12,500 alumni (11).

These struggles of the younger student opinion against the old drinking traditions in the large and conservative universities from 1910 to 1918 reflected what already had taken place or was taking place in more decisive ways in the state institutions and smaller colleges. In the latter the attitudes of students and professors in large numbers were now one of aggressive action against the liquor traffic and the saloon as sources of the trouble in college and the community. An organized college anti-liquor movement was promoting study and discussion of the problem in hundreds of colleges each year, conducting a great series of public speaking contests, reaching with its student secretaries three hundred colleges and more than 75,000 students each year, and enlisting young men and women for intelligent service in anti-liquor activities. Under its leadership students in large numbers gained a realistic knowledge of liquor in the community by sharing in the various activities that were seeking solutions.

During the summer of 1914, for example, more than 500 students gave time as volunteers, speaking, singing, in teams and groups, going out independently or under the temperance organizations into the town and country communities in many forms of anti-liquor activity. In 1915, 1,346 from 78 colleges shared in the local, state, and other anti-saloon and prohibition campaigns. In 1916, 2,330 from 114 colleges were at work during the summer and early fall months. The interest and its distribution are shown by the fact that Michigan had 568, 44 of whom were faculty members, in such activities; Ohio, over 1,000; California, 450; Missouri, 275; Nebraska, 94; Montana, 53; New York, Pennsylvania, Virginia and Texas also had part in the program. Students shared gladly in this work. It was an adventure as well as a public service. In one state it was so popular that 100 more volunteered than could be used. Few, if any, received salaries.

The custom of depending on alcoholic feelings to heighten social enjoyment was being questioned as unscientific and set aside rapidly in these pre-war days in college circles. Dinners, banquets, and parties were no longer necessarily alcoholic; even wines and beer at college functions lost prestige among students and faculty, and more slowly at alumni gatherings as well. The universities in the Central and Southern states joined with the church-related and smaller colleges in adopting new standards.

But even during this high-water mark period in the college anti-liquor movement, there remained in the Eastern universities and colleges, those attended by young people from the so-called "privileged" families and groups, drinking traditions which continued with little or no change.

The questioning attitude toward alcoholic drink that had grown for three-quarters of a century in American colleges became aggressive opposition in the average college and in vigorous groups in the universities by 1918 when the prohibition movement reached the point of national decision. Many forms of alcoholic indulgences were losing caste, except in limited circles. In the older colleges, though the trend was in the same direction, as shown by the vote of Yale seniors in 1918 to discontinue liquor at class and reunion parties, the hold of established customs and the influence of alumni and wealthy families with well-stocked wine cellars, who regarded themselves as privileged, continued as a restraining force in opposition to the anti-liquor trend and the laws after their adoption.

IV. *The Legal Banishment Period*

Writing about the situation as it developed in the colleges after the adoption of national prohibition, Professor Charles H. Warren of Yale reported in 1926 after six years' observation, that "the fraternities have never been so dry as they are today. The last prom dances were the cleanest I have attended in many years. I think there is less drinking now than ever in the history of the university" (12, p. 76). "The effect at Yale has been good," said Professor Charles C. Clark who makes it clear that he is not a prohibitionist. He adds, "I know for I have been a member of the Committee on Discipline. . . . In the old days our Committee was constantly busy with cases involving intoxication and the disorders originating from it. Now we have practically no business of the kind at all . . . in spite of the fact that in the old days we rarely troubled ourselves with a case of mere intoxication if it had not resulted in public disorder (12, p. 76). These changes had occurred in a college in which the prevailing sentiment continued to be wet, the senior class of that year recording its sympathies as 80 per cent on that side (12, p. 72).

"Out of 7,800 students, 88 per cent are in favor of prohibition," comments the *Chicago Post* (13) on a 1926 referendum by Professor R. L. Mott of the University of Chicago. The survey covered 37 colleges and universities; 12 per cent favored repeal and 41 per cent modification. "This overwhelming proportion is divided only on the question of how its enforcement may be made most effective" (14).

A poll of 100 college editors in 1926 concludes that, in the opinion of the majority "drinking among students has declined in recent years," and that such as remains is by those who "think to put feathers in their caps if they can bespeak a bootlegger" (15).

"My observation twenty-five years ago was that it was the exceptional student who did not take a drink now and then," said a Dean of Men at West Virginia University in 1925. "Today conditions are reversed and it is the exceptional student who drinks. The few who break over cause the talk" (16).

"It has been six months since a student has been before me for violating the liquor laws. . . . there is not one one-hundredth the drinking among the University [Michigan] students today that there was during the days of the saloon," said a judge of the Circuit Court at Ann Arbor in 1927. A barber at the edge of the campus who shaved students thirty-five years reported, "Students used to come into my shop drunk, would have to be taken out of the chair. . . . It has been three or four years since there has been a drunk student in my shop."

The colleges of the United States on the whole accepted prohibition as a social welfare advance. There were exceptions, decided and outstanding, but they are exceptions. Secret drinking continued as well as much bootlegging at some of the universities, especially those in large cities, near the Canadian line or the moonshine stills of the mountains, and the purchase from illegal sellers in time became an adventure to those who had seen little of the legal saloon. Student drinking and law evasions were exploited and publicized as student escapades and carousals had been in saloon days, because they appeal to public feeling. Yet, as in license days, drinking and law violation in colleges were much less than outside. The great body of college students accepted the purposes of the new situation, agreed that alcoholic indulgence was not necessary and that it was being outgrown in forward-looking nations. "The colleges, universities and schools, with rare exceptions, are fully in line," wrote James J. Britt, Chief Counsel of the Bureau of Prohibition in 1928 (17).

Evidence of this trend is found in surveys and tests of opinion and practice, the most scientific, though not the earliest, of which was by Professor E. E. Cortright, Education, of New York University, in 1926. His "objective evidence," Professor Cortright believed had "more than the average amount of legitimate findings in it . . . because of the manner in which it was collected" (18). Two questions were merged with 34 others of large social importance. The method was one of sampling by classes from one to four classes each of the colleges listed.

1. Should the Eighteenth Amendment be rigidly enforced?

Mt. Holyoke College group	97%	YES
Stanford University group	94%	YES
University of Minnesota group	88%	YES
Connecticut College group	87%	YES
University of Michigan group	84%	YES
Washington Square, N.Y.U. group	80%	YES
Smith College group	70%	YES
Education, N.Y.U. group	68%	YES
Amherst College group	64%	YES
University of Texas group	64%	YES
University of North Carolina group	72%	YES
Commerce, N.Y.U. group	72%	YES
Average, all college groups surveyed	77%	YES

2. Should the Eighteenth Amendment be abolished?

University of Minnesota group	90%	NO
Mt. Holyoke group	83%	NO
University of Michigan group	82%	NO
University of North Carolina group	81%	NO
Connecticut College group	70%	NO
Smith College group	70%	NO
Stanford University group	69%	NO
Education, N.Y.U. group	68%	NO
University of Texas group	68%	NO
Commerce, N.Y.U. group	56%	NO
Amherst College group	50%	NO
Washington Square, N.Y.U. group	57%	NO
Average, all college groups surveyed	69%	NO

"Analysis of the vote shows two distinct things. First, the wide range of regional opinion . . . the Atlantic seaboard wet . . . great Saharas in the western part of the country . . ." Second, the effect of sex opinion upon the decisions, for to produce the average of 77 per cent YES on the first question, the men gave a 66 per cent YES vote, and the women an 83 per cent YES. On the second question, to produce the 69 per cent NO average, the men voted 56 per cent NO, and the women 72 per cent NO (fractions disregarded). The sex balance of all students recorded is practically identical with the proportionate number of men and women students in the country."

The first attempt to obtain a comprehensive view of college attitudes after 1920 was made March 7, 1922. It was a letter to presidents asking their opinion of prohibition "in theory and fact," after observing it in operation two years. This approach, while limited, was significant as to official attitudes and opinions. Answers were received from 158 college and university presidents in 40 states. Of these 136 were distinctly favorable, 10 non-committal or indifferent, and 8 unfavorable; 4 were favorable to the theory, but not to the enforcement measures. The replies showed analysis of varying conditions. Almost universal was the opinion of the presidents that drinking was less than in pre-prohibition days, including several who were opposed to prohibition. "The whole problem of discipline has been both simplified and lessened," wrote the head of a great school of technology. A New England university president, in a state that did not ratify the Amendment said, "There is less drinking by students in this part of the country than ever before in the history of man" (19).

A survey of college deans, April 20, 1922, by Professor F. S. Southworth, brought answers from 471 of the 486 addressed. Of these 308 reported that there had been no increase in the consumption of liquor under prohibition, 134 reported a marked decrease, 16 that there had been no drinking before or since, and 13 that there had been an increase. Professor Southworth concludes, "Over 95 per cent of the colleges with over 87 per cent of the students thus reported a marked decrease or at least no increase, and of those reporting an increase not a single one attributed it exclusively to prohibition" (20).

To obtain a direct expression from students Dr. Samuel Plantz, President of Lawrence College in 1923, sent a list of 12 questions to 500 fraternities in 350 colleges and all parts of the United States (21). "To my questionnaire," he reported, "I received 112 replies. Of these 62 said there had been a decrease in the use of intoxicating liquors since prohibition; 14 said there had been no decrease; 9 said there had been an increase; 7 said they did not know, and the rest gave no answer. The 30 who claimed an increase, or no decrease, or that they did not know were in large universities mostly in the East and South, although the far and Middle West were represented.

"To the question about what proportion of the men in your institution, according to your best judgment, use intoxicating liquors, 33 gave 10 per cent or less; 16 gave between 10 and 30 per cent; 17 gave between 40 and 50 per cent; 5 gave between 50 and 60 per cent, and 14 gave between 60 and 90 per cent. In the higher percentages it was usually added that this meant not habitual drinkers, but those who indulged occasionally as at banquets and jollifications. It will be noted that the information derived from the fraternities is not nearly so favorable as that derived from the college deans and presidents; and I do not know that it is nearer the facts."

The attitude of student bodies at this period in the prohibition era was interpreted as follows by these fraternity men. To the question, "What is the attitude of your student body toward a strict enforcement of the 18th Amendment? 35, or one-third were favorable; 23 were opposed; and 12 favored the Amendment, but not the Volstead Act; 6 reported sentiment about equally divided; 13 said the student body was indifferent; and the remainder were evasive or gave no answer."

Explaining the background to his survey of college fraternity opinion President Plantz said, "College drinking in the past has been largely in the homes of fraternity men, where it was considered quite the thing to flavor their good times with liquor. Not infrequently there were orgies of drunkenness, almost like the German university *kneipe,* to celebrate a victorious football season, a homecoming, or some important college event which the boys wanted to honor. The drinking student was not a *persona non grata.* But this has been largely changed. In nearly all colleges, the frats have rules against bringing liquor into the houses and about members being found in a state of intoxication. Often these rules are enforced by fines, usually from five to twenty-five dollars, and sometimes by suspension or expulsion from the fraternity. It is now felt to be a disgrace to have a drunken spree, or to have drunken members. When such things have occurred, it has sometimes been taken up by the student council, the whole fraternity [put] on probation for good behavior, or required the expulsion of drinking members, or in a few cases, recommended to the faculty that the fraternity be suspended for six months or a year. There is no doubt that there is a marked toning up of fraternities since the enactment of the prohibition law."

And checking his survey of fraternities with those among college deans and presidents and a wide clipping of newspaper reports, Dr. Plantz concludes "that in the great majority of our small colleges, so-called, there is very little drinking; that in our large institutions there is a great deal of drinking on particular occasions, but that in some of these sentiment is changing."

After 1920 many colleges and students shared with others the impression that on the liquor problem little remained to be done. But as the difficulties of enforcement, the changes implied in social customs and conduct became clear, and illegal dealers extended their technique for obtaining profits out of bootlegging, rum-running, moonshining, and other old and new forms of illegal traffic, renewed interest became active. This naturally took opposite forms: (1) support for the outlawed drinking and customs and desires, evasion and disregard of the new laws, and exploitation of the weakness in prohibition enforcement; (2) support of the new regime, discontinuance of old traditions and customs, and efforts to strengthen public, and especially college opinion toward non-alcoholic sociability and law observance.

The picture of what happened in the colleges under prohibition has two sides both of which contain facts and truth in varying degrees.

1. On the one hand was the drinking, at first more or less surreptitious, later more open, the purchase of liquors by fraternities and clubs from bootleggers, the pocket flasks at celebrations, games, dances, and clubs. Much of this put into new forms, practices and customs of long standing in the old saloon days. The newspapers of 1921 to 1930 were full of sensational reports about student drinking after the big games, of bootleggers pushing their trade to the campus, of drinking parties in the fraternities and student houses, and of flasks at the dances. The stories of carousals on the special trains carrying students to the

inter-university games, federal agents in the guise of college fans, students within a short drive of the Canadian border who helped pay college expenses by importing and bootlegging were among the spectacular news features of the period.

After the 1928 game, for example, between Wisconsin and Minnesota the *Wisconsin Daily Cardinal* printed the following:

> The annual drunk is over. Practically every student is once more sober. The grand old home-coming spree has become a mere matter of history repeating history. Little Italy is quiet for there are no more dozens of students down there laying in a supply of home-coming cheer. Drunken students have ceased their maudlin wanderings up and down the streets. Respectability and decency are returning and the quiet air of scholasticism is once more beginning to reign. Impossible was it to walk down the street under night without meeting one drunken maudlin student after another. Impossible to go to the theater without being in the company of intoxicated students. Impossible to go even to a fraternity party without finding a number of students in various stages of intoxication and similar cases in non-fraternity rooming houses. Graduates and undergraduates, alumni, and visitors, many of them in all stages of intoxication, enjoying the annual homecoming. (22)

2. On the opposite side, with little or no publicity, but widespread in fact was the action taken by students themselves. At the University of Illinois, October, 1923, a meeting of 3,000 students voted to sustain prohibition, oppose drinking, and petition alumni, in anticipation of annual homecoming games, to leave hip-pocket flasks home. The declaration, signed personally by students, was sent with the usual invitation to alumni. The *Illini* wrote, "We want to look back on the Homecoming not only as the best in spirit and crowds, but as the cleanest." Student bodies at three other great universities took similar action as to their own practices and those of the "old Grads." A Yale meeting of 2,000 in 1923 in behalf of liquor law observance was sponsored by *The Yale News*, Admiral William L. Sims, the speaker. On February 8, 1924, *The Yale News*, stating editorial policy, listed as "No. 1," "The 18th Amendment should be strictly enforced throughout the university."

A national student conference with delegates from leading Eastern universities in 1923 (23) called on student bodies

throughout the country for positive expression of opinions on
the question. Approving this action, the *Brown University News,*
January 22, 1924, reported, "Already over 100 important educational institutions have voiced their approval of the enforcement
of the 18th Amendment. Brown University should be added to
this continually increasing list," and *Hoya,* Georgetown University, editorially challenged collegians to set a national example,
saying "The work might well begin in our schools, colleges, and
universities." A Princeton student forum after a two-hour discussion voted support, 192 to 42. The University of Pennsylvania
class of 1925 voted dry festivities for junior week, the secretary
stating that this voiced "not only its policy but that of the entire student body." At the University of Michigan a constructive
program sponsored by student leaders in anticipation of the junior
prom, included a conference of representative students, a mass
meeting with student speakers, and the cooperation of fraternities. "The campus was so dry," said the *Michigan Daily,* "that
they had to get out the lawn sprinklers." A straw vote by the
Daily "showed comfortable majorities against repeal, against
sale of beer and wine and in favor of strict enforcement."

At Illinois College, the student body put the college on record
as opposed to the current jokes on drinking in the movies, on the
stage, and in student and other publications. It expressed strong
support of the laws and sent the statement to President Coolidge.
Three fraternities at Rutgers filed voluntary statements favoring
prohibition and expressing intention to do all in their power to
stop the use of liquors in their groups and the college. Every fraternity reported regulations against liquor. The student self-
governing body at the University of North Dakota took action
against illegal selling on the campus and reported violators to
the officials, and the fraternities cooperated. Massachusetts
State reported a decided growth in student opinion against
drinking, the movement originating in one of the fraternities.
At Kalamazoo College in a student referendum of 300 votes, 3
were for repeal, 64 for wine and beer modification, and 263 for
a stricter enforcement. A mass meeting of 2,000 women at the
University of Wisconsin voted opposition to drinking. They cir-
culated a petition to Federal authorities for action against the
sources of intoxicants for students. A Mt. Holyoke student referendum expressed college opinion as opposing student drinking
and favoring prohibition; 765 votes were cast, 82 per cent of the

student body. Results: 669, 88 per cent "dry"; 53, 7 per cent, favoring wine and beer, and 41, 5 per cent, "wholly wet." The Russell Sage student governing association took a "decided stand against violation and use of intoxicants at social affairs." At Michigan State Normal the 450 men in a student body composed largely of women took a collective pledge of abstinence.

The idea of student women drinking hardly existed. A poll of 100 college editors, July 17, 1926, indicated "that drinking among students has declined in recent years" in the opinion of the majority of student editors. In one university five fraternities ejected from chapter houses visiting alumni who brought in liquor. At Carnegie Institute of Technology the Student Council recorded itself as favoring the 18th Amendment. The Student Council at the University of Arizona took action against booze parties, a student found drunk being expelled. At Macalester College 425 students in assembly voted to let their anti-liquor attitude be known in no uncertain terms. The Wooster College self-governing association voted a $25.00 fine for first offense drinking, and dismissal for second. The Indiana Interfraternity Association voted unconditional support of the 18th Amendment. University of Southern California students at the 1925 Washington's Birthday celebration, 3,000 attending, adopted a resolution for prohibition and for student action against disregard of the law. Pennsylvania State Student Council, 50 members, representing a student body of 3,400, heartily endorsed the public enforcement officers. Dartmouth governing body announced that it was "Vigorously opposed to drinking in Hanover and wherever the name of Dartmouth is concerned." University of Tennessee's men's mass meeting voted, "Not to tolerate drinking by students at public or private social functions." Denison student association, 1,000, expressed hearty accord with the law and condemned all attempts to violate it on the campus or country at large. Brown University student governing body stated, "Emphatic and vigorous opposition to bootlegging and drunkenness." Washington State association of students recommended to the administration the expulsion of students having intoxicants in their possession or under influence of such. Brigham Young student body, with 1,100 voting, except for 1%, favored the 18th Amendment. The editor of the University of Nevada *Sagebrush* reported, "It would be safe to say that approximately 3 per cent of Nevada

men drink. . . . In four years of observation I have known only
five women out of a student body averaging 700 who drank."

At Wesleyan University "The college authorities state that
there has been an entire change in the attitude of the students
and the faculty toward drinking, so that at the present time,
1924, they have only about one disciplining case a year in a body
of 600 students. And for a student to be known to drink liquor
at all is immediately followed by serious disciplinary measures.
. . . There is, however, some clandestine drinking, especially
associated with returning alumni and the fraternity life" (24).

A national student conference at Washington, April 5-6, 1924
(25), was the culmination of a series of student citizenship conferences throughout the country during the previous eight
months. Attended by 155 undergraduates representing 80 colleges from Texas and Colorado to New England, the conference
discussed such subjects as "The Situation in the Colleges Today,"
"Shall the 18th Amendment be Nullified by a Law-Defying
Minority?", "Shall the Law be Modified, or Repealed?" and "Can
a Government of Free Men Secure Obedience to Laws Legally
Passed by a Majority?" The theme of the conference was "Law
Observance," and the aim was to formulate and give national
expression of the average opinion on the liquor problem as
found at that time. A strong stand was taken in support of existing laws. One of the keenest observers, listening to the student
discussion, said: "The most disheartening thing was to hear the
undergraduates discuss the problem of the bad effects of the
Alumni when they came back for reunions, social events, and the
big games. The average undergraduate is a more law-abiding
citizen than the average father or older brother."

A careful newspaper survey at the end of the college year in
1924 (26), reaching two responsible sources in each college, the
president of the student body and the leading dean, was made
among 224 colleges and universities in all sections and nearly
every state. The survey sought to gain from the most dependable
sources reliable information that would contrast conditions before and after the adoption of national prohibition. The question
as to drinking among students was answered as follows: More,
5; Less, 128; Never a problem, 90. The question as to Law Observance by students: Better, 107; Worse, 14; Never a problem,
97. The conclusions were that student opinion was overwhelm-

ingly in support of prohibition; that the use of liquor was steadily
on the decline; that student drinking had been reduced since
prohibition; that better enforcement was demanded.

These views were supported from a different angle by the
representatives of a large book company constantly visiting colleges for purely business purposes, who said in 1925, "Boozing
is decidedly not popular on the college campuses today. College
sentiment is against it. In many universities it is emphatically
taboo, not because the faculty forbids it, but because student
leaders themselves will not have it."

On the whole, it seems clear that there was a very decided
reduction in the use of alcoholic liquors in colleges during the
first six or eight years of national prohibition, that the situation
was less favorable after about 1928, that after that date and
before repeal the change in attitude and opinion was far greater
than in personal and group practice, however spectacular the
claims of some about student resort to "hard liquors." There can
be no reasonable conclusion, taking into account all dependable
sources of information, but that alcoholic drink and drinking
customs were more nearly removed from American college life
from 1918 to 1930 than at any other period in the entire history
of the country.

V. *Reaction Period*

By 1932 wide questioning in connection with alcoholic drink
again had become prominent among students and colleges
throughout the country. But this time it related to a method for
handling liquor problems, to prohibition and its enforcement
rather than to alcoholic intoxication and its consequences in
life and society. Law evasion, bootlegging, rum running, home
brewing, and organized racketeering with large profits to shrewd
manipulators were the spectacular and powerful factors in the
experience of the young men and women at that time.

Under these conditions interest centered in the law, its modification or repeal, in the adventurous interest of trying the forbidden article, and a romantic turn toward social drinking customs and traditions of earlier days. An increasing number of
younger people first in the colleges of the East, near the Canadian border and in large cities, encouraged or extended illicit
practices. But the main change, at this period, was not in student drinking but in student thinking; it was a change in atti-

tudes more than in practices. Youthful drinking often seemed to those who were doing it to be much greater than it was.

But the changes in attitude, whatever the cause, were extensive, as shown in the 1932 survey by J. H. Barnett (27) with the cooperation of scientific experts and college authorities. It was a test of college opinion that included practically all of the colleges of the United States, that is, 409 out of the 426 accredited higher institutions. A carefully prepared questionnaire sent to each fifth name in the senior class was strictly anonymous and designed to procure the opinions of the students then in college, and to include all types of colleges in proportion to enrollment. The returns, 3,250, constituted 40 per cent of those sent out, proving a high degree of interest.

The question, "What is your attitude toward the Eighteenth Amendment and supplementary legislation?" showed answers as follows:

578	(a)	In favor of the present law
1,166	(b)	In favor of legalizing the sale of wines and beers
635	(c)	In favor of provisions to make the law more severe
1,301	(d)	In favor of repeal of the law
88	(e)	Indifferent toward the Amendment and its legislation

The result indicated that by 1932 college seniors in the ratio of about 2 to 1 were opposed to prohibition, or favored such changes as would be equivalent to reversal. This change doubtless corresponded to that throughout the country. But it is in striking contrast to the attitude shown by many of the largest universities, by the no less scientific survey of Professor Cortright in 1926 at which time the vote of seniors, except in one or two Eastern colleges, was strongly in support of the prohibition policy. And it was in contrast, also, with the survey made by Professor Mott, University of Chicago, in 1926, who found 88 per cent of 7,800 students in typical colleges as favorable to prohibition.

But the information brought out by the Barnett survey as to student drinking practices during this transition period is no less interesting. It shows an increasing spread of personal drinking, but a spread that does not at all correspond with that of wet student opinion.

For example, quoting from the survey, "Of the 1,280 males who drink, 328 list themselves as drinking once a week or more frequently, and 74 out of 309 females who drink, list themselves as drinking frequently. This gives a total of 402 Seniors drinking once a week or more frequently out of 3,250 who replied. This group is 12 per cent of the total, which is a relatively smaller proportion than has been commonly accepted as representing the facts." Or, briefly, in this last and very worst year of the national prohibition policy only 1 out of 8 college students was drinking as often as once a week, while more than 50 per cent were non-drinkers. To this may be added the statement of the compiler that the reports "reveal that Seniors who drink relatively infrequently are apparently anxious to be considered drinkers."

It is significant to note opinions of representative college deans in 1930, on the edge of the repeal movement, who had been continuously in college as students or teachers both during the open saloon and the prohibition periods. They probably more than any other group had dependable, first-hand observation and experience on which to base their conclusions. Representative statements, omitting colleges in which drinking problems were few in both periods, are as follows (28):

"There is much less drinking among students than there was fifteen or twenty years ago. But the results cause more comment," said C. J. Sambower, Dean of Men at Indiana University. "Out of a student body of four thousand not more than one per cent are habitual drinkers. Moreover, drinking among students is declining. The amount at present is distinctly less than it was five years ago."

At Illinois, Dean of Men Thomas Arkle Clark said that drinking in saloon years was "much more general" and "much less talked about." The saloon was the rendezvous for large numbers who made it a weekend loafing place. More general drinking produced more drunkenness, though the illegal liquor of this period was stronger. He adds, "Not many students learn to drink after they come to college."

"There is perhaps more talk about drinking in colleges now than twenty-five years ago," said President Arthur S. Pease of Amherst, but "the frequency and degree of drunkenness has been greatly reduced." And Dean William L. Machmer, of Massachusetts State, on the strength of his connection with the student discipline committee for thirteen years said that conditions were better in 1930 than in 1920, adding: "A drunken student is seldom seen on the campus today. . . . Our formal dances are so free from liquor that the administration does not view their coming with anxious concern. This was not true before prohibition" and "class and fraternity banquets now are absolutely free from liquor."

"During the eight years that I have been Dean of Men at West Virginia I have attended more than 300 dances. There has been a steady decline in the number of students who drink at these affairs. There has been a decided improvement during recent months. In 1922 some students 'passed out' at a few dances. Now the liquor breath is a decided exception at even our big dances," said Dean H. E. Stone. "Every one of the older faculty members and citizens with whom I have talked is positive that conditions have improved greatly both as to the town and the university."

"As a source for cases of discipline drinking has fallen from a major problem to one that is almost negligible," wrote Professor Clarence P. Gould, Western Reserve.

"Drinking today is not frowned upon by students to any extent—not even by women students," says a young dean, William D. Ramsey, Indiana University. "I am absolutely sure there is less drinking today than when I entered school. . . . My experience goes back six years. During most of my time as a student I lived in a fraternity house. . . . There are still numerous men who drink occasionally, but the number who do so habitually is very much smaller. Not only are fewer men drinking, but I think the amount consumed is smaller."

"Twenty years ago, when I was in college, our college banquets had wine served with the meals, and the pastime of drinking a man under the table was frequently indulged in. As one of the few abstainers, I regularly expected to take some intoxicated friend home and my expectations were seldom disappointed. I recall the surprise I felt when I first attended a 'dry' banquet, the 1910 national convention dinner of my fraternity, the first occasion that I recollect when there was no wine on the table and no public drunks. Several of my classmates drank themselves out of college, and the practice of students casually drinking in saloons was common. . . . Now there is some drinking, of course. But the banquets are dry, the dances are dry, I know of no student who has seriously injured himself in the four years I have been here," said Charles J. Turck, President of Centre College, Kentucky.

College presidents, notwithstanding their strong desire to uphold the reputation of their students and their own administrations, are scientific men and educators who know how to sift evidence. The following, therefore, is of merit as showing the situation in the colleges in 1930, when "prohibition at its worst" was soon to be followed by repeal and other methods of attempted handling of the liquor problem.

A questionnaire, in February, 1930, exclusively to presidents of state universities and the larger colleges, brought replies from 31 universities. Of these 26 presidents stated their belief that student drinking was not general; 1 said that there was more drinking at that time than before prohibition; 17 recorded themselves against repeal; 1 favored repeal; 5 desired some form of modification of the laws; 1 was for modification after prohibition had been given a fair trial; 1 said that though drinking had decreased, the students of his institution drank hard liquors almost exclusively; 1 declined to answer. The conclusion seemed clear that there was decidedly less drinking among colleges under prohibition than before.

But the college generations, freshmen in 1926 to 1928, the graduates of 1930 to 1932 were children in 1918. They had experienced nothing of the saloon and its social consequences; they knew nothing of the organized liquor traffic and how it promoted law evasion and vicious politics in the years of the saloons. Nor had there been public discussion, scientific instruction, or other education on the action and consequences of alcoholic liquor during their life experiences at all comparable with that which prevailed earlier. It was a new situation, a new generation facing a different alcoholic drink problem in the midst of an experiment not yet completed.

VI. *College Drinking Epidemic*

In the period of unrestricted distribution of intoxicating liquors that has followed the reversal of the prohibition policy, the renewed availability, easy access, and promoted sale of alcoholic pleasure have resulted in wider and more popular use by nearly all classes and groups, especially by young people, including college students, than can be found in any previous period. Individuals and groups among whom drinking formerly was disapproved and others to whom it was a matter of occasion in the saloon and during prohibition eras have accepted freely the present sense of release from social, moral, and legal restraint. The "bottle" and the "cocktail" have gained approval. Social drink customs and ways of extending the use and popularity of alcoholic beverages are promoted widely by trade propaganda. Never before has a generation of young people been brought so fully into contact with free-flowing quantities of liquor in the many ways in which it is now available to all in the grocery, the restaurant, the soda fountain, the roadside lunchroom, the tavern, the saloon, and the hotels. It is sold for home use and distributed to homes more extensively than in any former period. In communities which would not tolerate a saloon liquor may be procured at the corner drug store. Both new and revived customs have social prestige and influence. To drink has become "the thing to do." It is the fad of the moment. The swing is so general as to suggest a tidal wave of alcoholic indulgence.

In college communities this swing is in sharp contrast to the trend in the preceding half century under both saloon and no-saloon conditions. Liquor customs are sweeping college communities, even some of the church-related and smaller ones in which they had been taboo for years, as well as the universities in which they retained popularity during the restriction period.

Seeking recent information as to the extent and character of present college drinking, a comprehensive 1937 survey calls it a "great boom in student drinking" (29). The report shows a wide drift away from the ideal of abstinence and toward alcoholic sociability both in conduct and in opinion. We read that 303 reports from colleges indicate that drinking has increased since repeal and from 60 that it has not; 373 to 111 state that liquor is more available in college communities than before repeal; according to 267 college sentiment is favorable to "temperate" drinking; 18, indifferent; and 185, "teetotal." Briefly, "student drinking is on the increase everywhere" but with "relatively less drunkenness"; in 24 colleges drinking is acknowledged to be a problem and in 483 it is not so regarded; and "to drink as a gentleman" rather than heavily, or not at all, is now the idea. The conclusions reached are based on a questionnaire sent to 1,475 colleges, including each faculty member and student, the head of the college, and the college editor. The 645 replies represented 581 colleges of every type, sectarian and non-sectarian, large university, small college, and junior college. Many of those answering regard it as the most comprehensive survey ever made of the problem. The reports indicate less open drunkenness in proportion to the number drinking now than formerly. This comes, doubtless, from the great number of new competing interests and activities that supply social enjoyment and changes in group opinion toward the restraint of excess.

Another survey of more limited range, but of scientific worth was made by Professor Paul Studenski, New York University, between November, 1936, and May, 1937 (30). It included college students, white collar workers, and settlement house youth in and near New York City, by far the largest share being college students. "Of the 2,379 persons covered in this study," says Professor Studenski, "83 per cent reported that they drank occasionally or regularly either hard liquor, or beer, or wine. Only 17 per cent were complete abstainers. No marked difference has been discovered between the percentages of drinkers among the young men and young women, respectively. This is rather surprising. For one might have expected to find a somewhat lower percentage of drinkers among the young women than among the young men."

A fairly comprehensive questionnaire was distributed, filled out, and collected at group meetings. Of the total number returned and analyzed, 928 were from college students in New York City, 984 from college students outside of the city, 179 from white collar workers in the city, and 288 from young people in settlement houses. Since so large a share, 1,912 out of 2,379, were from college students, the facts and trends disclosed are of special significance as to the situation and attitudes among the students in that part of the country.

Among students of all ages and both sexes in New York City, 89 per cent were reported as drinkers and 11 per cent as non-drinkers; among students outside of New York City, 76 per cent as drinkers and 24 per cent as non-drinkers. The proportion of drinkers to non-drinkers, however, was higher among the white collar workers, 94 to 6, probably because of larger income and more time for indulgence of this sort.

The proportion of regular drinkers of hard liquor among the drinking young men appeared to be small. The proportion of occasional drinkers of hard liquor, on the other hand, was very large, about two-thirds in the younger group, of 18 to 21 years, and three-fourths in the older, of 22 to 25 years. Most of the hard liquor drinking was in the form of cocktails, highballs, etc. And most of it was done at parties and in homes, rather than in restaurants or at bars.

Nearly half of the young men reported increased drinking of hard liquors during the past two years. A somewhat larger proportion reported increased beer drinking. The proportion of young women reporting increased drinking of hard liquor was considerably larger than that of young men.

The reasons assigned for drinking were 1. Like the taste of liquor. 2. It makes one gayer and more entertaining. 3. Other people drink, and one desires to be sociable. 4. To forget trouble. 5. To brace one's self physically.

Eighty-five per cent of the students of colleges located in smaller cities and 75 per cent in colleges in New York reported that they have less respect for steady drinkers than for occasional drinkers, an opinion found predominantly among the young women. The majority expressed a more negative attitude toward a girl who is a steady drinker than toward a boy of that type.

The overwhelming majority demonstrated lack of scientific information by reporting that alcohol is a stimulant and that it warms one up in cold weather. The majority was correct on two questions: the uselessness of alcohol in warding off or curing disease, and the lesser harm of alcohol when consumed with food.

Approximately 75 per cent of the drinking youth favored a minimum age requirement of 18 years for the purchase of liquor; a minority of those 18 to 21 and a majority of those 22 to 25 favored raising the minimum age to 21. Three-fourths reported that they had no difficulty in purchasing liquor when under 18.

A majority reported that bars promote excessive drinking. Male college students were equally divided in opinion on allowing women to drink at bars; female students voted by a preponderant majority in favor of it. Settlement house youth, male and female, opposed bar drinking for women. An overwhelming majority of the young men in all groups voted against permitting unaccompanied women to drink at bars, as did the young women in all but one group.

But the outstanding changes in college "drink" traditions are those which include college women. The rush of young women to observance of "the cocktail hour" seems to be greater in some places at least than is the tendency of college men to renew drinking customs. Certainly for the moment it is more noted and spectacular. It may well be called the new liquor trend of the day. Of all the variations and new aspects that characterize the present expanding indulgence in intoxicants, none is in more sharp contrast with the trends of the past, or more unexpected than is this.

Quoting *The Literary Digest* survey of tendencies, "Co-eds and women students in general have lost their moral revulsion against drinking. Women's colleges are most liberal because so many of their students come from cosmopolitan areas." Of 36 New England colleges, 16 men's and 6 women's were reported as wet; 11 men's and 2 women's as having occasional or no drinking. The proportion in New England of women's colleges thus "taking to drink" since repeal seems to be larger than of the men's colleges. In the Middle Atlantic states, "women's colleges are the drier group." In the South, where they are numerous and smaller, all reported themselves as dry. Yet everywhere the "teetotal" idea "appears to be crumbling."

The increase among women students seems to be greater in the stronger liquors, especially cocktails, than in those of lower alcoholic content. Among the colleges of all kinds reporting, one-third see "a greater increase in cocktail and highball consumption." The tendency of girls to take cocktails rather than beer is explained, in part at least, by a women's college president who says that "girls will never drink much beer, because they are afraid it will make them fat."

In the past the influence of young women was a powerful restraining force against heavy indulgence by young men. Now they drink freely together anywhere. As a college editor expressed it, "Instead of holding men back, co-eds are saying, 'Let's have another.'"

Increasing use creates a demand for more opportunities to drink. Some college groups, limited in number, to be sure, but influential, are calling for enlarged drinking facilities on the campus. A student publication at a great central university editorially advocates the removal of restrictions against drinking at dances, saying that "perhaps the chief objection to holding dances on the campus is that drinking facilities are not provided. This is best met by a realization that a very large proportion of the students demand alcohol to produce a synthetic rapport . . . and that drinking on the campus would be better than drinking down town."

A poll of college editors by a brewers' association (31) developed the information that 40 editors out of 52 replying found more drinking in college today, but that, according to 41 of these, conditions had improved. The "improvements" listed included such as "we have less surreptitious drinking"; "We know what we are getting"; "We drink for pleasure and not for oblivion." A university daily wrote, "Taverns are coming to be places of serious discussion, just as were the coffee houses of the eighteenth century." Of the 52 colleges questioned in the brewers' poll, 16, and the largest, permit beer or other liquor on the premises.

An advertising service reports that 91 undergraduate publications out of 868 for which they handle advertising, are permitted to print beer and 39 "hard" liquor ads. At Harvard a state license permits the sale of beer in the lounge of a student house named for a former president who led in the local efforts to keep saloons out of Cambridge; Columbia serves beer in the university lounge; Yale has dropped a restriction against keeping alcoholic drinks in students' rooms; *The Yale Alumni Magazine* of November 12, 1937, shows pictures of members of the class of 1913 entertaining sons of their class, now students, at a smoker and beer party. The pictures are of students and professors drinking together. Princeton proctors assigned to enforce a regulation against use and possession of liquor on the campus are said to wink at infractions except when noisy disturbances result; at California beer only is allowed within a mile of the campus, but fraternity houses off the campus do a thriving trade unimpeded; Northwestern is reported to have relaxed its customary regulations to please alumni on a homecoming day.

Drinking at the big games and in the celebrations following is popular. "A gala football crowd," wrote Dean Christian Gauss of Princeton, "has become an ideal setting for the drunken exhibitionist. In many universities the authorities have instructed their police to evict drunkards, yet almost never can one be evicted. The crowd's sympathies are with the drunkard; he has become part of the spectacle, the clown of the circus" (32).

In contrast is the report of the following incident at Yale in 1923: "While the thousands crowded the Bowl for the Yale-Army contest, a youth stood erect from the crowd and tilted a bottle to his lips. Instead of envious glances that formerly accompanied such a move, there was a roar from the surrounding multitude. . . . Cries of 'put him out' were heard echoing over the field. . . . A policeman suddenly appeared . . . the drunken boy and three companions were ejected . . . the crowd cheered the bluecoat" (33).

In various directions it is evident that university authorities now often base their regulations on the assumption that intoxicating liquors among students are serious enough for consideration only when disorders and public disturbances result. The impression is that the amount consumed is best controlled by the pressure of the students against their friends who tend to become disgustingly intoxicated. This attitude is in marked contrast with that of the deans of colleges, generally, and of disciplinary officials during much of the license and all of the license and all of the prohibition period.

As to direction that these enlarged drinking habits may take in the future, it is a question whether the present generation of youthful drinkers will be able to gain greater control over themselves than did youth of similar age in the former saloon days. Most of them believe that they can. But Dean Paul Nixon, Bowdoin College, reports that a survey of a recent graduating class on a variety of subjects including "temperance" shows that in one year 10 per cent had gained in that respect, 30 per cent had remained unchanged, 40 per cent had lost a little, and 20 per cent had lost greatly—that is, that 60 per cent actually had increased their intemperance during the first year out of college.

This means about the same as the statement in the Studenski survey that "nearly half of the young men reported increased drinking of hard liquors during the past two years. A somewhat larger proportion reported increased beer drinking," and that "the proportion of young women reporting increased drinking of hard liquor was considerably larger than that of the young men."

VII. A Survey of the Surveys

But what is significant, if anything, about the prevalence of alcoholic customs in college communities which stand out as the sources of higher education in the life of the nation? What may be gained in a constructive way from a comparison of the attitudes and customs relating to alcoholic pleasure in this special group during the three periods—license, prohibition, repeal—in the recent history of the United States? The following conclusions may stimulate further study:

1. College alcoholic pleasures, customs, and consequences are not different from those elsewhere in influential society. They are a cross-section, a spectacular exhibit of the rapidly moving life and thought of the day. Notwithstanding age-old traditions peculiar to colleges, honored and retained here and there, and the outbreaks of enthusiasm moistened with alcohol after the big games, at fraternity, alumni, and other group affairs, liquor enjoyment is not "collegiate." Resort to it and dependence upon it follow social, class, family, and community standards. But as a feature in publicity and public interest student drinking has a clear place of its own.

2. The pressure of dignified and conventional social customs more than any other factor gives alcoholic indulgences a continuing place of influence in college life. This is evident from the study in all of the three main periods. The desire to share with others in what they are doing, to be a "sport" not a "wet blanket," to follow practices that are socially approved and to avoid those that are disapproved by the social hostess, the upperclass, or alumni, or those in positions of toastmaster, and the leaders of the party is a dominating social force with most people, young or old. The continual seeking after alcoholic pleasure in the face of scientific and practical experience and the objective evidence of tendencies toward excess are due largely to the operation of customs accepted almost unconsciously from generation to generation.

3. Frequent social drinking, in the college group or outside, is a source of the later drinking habits often overlooked, or ignored, or undiscovered until the desire has been fixed in the habit patterns of life.

4. A certain amount of "adventure drinking" comes from the tendency of college youth to "try anything once" and to learn by the experimental approach encouraged in modern education. This may result in hilarious or spectacular indulgence, but it as often ends with a few experiments. This form of drinking was unusually prominent during the prohibition period, and freely exploited by those opposed to that policy. Yet it does not tend to the establishing of life habits with their danger of heavy

drinking as do the pressures of social custom and profit-seeking promotion.

5. Another type is reported by the student whom Professor Slosson calls the "natural rebel, the Bohemian, the self-assertive collegian, just old enough to feel social restrictions as intolerable." He is the one who "began drinking under prohibition, and because of it, obtaining more thrill from the thought that he was breaking a law than from the drink itself." But this sort of individual facing social drink pressure may as readily defy it and adopt personal "dry" practices because he is individualistic. His position is more promising than that of the overwhelming majority who accept the "goose step" of college or community traditions.

6. The seeking of release that prompts many in the general community to drink for emotional expression, escape from irritations, self-consciousness, or misery, probably is not so frequent and has less excuse among normal young people in college than it has outside where weak personalities have to face the problems of life.

7. The more dangerous forms of social drinking, such as "the cocktail hour," are growing in popularity. The trend of a century of increasing criticism of these practices has been reversed. To drink is the expected thing. And this reaction now includes young women as well as men. Such customs spread liquor more widely and among far greater numbers than did the "forbidden fruit" psychology in the days of legal restraint, or the open invitation of the saloon years. Heavy drinking is not openly evident, but the appeal of social smartness and of easy access constantly adds to the number of drinkers and the frequency of their use. Out of the new situation is certain to come an increasing number whose lives cannot be happy without satisfaction of the sensations that come from alcohol.

8. The facts of this survey emphasize the importance of comprehensive study of the entire problem of alcoholic indulgence in life today; of the separation of scientific truth from socially inherited or propaganda-made opinions; of the trends in the different periods and their meaning; of the satisfactions and dissatisfactions that are connected with narcotic pleasure; and of the place that intelligence and educated leadership may take in efforts toward understanding and solution in coming years.

9. The broadening of liquor customs in college communities

has a meaning of its own, since it occurs in that group from which most of the future leaders of social prestige and public opinion will come. Not all the youth in college become leaders; not all who become leaders attend college; but the ratio of those with leadership ability and opportunity in college is decidedly greater than elsewhere among young people. Therefore the growth of drinking approvals among students is of far greater significance to the country than among youth in general.

10. For a hundred years after 1830 thinking people were increasingly critical of liquor and its customs. The ratio of non-drinkers and rare-occasion drinkers increased, and the ratio of frequent drinkers decreased. For twenty years, previous to 1930, liquor use was seriously disapproved. Less drinking existed in colleges in proportion to attendance, notwithstanding heavy criticism of legal restraint, and an increase of "wet thinking," in the prohibition period than at any previous period in the history of the country.

11. The present trend is a reversal of the trend of 100 years. It is toward a wider diffusion of drink practices and greater regularity of use among larger numbers. For a comparable situation one must turn back, not twenty, nor thirty years, but to the conditions that prevailed more than a century ago.

REFERENCES

1. Thayer, W. R. *Universities and Their Sons* (1898), Vol. 1.
2. "College Customs," *Standard Encyclopedia of the Alcohol Problem,* Vol. II, pp. 646-52.
3. Crane, Richard T. *The Demoralization of College Life* (1911).
4. Crane, R. T. *Boston American* (September 11, 1911), p. 36.
5. *Washington Star* (November 15, 1913).
6. *Intercollegiate Statesman* (April, 1909).
7. *Intercollegiate Statesman* (April, 1913).
8. "Michigan College Dry Campaign," *Intercollegiate Statesman* (May, 1916).
9. "Fighting Beer-busts at California," *Intercollegiate Statesman* (May, 1912).
10. "Yale Seniors Banish Booze," *Intercollegiate Statesman* (March, 1917).
11. "Drink Traditions at Yale," *Intercollegiate Statesman* (April-May, 1917).
12. Fisher, Irving. *Prohibition at Its Worst,* pp. 72-82.

13. *Chicago Post* (June 4, 1926).
14. *Intercollegiate Statesman* (October, 1926).
15. "College Student Editors on College Drinking," *Literary Digest* (July 17, 1926).
16. "Changing Student Customs," *International Student* (May, 1927).
17. *Current History* (April, 1928).
18. CORTRIGHT, E. E. "Objective Evidence of Student Opinion," *International Student* (May, 1927).
19. "American Colleges and Prohibition"; survey of opinion, *Intercollegiate Statesman* (April, 1922).
20. *Scientific Temperance Jr.* (September, 1922).
21. Samuel Plantz, manuscript.
22. *Intercollegiate Statesman* (October, 1923).
23. *Intercollegiate Statesman* (November, 1923).
24. *Intercollegiate Statesman* (May and June, 1924).
25. "National Student Conference Takes Action," *Intercollegiate Statesman* (April, 1924).
26. "American Student Attitudes," *Christian Science Monitor* (June, 1924).
27. BARNETT, J. H. "College Seniors and the Liquor Problem," *Annals American Academy* (September, 1932).
28. "Drink in Colleges, 'Before and after,'" *International Student* (April 30, 1930).
29. "Great Boom in Student Drinking," *Literary Digest* (March 6, 1937).
30. STUDENSKI, PAUL. "Liquor Consumption Among American Youth," Social Study Committee, National Conference of State Liquor Administrators, 1937.
31. THEIL, LEON S. "Must Drinking Be a College Sport?", *Allied Youth* (February, 1937).
32. GAUSS, CHRISTIAN. "Will the Football Bubble Burst?", *Saturday Evening Post* (September 14, 1935).
33. *New Haven Union* (1923); quoted in Plantz survey.

Chapter 3

EDUCATION AND DRINKING BEHAVIOR

HAROLD A. MULFORD

University of Iowa

BEHAVIORAL SCIENTISTS have found that much behavior in our society varies according to educational level. They have also found that the concept "education" can be operationalized conveniently as the number of years of formal schooling completed. Therefore, it is not surprising that investigations of drinking behavior often employ education as a variable. Usually, however, the concept education is employed as merely one of several background factors examined for possible association with drinking patterns. The concept has received little attention as a major explanatory variable. This state of affairs undoubtedly reflects the fact that researchers have not agreed upon the logical content of the concept—if indeed they attend to it at all. It is not certain what phenomena are subsumed by the rubric "education."

The studies that have investigated the association between educational level and drinking behavior mostly fall into two categories: first, general population surveys which examine the association between education and (a) the prevalence of drinkers, (b) the extent of drinking and (c) extreme deviant drinking; and secondly, studies of the educational attainment of institutionalized alcoholics.

This chapter draws from surveys of general population samples but will not attend to studies of institutionalized alcoholics. Lemert (8), in 1951, reviewed the investigations of hospitalized and jailed alcoholics and concluded that the study populations were too highly selected in too many known and unknown ways to permit generalizations beyond the specific populations under study or to permit conclusions regarding educational differences between alcoholics and the general population. We concur. Since subsequent studies of institutionalized alcoholics suffer the same methodological shortcomings, we will give little attention to them here. Instead, we shall review current knowledge regarding rates of drinkers, rates of heavy drinkers, and rates of deviant or problem drinkers as they vary by education in the general adult population.

Education and Rates of Drinkers

Table 1 presents the rate of drinkers[1] by education found in the several state and national general population surveys that have been reported. Without exception, these surveys have reported a positive association between rates of drinkers and edu-

TABLE 1.—Per Cent Who Drink, in Selected Social Segments

	Riley-Marden USA (1946) (N=2677)	Washington State (1951) (N=478)	Iowa (1958) (N=1185)	Iowa (1961) (N=1213)	Mulford USA (1963) (N=1509)	Cahalan, Cisin, & Crossley USA (1964-65) (N=2746)
Adult Population 21 years and older	65%	63%	59%	59%	71%	68%
College	70*	64	63	66	80	77%
High School		66	60	64	75	71%
Grade School	62†	61	51	45	53	53%

* At least graduated from high school.
† Less than high school graduate.

[1] To distinguish "drinkers" from "abstainers" the two Iowa surveys (12, 15) and the 1963 national survey (11) used a question originally developed by the Gallup Poll: "Do you ever have occasion to use alcoholic beverages such as liquor, wine or beer—or are you a total abstainer?" The response alternatives were: (1) "Yes, I have occasion to use," and (2) "No, I am a total abstainer." The term *drinker* as used in this paper means persons who responded positively to the question.
Riley and Marden (19) asked, "Would you mind telling us which of these you sometimes drink?" The response alternatives included different types of beverage alcohol and "none" category. Maxwell (9) did not report the question wording used in the Washington state survey. Cahalan, Cisin and Crossley asked a separate question for each type of alcoholic beverage and defined drinkers as those who usually drink some alcoholic beverage at least once a year.

cational achievement. In every case, the grade school educated have the lowest rate of drinkers; and, with the possible exception of the Washington study, the college educated have the highest rate. However, the rate for the high school educated is only slightly below that of the college educated.[2]

Riley and Marden (19) in 1946 reported the first systematically gathered evidence that the use of beverage alcohol in the United States varies according to educational attainment. They studied 2,677 respondents, chosen to represent the adults[3] of the nation, and found that 70 per cent of those with at least a high school education said they sometimes drank alcoholic beverages. This compares with 62 per cent of those who had not graduated from high school. These are the only two educational categories reported by these authors.

In 1951, Maxwell (9) studied the drinking behavior of 478 respondents representing the adult population of the state of Washington. Although, as shown in Table 1, the prevalence of drinkers varied little by educational level, still, consistent with the other studies, the grade school educated had the lowest rate.

In 1958, Mulford and Miller (12) surveyed the drinking behavior of adult Iowans by interviewing a representative sample of 1,185 respondents. While they found little difference in rates of drinkers between the college and high school educated, the grade school educated had the lowest rate and the college educated had the highest rate. These findings were again confirmed in 1961 by a replication study involving a sample of 1,213 adult Iowans (15).

In 1963, Mulford (11) investigated the drinking behavior of 1,515 respondents, chosen to represent the nation's adults. Again, the college educated had the highest rate of drinkers while the grade school educated had the lowest rate and, again, the difference between the college educated and the high school educated was relatively small.

In late 1964 and early 1965, and after five years of preliminary studies to develop refined methodological procedures, Cahalan, Cisin and Crossley surveyed a national sample of 2,746 respond-

---

[2] "College educated" is here defined as one or more years of college. "High school educated" means one to four years of high school and "grade school educated" means one to eight years of elementary school completed.

[3] "Adults" refers to persons 21 years of age or older.

ents and, as seen in Table 1, obtained very similar results (4, p. 45).

Finally, several community surveys also show the same relationship between education and prevalence of drinkers. This includes studies in Berkeley, California (7, p. 80), Hartford, Connecticut (3, p. 16), and Cedar Rapids, Iowa (18, pp. 22-25).

Although these several studies span a seventeen-year time period, they permit few, if any, conclusions regarding trends in the relationship between drinking and education. A comparison of the findings of the 1946 Riley-Marden study and the more recent national studies does, however, suggest an increase in the rate of drinkers for all educational levels.

In summary, it is safe to conclude from the findings presented in Table 1 that Americans with more education have a higher rate of drinkers than do those with less education. However, the difference between the college educated and the high school educated is relatively small as compared with the greater difference between the grade school and the high school educated. These conclusions are strengthened by the fact that these studies span a fairly long time period and involve different study populations, as well as variations in methodological procedures.

Specifying the Relationships

While the consistency of the above findings leaves little doubt that the prevalence of drinkers is higher among those with more years of schooling, the nature of the relationship between education and drinking behavior remains to be specified. A step in this direction was taken by Mulford and Miller (12, see Tables, pp. 717, 719) who examined the prevalence of drinkers by education while controlling several other sociocultural factors, namely, sex, religion, age, and rural-urban residence.[4]

The pertinent findings of this state survey are summarized in Table 2:

1. *Sex and education.* Table 2 shows that for both men and women the grade school educated had the lowest prevalence rate; but, whereas the rate for men increased monotonically with increased education, for women the high school educated had

---

[4] Cahalan, Cisin and Crossley ran certain measures of drinking behavior against education while controlling sex, but otherwise made little use of education as a variable in their analysis (4, Tables, pp. 45, 332, 334, 338).

TABLE 2.—*Per Cent Who Drink, by Education and Other Selected Factors*

	Grade School		High School		College		Total	
	Per Cent Drink	N	Per Cent Drink	N	Per Cent Drink	N	Per Cent Drink	N
A. Sex								
Male	60	165	67	288	79	121	66	574
Female	37	121	54	326	49	132	49	579
B. Residence								
City	60	118	66	292	72	134	66	544
Town	46	71	56	126	60	67	55	264
Farm	42	97	53	197	49	51	49	345
C. Age								
21-35	61	39	67	254	75	100	69	393
36-45	51	64	64	177	64	62	62	303
46+	48	184	46	182	50	90	48	456
D. Religion								
Catholic	74	55	76	134	92	38	79	227
Lutheran	56	39	66	67	50	20	61	126
Methodist	36	36	50	100	59	39	49	175
P.D.U.*	48	77	61	169	60	83	58	329

* Protestant, denomination unspecified.
Source: (12, tables: (12, tables, pp. 717 and 719).

a higher rate than the college educated. However, Cahalan, *et al.* (4) found the relationship monotonic for both sexes.

2. *Residence and education.* Regardless of residence (city, town or farm), the grade school educated had the lowest and the college educated had the highest rate of drinkers, except that for farm dwellers the high school educated had the highest rate.

3. *Age and education.* When age was controlled, again, those with less education tended to have the lowest prevalence rate. However, educational differences decreased with increasing age and virtually disappeared for the age group "46 years and older." Approximately one-half of this age group drank regardless of educational level.

4. *Religion and education.* Drinking prevalence was positively associated with education within each of the four religious categories which had Ns large enough to justify examination. These were Catholics, Lutherans, Methodists, and Protestants who did not specify a denomination. However, education was not uniformly related to prevalence rates within the various religious groups. Among Catholics the prevalence rate differed little between the grade school and the high school educated, but rose sharply for the college educated. Among the "unspecified" Protestants the greatest difference was found between the grade school educated and those with more education.

A replication of the 1958 Iowa survey (15, p. 46) conducted three years later (1961), supported the reliability of the originally observed prevalence rates for the total population and for each of the three educational categories. The replication also confirmed the original findings that when the several factors of sex, residence, religion, and age are each controlled none erased educational differences except for the age group "46 years and older," as noted above. Nevertheless, the degree and meaning of these associations remain problematic. Further efforts to specify the relationship between education and drinking behavior must await studies using a much larger sample.

Moreover, the sample used in the Iowa studies was not large enough to examine variations in drinking behavior by educational level when *simultaneously* controlling more than one other factor. Conceivably, a study involving a very large sample, permitting the simultaneous control of sex, age, religion, residence and other background factors, would magnify educational differences in drinking behavior for certain social segments whereas in other segments the differences would disappear or the direction of the relationship would change. This is a much-needed step toward resolving the concept "education" into its components.

Education and Extent of Alcohol Consumption

Studies to date yield few conclusive answers but raise many questions about the relationship between the extent of alcohol consumption and educational level. This relationship is not so clear as the relationship between rates of drinkers and education.

Riley and Marden (19) found no difference in the rate of "regular" drinkers (drink three times a week or more) when the rate for those who had not graduated from high school (17 per cent) was compared with the rate for high school graduates (18 per cent). Maxwell (9), using the same definition for "regular" drinker, distinguished between the college, high school and grade school educated, and reported that 6 per cent of the college educated as compared with 12 per cent of both the high school and grade school educated were regular drinkers. In a later report based on the same data, Maxwell (10) reported that the high school educated respondents also had a higher proportion of heavy drinkers (Q-F Index types 4 and 5)[5] than did the college educated.

Cahalan, *et al.* (3, p. 16), using data collected in a Hartford, Connecticut, survey in 1964, found that the rate of heavy drink-

---

[5] The Quantity-Frequency (Q-F) Index originally developed by Straus and Bacon (20) was adopted for use in the Washington state survey, the two Iowa studies, and the 1963 national survey. The Q-F Index is based on the respondent's report of the number of drinks (converted to absolute alcohol) which he ordinarily consumes at a sitting, combined with the reported frequency of such "sittings" in a given period of time. Various response combinations yield the following five Q-F Index types:

Type 1. Drinks infrequently (once a month at most) and consumes small amounts (not more than approximately 1.6 ounces of absolute alcohol).

Type 2. Drinks infrequently (once a month at most) and consumes medium (1.6 to 2.88 ounces of absolute alcohol) or large amounts (more than 2.88 ounces of absolute alcohol).

Type 3. Drinks more than once a month but consumes small amounts.

Type 4. Drinks two to four times a month and consumes medium or large amounts.

Type 5. Drinks more than once a week and consumes medium or large amounts.

For a further description of the Index, see Mulford and Miller (13).

ers among drinkers was considerably lower for the grade school educated (4 per cent) than for either the high school or the college educated, both of whom had a rate of 17 per cent. However, their findings are contradicted by the Cahalan, Cisin, Crossley national survey findings (4, p. 45) where the highest rate of heavy drinkers was found among those with "some college" (15 per cent) and the lowest rate was found among those with "some high school" (10 per cent). Otherwise they found little association between education and rates of heavy drinkers. The latter findings are more consistent with the Iowa study findings, as well as the findings of the earlier national survey by Mulford (11). The two studies by the Cahalan group (3, 4) both used a very complex procedure to define "heavy drinker." They gave as typical examples of a "heavy drinker": "Drank nearly every day with five or more drinks at a sitting at least once in a while; or drank at least weekly with usually five or more drinks in most occasions of drinking" (4, pp. 8, 21-28; compare 3, p. 12).

Mulford and Miller in the first Iowa survey (13) examined rates of heavy drinkers[6] (defined as Q-F Index type 5) and related these rates to educational level. There was no significant association between rates of heavy drinkers and education until other factors were controlled. This is seen in the first row of Table 3 where the rate of heavy drinkers varies only one percentage point for the three educational categories. However, the table also shows that, when other background factors are controlled, educational differences in rates of heavy drinkers do appear.

Sex and education. The association between education and heavy drinking goes in opposite directions for the two sexes. While the rate for women decreases, the rate for men increases with increased education. It is interesting to note that among men both light drinking and heavy drinking increase with increased education, which means that the proportion of moderate drinkers among men decreases with increased education. The Cahalan, Cisin and Crossley study (4, p. 45) reveals no association between education and heavy drinking using the educational categories employed throughout this chapter. However,

[6] Here the base for the rates of heavy drinkers is drinkers only. This is true of the Cahalan, *et al.* national study also.

TABLE 3.—*Distribution of Light and Heavy Drinkers among Drinkers in the Iowa Adult Population, by Education and Other Selected Factors*

| | GRADE SCHOOL | | | HIGH SCHOOL | | | COLLEGE | | |
	% Light	% Hvy	N	% Light	% Hvy	N	% Light	% Hvy	N
Totals	44	16	135	47	16	357	51	17	157
A. Residence									
City	46	15	68	41	18	190	41	22	92
Town	40	17	30	48	18	67	65	13	40
Farm	47	17	36	59	11	99	64	4	25
B. Religion									
Catholic	34	21	38	41	21	96	34	17	35
Lutherans	50	10	20	48	14	44	40	20	10
Methodists	50	8	12	56	17	48	64	18	22
P.D.U.*	50	8	36	52	7	99	59	12	49
C. Age									
21-35	61	13	23	48	15	165	55	16	75
36-45	35	19	31	43	17	111	44	15	39
46+	43	15	81	49	18	78	52	17	42
D. Sex									
Male	35	18	91	38	23	185	41	25	93
Female	65	12	43	56	9	171	66	5	64

* Protestant, denomination unspecified.
Source: (13, tables, pp. 30-31, 33).

using finer categories of educational attainment which distinguish "some high school" from "completed high school" and "some college" from "college graduate" their data indicate that men who have completed high school but have no college stand out with the heaviest rates of heavy drinkers (28 per cent). Women who are prominent for their low rate of heavy drinking are those who are college graduates (2 per cent) and those with no more than a grade school education (3 per cent). This is consistent with the Mulford-Miller findings that women with more education have lower rates of heavy drinkers.

Residence and education. Controlling rural-urban residence also yields a reversal in the direction of the associations. Among city residents, the proportion of light drinkers decreases and the proportion of heavy drinkers increases with increased education. The reverse of this is found among town and farm dwellers. The increase in light drinking and decrease in heavy drinking with increased education is most pronounced among farm residents.

Religion and education. When religion is controlled, the association between education and rates of heavy drinkers differs for Protestants and Catholics; i.e., the rates of heavy drinkers tend to increase with increased education for Protestants but the relationship reverses direction for Catholics.

Age and education. The proportion of light drinkers varies with education in each age category in a complex way. In the youngest age group, the grade school educated have the highest proportion of light drinkers, while the opposite is true in the older groups. Variations in the proportion of heavy drinkers by education virtually disappears when age is controlled, which undoubtedly reflects the high association between age and education attainment.

In the Iowa replication study, of the several sociocultural factors investigated for their association with the extent of drinking in the original study, education had the most questionable reliability. Whereas in the 1958 study there was no total association between education and rates of heavy drinkers, an association did appear in the replication. For example, heavy drinkers comprised only 5 per cent of the grade school educated drinkers compared with 15 per cent of the college educated. It was also observed in the replication that, whereas the association between heavy drinking and education was stronger for men than it was in the original study, it disappeared for women. Moreover, in the 1963 national survey, Mulford (11, p. 640) found that while the rate of heavy drinkers was lowest (9 per cent) for the grade school educated, it was only slightly higher (11 per cent) for both the college and high school educated. This lack of strong total association between education and rates of heavy drinkers is consistent with the original (1958) Iowa study findings.

The above findings regarding the association between extent of drinking and education only whet our curiosity. Because the associations run in different directions for different segments of the population, the total association is cancelled. But, apparently, the extent of alcohol consumption does vary by education for certain sociocultural segments. Again, we note the need for a sample large enough to determine the variations in drinking behavior according to the several sociocultural factors.

Nevertheless, we may draw the following tentative conclusions. The extent of alcohol consumption appears to *increase* with increased education for men, unspecified Protestants and city dwellers, but it *decreases* with increased education for women, Catholics and farm residents. However, caution is in order. All of the apparent associations mentioned might look quite different if, for example, age and one or more additional factors were controlled simultaneously.

Education and Extreme Deviant Drinking

Another measure of drinking behavior that has been examined for its association with education is extreme deviant drinking behavior manifested by those who are commonly labeled "alcoholics." Whether alcoholics differ from the general population with respect to educational status is not yet known. However, there are some relevant study findings which warrant review here.

Since Lemert (8) has pointed out the fallacy of drawing conclusions about educational differences between alcoholics and non-alcoholics based upon institutionalized populations, here we shall consider only the general population studies which have attempted to isolate the most extreme deviant drinkers for comparison with the remainder of the sample. There have been several such studies, the findings of which provide useful hypotheses for further research.

The first such study was conducted in Kansas in 1954 (1). In this field survey appropriate county authorities—usually the judge, county attorney, and police—were asked to list members of the community whom they considered problem drinkers and to describe them in terms of several sociocultural attributes. Problem drinkers were defined as persons whose drinking had led to a personal or family problem in health, work or income, marital or domestic relations, or in community relationships. This was done in several communities chosen to be roughly representative of the state of Kansas. The respondents were unable to estimate the educational level of many of the problem drinkers whom they reported. However, among the cases reported, the less educated appeared to be overrepresented (1, p. 59).

Neither Riley and Marden (19) nor Maxwell (9) distinguished "extreme deviant" drinkers in their general population surveys. However, Mulford and Miller, in the 1958 survey (14), using the Iowa Scale of Preoccupation with Alcohol did attempt to isolate the most extreme deviant drinkers for comparisons with the balance of the sample. Whether we consider the 35 respondents with Preoccupation Scale scores of I or II or the 73 with scores I-III (that is, the most preoccupied), the grade school educated were overrepresented and the college educated underrepresented. Only 9 per cent of those who scored I or II as compared with 22 per cent of the total sample were college educated. On the other hand, 44 per cent of the highly preoccupied as compared with 25 per cent of the sample had a grade school education (16).

In the 1963 national survey, Mulford (11) used two indexes to isolate the most extreme drinkers: the Preoccupation Scale and the Trouble-Due-To-Drinking Index. Deviant drinking as measured by both of these scales showed only a slight decrease with increased education. The rate of trouble-due-to-drinking was 13 per cent for the grade school educated, 10 per cent for the high school and 9 per cent for the college educated. The rate preoccupied for the three educational categories was 11 per cent, 10 per cent and 9 per cent, respectively.

In a community survey (Cedar Rapids, Iowa), Mulford and Wilson (17, pp. 22-25) found a similar but stronger association. Among the 46 persons high on the preoccupation scale (scores of I, II, or III) the college educated were underrepresented. Only 13 per cent of the preoccupied drinkers had a college education as compared with 24 per cent of the general population sample of Cedar Rapids. The grade school educated were slightly overrepresented among preoccupied drinkers, 24 per cent as compared with an expected 21 per cent. On the other hand, the high school educated were considerably overrepresented among the 46 highly preoccupied drinkers, 63 per cent compared with an expected 54 per cent. The Cedar Rapids study also found that the grade school educated as well as the high school educated were both overrepresented among persons reporting trouble due to drinking, while the college educated were considerably underrepresented. Bailey et al. (2, p. 27), in a survey conducted in New York City, isolated 132 "probable alcoholics"; the individuals so classified were identified on the basis of the drinking problems they or family members reported, plus indications of gross drinking behavior noted by interviewers. The study found that the rate of "probable alcoholics" was highest among the least educated. Finally, Cahalan, Cisin and Crossley isolated a category of extreme drinkers which they called "heavy escape drinkers"; and it appears that again the college educated are underrepresented and the grade school educated are overrepresented among such deviant drinkers, at least as compared with other heavy drinkers and moderate drinkers. This was true of both men and women except that the college educated are underrepresented among all women heavy drinkers whether or not they drink to escape life's problems (4, p. 338).

In summary, the several surveys of national, state and local community populations which have attempted to isolate the most extreme deviant drinkers have consistently found the grade school educated to have the highest rates, while the college educated have the lowest rates. The consistency of this finding is more impressive when one considers the variety of study populations and methods employed, especially the methods of identifying the presumed alcoholics.

We believe, however, that this major conclusion remains problematic. All of the criteria used to isolate the presumed alcoholics in these several studies, with the exception of the Cahalan, Cisin and Crossley criteria for heavy escape drinkers and possibly the preoccupation scale developed by Mulford and Miller, rest heavily upon the amount of trouble the respondent encountered because of his drinking. Any index of trouble-due-to-drinking is likely to be biased in favor of the better educated and against the less educated. The better educated (higher SES) persons have certain built-in protections against trouble due to drinking. They are likely to be treated more gently by the police. They are less likely to have financial trouble, which is often indirectly related to domestic family trouble. Furthermore, the better educated are more likely to be married to a spouse who is a drinker and who will, therefore, be more tolerant of drinking and heavy drinking at home rather than in public. That is, the more tolerant spouse is not so likely to force the heavy drinker to do his drinking in public where there is a greater chance of encountering trouble. Some of the items constituting the preoccupation scale may also be biased in a similar fashion. For example, a person with more education is more likely to have enough financial resources that he need not worry about his supply or be concerned about having enough to drink at a party. And, perhaps he can afford to be very discriminating about the brand and type of beverage he drinks. Moreover, the scale may be biased against the higher educated because its origin lies in studies of AA members and institutionalized alcoholics (5, 6, 18). The higher educated very heavy drinkers are more likely to escape the institutionalization process and thus would be underrepresented in institutions, including AA groups.

Summary and Discussion

Any conclusions regarding differences in drinking behavior according to educational attainment must be treated as highly tentative. The studies to date have laid valuable groundwork and provide useful hypotheses. One of the strongest conclusions is that persons who have completed more years of formal education are more likely to be drinkers. However, even this relationship partly reflects the association between age and educational level.

The conclusion that the extent of drinking increases with increased education for men, unspecified Protestants and city dwellers, but decreases with increased education for women, Catholics and farm residents, is worthy of further study. But, again, age must be controlled since this factor tends to reduce or erase educational differences in rates of heavy drinkers. And the conclusion that the rate of extreme deviant drinking is highest for the grade school and lowest for the college educated should be treated as a working hypothesis until our society reaches more consensus regarding the classification and labeling of drinkers.

While we still are in the process of defining the alcoholic as a social object, there is also the problem of more clearly defining the concept "education." A major difficulty with the concept as a useful scientific tool is that so many factors are subsumed by it. The deceptive ease of defining the concept operationally may have deterred a thorough conceptual analysis. In brief, we do not know all the factors implied by amount of education.

Number of years of school completed reflects a host of factors which must, ultimately, be distinguished and separately related to drinking behavior. It is likely that not all of the associations will be found to be in the same direction. The component elements of the concept education as presently defined, which are most likely to modify the meaning of exposure to education, would include at least age, financial and class status, religion, sex, and probably many more. The older age groups in our population have, on the average, a lower number of years of formal schooling. In addition, it appears that there has been a trend toward a more liberal attitude toward alcohol use over the past generation or two. Number of years of schooling also is often dependent upon financial status. Moreover, certain religious groupings tend to have a higher level of education, and males are more likely than females to acquire more years of schooling. Years of schooling also reflect physical and social maturation, not to mention changes in role obligations and self-definition. These are only some of the variables which must be considered in interpreting the number of years of education reported by an individual.

It is meaningless to think of education as a casual variable until the elements of the concept have been specified. To operationalize education as years of formal schooling completed is justifiable, therefore, primarily as a matter of convenience. It is not at all clear that anything taught in school greatly affects drinking habits. Straus and Bacon (20, p. 63) report, for example, that college students pay less attention to teachers' than to parents' advice to abstain. What is learned informally about drinking by participants in the educational system that might explain the association between educational attainment and differences in drinking behavior, remains a matter for conjecture. We suspect that when the concept is resolved into its component elements we will find ourselves dealing with the attitudes or plans of action toward alcohol and several other objects including oneself, which the individual learns in interaction with significant other persons, and that this interaction and learning is only indirectly a function of educational attainment.

A great deal of work remains to be done at both the conceptual and the empirical levels if the concept *education* is to be useful in understanding drinking behavior. One valuable next step would be a general population survey involving a number of cases great enough to permit a finer analysis than has been possible to date.

REFERENCES

1. *Alcoholism Survey, State of Kansas.* Topeka, Kansas: Kansas State Commission on Alcoholism, 1954.
2. BAILEY, MARGARET, PAUL W. HABERMAN, and HAROLD ALKSNE. "The Epidemiology of Alcoholism in an Urban Residential Area," *Quarterly Journal of Studies on Alcohol,* 26: 19-40, 1965.
3. CAHALAN, DON, IRA H. CISIN, ARTHUR D. KIRSCH and CAROL NEWCOMB. *Behavior and Attitudes Related to Drinking in a Medium-Sized Urban Community in New England.* Social Research Project, Report 2. Washington, D. C.: George Washington University, 1965.
4. CAHALAN, DON, IRA H. CISIN, and HELEN M. CROSSLEY. *American Drinking Practices, A National Survey of Behavior and Attitudes Related to Alcoholic Beverages.* Social Research Project, Report 3. Washington, D. C.: George Washington University, 1967.
5. JACKSON, J. K. "The Definition and Measurement of Alcoholism, H-Technique Scale of Preoccupation with Alcohol and Psychological Involvement," *Quarterly Journal of Studies on Alcohol,* 18: 240-262, 1957.
6. JELLINEK, E. M. "Phases of Alcohol Addiction," *Quarterly Journal of Studies on Alcohol,* 13: 673-684, 1952.
7. KNUPFER, GENEVIEVE. *Characteristics of Abstainers; a Comparison of Drinkers and Non-Drinkers in a Large California City,* California Drinking Practices Study, Report No. 3, 1961.
8. LEMERT, EDWIN M. "Educational Characteristics of Alcoholics," *Quarterly Journal of Studies on Alcohol,* 12: 475-478, 1951.
9. MAXWELL, M. A. "Drinking Behavior in the State of Washington," *Quarterly Journal of Studies on Alcohol,* 13: 219-239, 1952.
10. MAXWELL, M. A. "A Quantity-Frequency Analysis of Drinking Behavior in the State of Washington," *Northwestern Science,* 32: 57-67, 1958.
11. MULFORD, HAROLD A. "Drinking and Deviant Drinking, U.S.A., 1963," *Quarterly Journal of Studies on Alcohol,* 25: 634-650, 1964.
12. MULFORD, HAROLD A., and D. E. MILLER. "Drinking in Iowa, I., Sociocultural Distribution of Drinkers with a Methodological Model for Sampling Evaluation and Interpretation of Findings," *Quarterly Journal of Studies on Alcohol,* 20: 704, 726, 1959.
13. MULFORD, HAROLD A., and D. E. MILLER. "Drinking in Iowa, II., The Extent of Drinking and Selected Sociocultural Cate-

gories," *Quarterly Journal of Studies on Alcohol*, 21: 26-39, 1960.

14. MULFORD, HAROLD A., and D. E. MILLER. "Drinking in Iowa, IV., Preoccupation with Alcohol and Definitions of Alcohol, Heavy Drinking and Trouble Due To Drinking," *Quarterly Journal of Studies on Alcohol*, 21: 279-291, 1960.
15. MULFORD, HAROLD A., and D. E. MILLER. "The Prevalence and Extent of Drinking in Iowa, 1961; A Replication and an Evaluation of Methods," *Quarterly Journal of Studies on Alcohol*, 24: 39-53, 1963.
16. MULFORD, HAROLD A., and D. E. MILLER. "An Index of Alcoholic Drinking Behavior Related to the Meanings of Alcohol," *Journal of Health and Human Behavior*, 2: 26-31, 1961.
17. MULFORD, HAROLD A., and D. E. MILLER. "Preoccupation with Alcohol and Definitions of Alcohol; A Replication of Two Cumulative Scales," *Quarterly Journal of Studies on Alcohol*, 24: 682-696, 1963.
18. MULFORD, HAROLD A., and RONALD WILSON. "Identifying Problem Drinkers in a Household Health Survey," U. S. Dept. of Health, Education and Welfare, Public Health Service, Publication 1000, Series 2, Number 16. Washington, D. C.: U. S. Government Printing Office, May 1966.
19. RILEY, J. F., JR., and C. F. MARDEN. "The Social Pattern of Alcoholic Drinking," *Quarterly Journal of Studies on Alcohol*, 8: 265-273, 1947.
20. STRAUS, R., and S. D. BACON. *Drinking in College*. New Haven, Conn.: Yale University Press; 1953.

PART TWO
EMPIRICAL STUDIES

INTRODUCTORY NOTE

THE EMPIRICAL STUDIES presented in Part II are organized around the themes of development, social structure, and meaning. Although any given chapter may include material which bears on more than one of these themes, Section A (chapters 4-9) focuses on the emergence of drinking patterns and style of drinking as a social process which both antedates and postdates the college years. Section B (chapters 10-14) emphasizes the relevance of social norms and groups in the emergence and regulation of alcohol use and abuse among collegians. Section C (chapters 15-17) calls attention to personal needs and cultural definitions of drinking behavior as factors which influence the ways in which individuals think about and use beverage alcohol.

In the typical case, a collegian does not learn to drink in college. Young people in the process of growing up in the United States, where most adults drink at least occasionally, expect to drink when they become adults and most eventually do. The motivations for drinking among youth in high school and the social characteristics of the majority who have established a drinking pattern before graduation from high school are essentially like the motivations and patterns of drinking found among the adults who serve as role models for youth (chapter 4).

Although most college students drink, established patterns of drinking are less commonly found among freshmen than among upperclassmen. And the proportion of abstaining college freshmen varies considerably with the different parental and community norms about drinking and abstinence to which students are exposed prior to entering college. Campbell (chapter 5) uses a sample of freshmen known to have been exposed to abstinence norms and who were in fact predominantly abstinent as seniors in high school to predict continued conformity to these norms under the changed normative and surveillance conditions which accompany entrance into college. He reports that identification with abstaining parents and, to a greater extent, internalization of abstinence norms predicts continued abstinence, a preference for abstaining friends, not joining fraternities, and the devaluation of alcohol and its use. Yet even in the freshman year, Campbell's students are well on their way to joining the majority of collegians who drink.

Maddox (chapter 6), following a sample of male Negro collegians through their first year in college, notes that, in contrast to Campbell's abstainers, the Negro collegians began college as drinkers. The drinking styles of most of these Negro students are, however, unstable. The abstainers who become drinkers and the drinkers who become ex-drinkers or reduce their drinking suggest that students have a great deal of negotiating to do before a stable drinking pattern emerges. Students appear to be searching for a drinking style which balances in a satisfactory if not optimal fashion parental norms, peer group expectations, and desirable alcohol-induced modifications of reality which are not overly threatening. Russell's collection of excerpts from autobiographical accounts of drinking in college illustrates the variety and complexity of the issues which students must negotiate. In their drinking students illustrate role playing, role taking, and, perhaps more important, role making. For many, if not most, students, there is a playful quality evident in their drinking. At one time or another they use parents and peers as models for their drinking behavior or abstinence. But, in the end, the typical student must make a role for himself as a drinker or an abstainer, and the particular role he makes always has complex determinants. Only subsequent research will determine whether, in the typical case, the graduating collegian has established a stable pattern of drinking.

Roman (chapter 8) focuses on a special but increasingly large category of collegians, the graduate student in arts and sciences. He notes the unobtrusiveness of drinking among these students and conjectures that those for whom drinking was a preoccupation probably would not make it to graduate school anyway. Moreover, economic restraints, patterns of social activity which are unlike those of the undergraduate, and normative constraints which define rather clearly appropriate and inappropriate drinking help keep drinking unobtrusive among graduate students for the most part. Roman speculates that, while the incidence of problem drinking would appear to be low among graduate students, potential trouble with drinking may be masked by the effective constraints of the college environment. Only with the removal of these constraints, as in the case of the graduate student who becomes a professor, would this potential become obvious. This suggestion only reminds us that we should know more than we do about the drinking behavior of faculty members in colleges and universities to match what we know about their students.

Roman's speculation about the masked potential for problem drinking among graduate students anticipates the interest of Trice and Belasco (chapter 9). Is there a relationship between drinking behavior in college and subsequent pathological drinking behavior? We do not have prospective studies on drinking behavior which follow collegians as they become alumni. Trice and Belasco have used the more common and admittedly risky procedure of retrospection in the characterization of drinking in college by a number of alcoholic executives. They suggest that little if anything in the descriptions of drinking in college by these executives seems especially significant as a predictor of their pathological drinking behavior as executives. The important factors in the development of alcoholism for these alumni appear to have been related to specific aspects of their career development after graduation from college. Trice and Belasco do not propose a systematic theory of alcoholism on the basis of their limited data. They do suggest, however, that drinking patterns among collegians may not be a very adequate basis for predicting pathological drinking among college alumni.

Section B shifts attention from the development of drinking patterns to the structural context in which drinking styles develop. Mizruchi and Perrucci (chapter 10) outline a perspective for the analysis of drinking norms. They note, for example, that such norms are sometimes prescriptive but more often proscriptive in our society. The absence of directives about how to drink, in contrast to a directive that merely states "Don't," is troublesome in a highly mobile society in which most people in fact drink. Mizruchi and Perrucci argue that drinking situations in this society are all too frequently characterized by normative ambiguity or permissiveness. This ambiguity, in turn, increases the probability of ambivalence toward drinking and the development of integrated and integrating drinking norms which ordinarily would keep drinking within socially approved bounds.

Peek (chapter 11) provides an illustration of proscriptive

norms in his review of formal college drinking rules. The rules in the typical college say "Don't." But the fact is that students in the typical college do drink and evidence found in other chapters of this volume suggests that collegians do not appear to take drinking prohibitions any more seriously than the administrators who announce and fail to implement them. This situation might be discussed with appropriately cynical remarks about human inconsistency. But the Mizruchi and Perrucci discussion indicates that college rules may encourage problem drinking, the very behavior the rules are ostensibly meant to preclude. Stable patterns of moderate drinking may develop in college in spite of campus drinking rules, not because of them. [Parental and community norms which students bring to the campus with them, as well as peer group norms developed on the campus, may provide the rules which actually direct drinking in college.]

Alexander and Campbell (chapter 12) indicate, however, that lack of consensus about drinking rules is found off as well as on the campus. Major segments of religious denominations have prohibitive norms in regard to drinking and these norms have an impact on the way in which even drinkers devaluate their behavior. College drinkers who are affiliated with churches which prefer abstinence handle the resulting dissonance occasionally by disaffiliation but more often by reduced participation and by selective inattention to the proscriptions. Although Alexander and Campbell only hint at the possible consequences of drinking by an individual who has been taught that drinking is morally wrong, loss of self-esteem is certainly one of the most likely consequences (chapter 6).

Gusfield (chapter 13) and Rogers (chapter 14) both concentrate on the importance of community and campus culture and social structure for understanding drinking among collegians. [Any given campus is a mixture of individuals whose drinking or abstinence reflects parental, social class, religious and ethnic preferences.] On the campus, fraternities and sororities represent the institutionalization of relatively heavy drinking which, in the cases of those exposed to them, sometimes intensifies existing drinking patterns and at other times reshapes these patterns to conform to the drinking style characteristic of these social groups. Colleges are typically drinking places and, within colleges, fraternities and sororities are relatively the places most dedicated to drinking. This is so even when it is recognized that dominant drinking styles vary from one campus to another and, on any given campus, among social groups.

[Drinking means different things to different drinkers.] This is the inference invited by Sections A and B of Part II and made explicit in Section C. Jessor, Carman, and Grossman (chapter 15) look specifically at the notions which students have about what drinking can do for them in relation to their expectation of fulfilling needs for achievement and affiliation.] The use of alcohol is seen by these authors as a socially learned way of adapting and coping with individual needs. And it is those students who do not expect their needs for achievement and affiliation to be met that are most likely to drink with the intention of narcotizing themselves and to experience trouble as a consequence of their drinking.] Jessor, Carman, and Grossman do not argue that most students drink to narcotize themselves or have trouble with their drinking. Their data would not support such a conclusion. Moreover, for the same reason, they do not argue that even those students who have come to use alcohol as a narcotizer and who have experienced trouble with their drinking are fledgling problem drinkers. Williams (chapter 16) is clearly interested in using configurations of personal needs to identify the pre-alcoholic among collegians, although he is appropriately aware of the limitations of his data. What Williams does demonstrate is that problem drinkers are plentiful on college campuses and that these problem drinkers present personality profiles which approximate the profiles of known alcoholics. But, equally important, Williams notes that the relationship between the personality profiles of known alcoholics and collegians who are problem drinkers is far from perfect. The predictive value of Williams' profiles remains to be demonstrated, as Williams himself is aware. Park (chapter 17), the originator of the problem drinking index used by Williams, is concerned with configuration of drinking behaviors rather than personality profiles. Through factor analysis he has identified a pattern of problem drinking, as distinct from social drinking and relief drinking, which apparently has some utility when applied cross-nationally. This work calls attention to the various nuances of drinking in different cultural settings. But more important, it suggests that, compared with Finnish and Italian students, Amer-

ican collegians appear to have a high incidence of problem
drinking. With this observation we have come full cycle. The
American collegian develops his pattern of drinking in a cultural and social setting designed to create trouble. It is hardly
remarkable that many of them do experience trouble with drinking. It is probably more remarkable that so many do not.

Section A. Development Patterns

Chapter 4

DRINKING PRIOR TO COLLEGE*

GEORGE L. MADDOX

Duke University

THE ADOLESCENT does not invent the idea of drinking. He learns it. The acceptability and desirability of drinking are continually suggested to him by the elaborate integration of the use of alcohol into American culture and adult social behavior. A majority of adults in the United States drink at least occasionally, and research indicates that the proportion of drinkers and their drinking patterns have remained relatively stable since 1943. Children, on the other hand, are generally assumed to be abstinent. Any attempt to explain the persistence of adult drinking therefore necessarily focuses attention on when and how the abstinence of childhood is transformed, for the majority, into the drinking patterns of adulthood.

Drinking Is Learned Behavior

The human offspring is not born a social being. This is a basic assumption in the behavioral sciences. Although the individual is born with the potentiality for becoming a social being, whether and how this potentiality is developed and channeled are largely matters of learning. An individual's expectations, his attitudes, and his behavior are developed through contact with adult members of the species over a long period of time. His responses to persons and other objects or events in his external environment can be adequately understood only as one understands the tra-

* Condensed from *Alcohol Education for Classroom and Community*, edited by R. McCarthy. © 1964 by McGraw-Hill, Inc. and used with their permission.

---

* Condensed from *Alcohol Education for Classroom and Community*, edited by R. McCarthy. © 1964 by McGraw-Hill, Inc. and used with their permission.

ditional meanings which persons, objects, and events come to have for him as a result of his interaction with those persons who are significant in his experience. The individual never views the external world entirely free from the influence which these culturally defined and socially shared meanings and expectations come to have for him.

The system of traditionally defined meanings which serve as potential guides for behavior, and which are shared with other members of a group, is what the behavioral scientist designates as culture. In becoming a social being the individual may be said to be socialized. He learns to play roles appropriate to a wide variety of social situations. When socialized individuals not only share similar expectations about social roles but also sanction conformity to these shared expectations, behavior patterns are said to be institutionalized. From the point of view of the behavioral scientist, most drinking behavior can be understood best as an aspect of culture; the use or non-use of alcohol is institutionalized behavior for particular groups within the society and is integrally related to a number of roles.

The availability of alcohol to members of a society does not in itself explain its use or non-use as a beverage. Whether one drinks—and what, how, where, when, and with whom—is institutionalized behavior for particular groups. Although the use of alcohol is obviously a part of the cultural tradition of the United States, so also is abstinence. And, while some drinking is obviously institutionalized for some persons in some groups, whether one is encouraged, permitted, or forbidden to drink reflects such social factors as ethnic background, socioeconomic position, religious orientation, age, and sex. Some use of beverage alcohol is institutionalized among Orthodox Jews, for example; total abstinence is institutionalized among Mormons. Drinking is more permissible for the male than for the female, more permissible for the adult than for the adolescent. Therefore, in becoming socialized, the individual is never exposed to culture in general; he is exposed to particular groups whose members introduce him to the institutionalized roles appropriate for him in that group. The male child, for example, does not learn only how to be a man. He must also learn what it means to be a child as distinct from an adult, or, perhaps, what it means to be a white middle-class Presbyterian as distinct from a Negro lower-class follower of a Father Divine. He must learn

whether drinking is ever appropriate and, if it is, when, where,
with whom, and to what extent it is appropriate. An individual's
drinking behavior typically conforms to the expectations of significant groups in his social environment.

Adolescence is of particular relevance to an understanding of
the emergence of drinking or abstinence in our society because
it is obviously the transition between the childhood and the
adult roles. The boundaries of adolescence are not clearly or
precisely defined for us. In general terms, introduction to this
age grade comes with puberty, i.e., about age 12 to 15. It is
terminated informally by the assumption of adult-like responsibilities such as marriage or a full-time job, or by entrance into
the armed forces, which occurs normally upon graduation from
high school at about age 19. It is terminated formally by attaining the age of 21. Adolescence, therefore, is roughly synonymous
with the teen years and the junior and senior high school grades
of our educational system. The precise determination of biological ages equivalent to the beginning and end of adolescence in
this society is neither possible nor particularly relevant. What
is important is the recognition that, in our society, the adolescent is in a transitional age grade in which he is no longer a
child but not yet quite an adult. Literally, the adolescent is in
the process of becoming an adult; he is permitted, and increasingly required with age, to play at the institutionalized roles
associated with adulthood. The adolescent consequently learns
the attitudes toward and the uses of beverage alcohol appropriate to adulthood as he has come to understand generally what
it means to be an adult.

A Review of the Research

What, in fact, adolescents in our society typically learn to
think about and to do with beverage alcohol is not merely a
matter of speculation. From 1948 to 1965 eleven studies were
made of drinking behavior and attitudes, involving well over
10,000 adolescents in high school (1-11). These studies have
been supplemented by several investigations of the older adolescent in college (12-14). In addition, limited information about
the dropout, the adolescent who is of high school age but not
in school, has been provided incidentally in another study (15).

It is not possible to summarize the findings of each investigation separately. Fortunately it is not necessary to do so, since the most striking conclusion to be drawn from a comparison of these various investigations is the similarity of their findings. It is therefore possible to summarize, without specific reference to relatively minor variations in the findings, some of our most basic information concerning what adolescents in our society are thinking about alcohol and doing with it.

1. The personal use of alcohol is not typically a childhood experience in this society. The first personal use tends to occur about the thirteenth or fourteenth year, that is, at puberty or upon entrance into high school. Some tasting commonly occurs before this time, however.

2. The probability is quite high that every adolescent in our society will have drunk an alcoholic beverage at least once before being graduated from high school. The establishment of regular patterns of alcohol consumption does not necessarily follow such experimentation, although regular use is modal among older youth.

3. There is marked variation from community to community in the proportion of adolescents who drink beverage alcohol, that is to say, those for whom drinking has not been confined to a single isolated experience or to religious situations only. Majorities ranging from 6 to 8 out of 10 adolescents have been found to be drinkers in some communities, both in high school and in college, while minorities of only 3 or 4 out of 10 have been found to be drinkers in other communities. These variations reflect regional and ethnic subcultures.

4. The first personal use of alcohol is typically reported to be in the home, with parents or other relatives present.

5. Adolescents who drink typically report that at least one parent drinks. The abstinent adolescent usually reports that his parents are also abstinent.

6. The proportion of drinking adolescents who claim parental approval is greatest among those who confine their drinking to the home.

7. Among adolescents, as among adults, the probability that an individual will drink varies with such social factors as sex, age, socioeconomic position, ethnic and religious background, and rural or urban residence. The probability that

the adolescent will drink increases with age. The drinker is more likely to be a male than a female; at the extremes of socioeconomic status rather than in the middle range; a Jew or Catholic rather than a Protestant; and living in an urban rather than a rural area.]

8. Adolescents typically associate drinking with adult role-playing and particularly with those situations in which adults are being convivial, celebrating a special event, or seeking relief from tensions and anxiety.

9. The probability that an adolescent will drink increases as he approaches the assumption of adult-like roles and responsibilities. Since in our society this comes, for the majority, with graduation from high school, this proposition may be restated: The probability that an adolescent will drink increases as he approaches graduation from high school.

10. Adolescents tend to perceive alcohol as a social beverage rather than as a drug; they tend to emphasize, in their descriptions of drinking and its consequences, what alcohol does for the drinker rather than what it does to him.

11. The prevalence of drinking among adolescents in a community is not demonstrably dependent on the legal restraints specifically designed to prevent or discourage drinking among minors.

12. Only a minority of adolescents, even when they themselves are abstinent, consider drinking, either among adults or among their age peers, to be morally wrong under all circumstances. Some subgroups of adolescents—for example, persons identified with certain Protestant denominations —are more likely than others to report personal abstinence and to express disapproval of all drinking by their age peers.

13. The incidence of problem drinking among adolescents appears to be low. The most commonly used beverages are typically those with low alcohol content. The best estimates of the proportion of adolescents who consume, on the average, at least one drink a day range between 2 and 6 per cent. Subjective evaluations of the consequences of intensive drinking suggest that perhaps 1 in 4 adolescents who drink becomes high or gay during a given month and that perhaps 1 in 10 experiences drunkenness.

14. Adolescent attitudes toward, and use of, beverage alcohol

are oriented toward, and to a large extent are imitation of, adult attitudes and behavior. The existence of a teen-age culture or of adolescent gangs within which drinking is primarily an expression of adolescent rebellion against, or hostility toward, adult authority is not supported by the evidence. This does not mean that drinking by adolescents never is an expression of rebellion and hostility toward adult authority, but that this is not typically the case.

15. There is little evidence based on carefully controlled investigation to indicate significant modifications in adolescent attitudes toward, or use of, beverage alcohol over the past two decades.

In brief, the available research on adolescent attitudes toward beverage alcohol and adolescent patterns of use or nonuse suggests the establishment of regularity by the time they are graduated from high school, if not before. Observed variations in attitude toward and in patterns of drinking are closely related to social factors such as family, religious affiliation, ethnic background, socioeconomic position, age, and sex. An adolescent's behavior reflects the institutionalized behavior patterns of the significant social groups with which he is identified and mirrors the complex cultural traditions of American society. In sum, he does not invent ideas of drinking or abstinence; he learns them.

Agents of Socialization

Since what the adolescent learns to think about and do about drinking reflects so basically his exposure to cultural traditions as interpreted by and channeled through significant groups and persons with whom he is identified, specific attention needs to be given to selected agents and agencies of socialization. The influence of parents, peers, the mass media of communication, and religious and secular educational agencies will be considered briefly here.

The most accurate basis for predicting what an adolescent will think about and do with beverage alcohol is to know what his parents think about and do with it. Such prediction is, of course, not perfect. Parents frequently have complex and contradictory attitudes toward adult drinking; this is even more likely to be true with regard to drinking by their adolescent children. Nevertheless, the evidence which we have just reviewed indicates that if both parents are drinkers, the probability is high both that the adolescent child will eventually drink and that he will be introduced to drinking by his parents. If only one parent is a user, the probability decreases. If neither parent is a user, the probability is high that the adolescent will be abstinent.

Theoretically, one would expect the observation that parents are the best key to understanding the behavior of their adolescent children. The parents have access to the child before, longer than, and more intimately than any other persons or social groups. Therefore, when adolescents report that they view drinking as typical adult behavior; that their first drinking experiences occur more often at home than any other place; that parental law frequently permits some drinking in the home; and that alcoholic beverages are frequently available in the home—then one would expect adolescent use of and attitudes toward beverage alcohol to be very much as they are in fact found to be.

Although the image of adulthood which parents provide is basic for the adolescent, it is not the only available image. Age peers, who have been socialized by adults who may have varying attitudes toward alcohol, become important quite early in the experience of the child and assume increasing importance with age. This is especially the case in our society, given its institutionalization of a relatively long transitional period between childhood and adulthood. A great deal has been written in recent years about youth cultures and adolescent peer groups which institutionalize patterns of behavior that are contrary to adult expectations and demands. Since in our society drinking is generally thought to be primarily the prerogative of adults, drinking by adolescents has sometimes been interpreted as behavior expressing hostility toward adult demands and expectations. From this point of view, the adolescent peer group or gang whose members drink is considered to be deviant and to be a constant source of temptation and seduction for the nondrinking adolescent. This point of view is encouraged by legislation which variously defines the purchase, possession, or use of alcohol by minors as illegal.

A review of the evidence indicates how distorted this perspective is. First exposure to use in the home, parental law permitting limited use in the home, the relationship between the assumption of adult-like roles and the probability of use—these data suggest that many adolescents would learn to drink if there were no contact with age peers whatsoever. The evidence does suggest that there is frequently more drinking in peer groups than parents know about. This is not difficult to understand when one remembers that adolescence in our society is an ill-defined period in which the individual is in the process of becoming an adult, a period in which he must play at being an adult without being allowed to play adult roles fully. With regard to drinking, as with smoking and sexual behavior, the adolescent perceives that what is appropriate for adults is not equally appropriate for himself, even though it may eventually be. Thus, while some drinking may be considered permissible for adults, the determination of when adulthood is achieved remains a persistent problem for both adults and adolescents. The task is complicated by the ill-defined limits of the adolescent age grade. In such a situation, some tensions and disagreement between adolescents and adults would be expected. It does not follow that all, or even most, adolescent drinkers are by definition in open rebellion against adults.

It does not follow, either, that groups of adolescent drinkers are irresistibly seductive to non-drinkers or that they place irresistible pressure on the non-drinker to become a user. Research has not clearly identified the mechanisms which help the non-drinking adolescent to remain abstinent. But the fact remains that a large minority, and in some communities a majority, of adolescents continue to be abstinent alongside groups of adolescents who drink. This is possible because the non-drinker is able to find support for his abstinence from age peers and adults who are important to him. Moreover, there is simply no evidence that the principal criterion by which adolescents judge the acceptability of one another is whether or not alcohol is used. In brief, the adolescent does not have to learn about drinking from his age peers; observation of adults, particularly parents, provides him with much of this information. Age peers do provide support for experimentation with drinking which is considered premature by adults; however, this experimentation involves behavior which is typically recognized as legitimate for those who have achieved adult status. The myth of inevitable and irresistible peer-group pressure to drink may well be one of those myths which tend to become self-fulfilling prophecies.

The impact of the mass media of communication on what the adolescent thinks about, and does with, alcohol also needs critical review. Like age-peer groups, the mass media have the characteristic of exposing the adolescent to alternative models of behavior which do not necessarily support the parental model. In a complex society this problem of confronting the adolescent with alternative and sometimes contradictory models of behavior is, of course, not confined to the use of alcohol alone. Books, magazines, newspapers, radio, and television continually suggest alternatives in religion, politics, ethics, speech, clothing, and style of life in general to the adolescent without necessarily being mediated through parents or other adults.

These observations have led some persons to conclude that mass media are agencies of evil aiming at the destruction of the moral fabric of society. The mass media, particularly advertising, are assumed somehow to be responsible for the prevalence and incidence of drinking, for example. There are no carefully controlled studies demonstrating a relationship between the prevalence of liquor advertising and the incidence of drinking. However, a close relationship would not be expected on inferential grounds. If the non-drinker could be incited to drink merely by exposure to sophisticated advertising, then the persistent portion of non-drinkers in our society who presumably are exposed to such advertising would be difficult to explain. The assumption that individuals can be manipulated simply by subjecting them to the mass media is overly simple and misleading. It is increasingly obvious that knowledge of the interpersonal environment of the individual is basic to an understanding of what exposure to mass media advertising means to him and of what his response to that exposure is likely to be (16, 17).

The effect of the mass media on drinking behavior cannot be totally discounted. At the very minimum, advertisement of beverage alcohol suggests the legitimacy and normality of some adult drinking. Such a suggestion would tend to confirm the impression of the adolescent whose interpersonal relationships have oriented him to drinking. It remains to be demonstrated that the mass media are crucial in transforming into a drinker the abstinent adolescent whose interpersonal relationships support his abstinence.

American churches do not exhibit a consistent position with regard to the use of alcohol. While there would appear to be

116   GEORGE L. MADDOX

general agreement among the various churches that some uses
of alcohol are misuses, there is obviously not agreement that total
abstinence is the only morally defensible way of life. Moreover,
as suggested in the previous discussions of the mass media, the
influence which could be exerted on the adolescent by a model
of adult behavior originating in and transmitted by a church
organization cannot be understood apart from the interpersonal
environment of the adolescent. For example, drinking is consistently found to be less among both adult and adolescent members of certain religious groups. Yet, since identification with
and participation in such groups is largely voluntary, it is not
always apparent that the observed behavior is to be explained
as a result of that religious identification and participation. It
is equally possible that a religious organization continues to
attract persons whose attitudes and drinking behavior are most
consistent with, or at least can be made compatible with, the
position assumed by that organization.* The evidence on this
point is not conclusive. Nevertheless, there is no indication that
religious organizations as socializing agencies can or do intervene effectively to increase the prevalence of abstinence among
persons whose interpersonal relationships otherwise support
drinking.

The conclusion which has been drawn about the church, as a
socializing agency with regard to the use of beverage alcohol
and attitudes toward it, is generally applicable to the public
school. There is no evidence indicating that the public school
has intervened successfully to increase the prevalence of abstinence among those whose interpersonal relationships otherwise
support drinking. The school, as a public institution based on
involuntary attendance, is typically more heterogeneous than
most church groups. A typical public school will include students whose parents and peers support the legitimacy of some
drinking and students whose parents and peers do not. Awareness of this diversity of background underlies the decision of
many schools to avoid altogether any discussion of the use of
alcohol. Other schools restrict their attention to emphasizing the
illegality of the use of alcohol by minors and in this way avoid
raising the question of the legitimacy of adult drinking. Thus,

* See chapter 12 in this volume.

while the public school may provide information and encourage attitudes and skills supporting temporary or even total and permanent abstinence, there is every indication that the public school is less important than parents and peers in determining whether or not the adolescent will drink.

In summary, parents and age peers, in that order, are the principal socializing agencies which appear to be crucial to an understanding of the emergence of attitudes toward beverage alcohol among adolescents in our society. The available evidence does not indicate that the incidence of drinking and abstinence has been or can be significantly modified by the intervention of the mass media, the church, or the school, independently of interpersonal relationships with parents and age peers.

Why Drinking Persists

The typical adolescent in our society eventually learns to drink. He learns to want to drink. He learns this in very much the same way that he learns to want to drive an automobile, to smoke, to be married; and he learns all these things primarily from the same people, his parents and age peers. Whether one approves or not, drinking is a culturally defined and institutionalized part of the strategy through which many adults relate themselves to the social environment. Adults have reasons for their drinking, as they have reasons for many of the things they do. Most adults develop a vocabulary of motives or reasons for their behavior in anticipation of answering the question: Why did you do this or that? When adults are asked why they drink, they typically speak of being sociable, of enjoyment, of celebrating special events, or of relieving tensions and anxiety. Thus, while modification of reality is one of the verbalized reasons for drinking among adults, it is not usually advanced as the principal reason, nor is there any reason to believe that it is in fact the principal reason. Alcohol is more commonly a symbolic means for relating oneself to the interpersonal environment.

When adolescents are asked why they drink, it is not surprising that they offer a vocabulary of motives similar to that of adults. Adolescent drinkers are generally agreed that they or their age peers drink to be one of the crowd, to celebrate special occasions, and to enjoy themselves. Reduction of tension and anxiety is recognized as a reason why some adults drink, but adolescents themselves seldom attribute their drinking to this motive.

Drinking or abstinence among adolescents, then, seems best understood as an integral aspect of growing up, of becoming an adult as they understand what adulthood means. For the majority, adulthood implies some drinking; for a persistent minority, it does not. For those who associate adulthood with some use of alcohol, the probability of use increases consistently as the assumption of adult roles and responsibilities is approached. Drinking with one's age peers—in contrast to tasting with one's parents or with other adults—is initially, for these adolescents, part of an improvised rite of transition which terminates their adolescent status and introduces them into the relatively autonomous world of the adult.

Drinking Involves Risks

The institutionalization of patterns of drinking tends to minimize the risks associated with its use. The drinking of most individuals stays within the limits prescribed by the groups in which they habitually participate. All risks, however, cannot be eliminated. The fact that alcohol is typically thought of and used predominantly as a social beverage does not ensure that it will never be thought of and used as a drug. Alcoholism and drunkenness are cases in point. The persistence of drinking patterns which deviate from the institutionalized expectations among adult drinkers is a source of legitimate concern in our society, even though such deviant behavior is characteristic of a minority of adult drinkers only.

For some adults any use of alcohol by an adolescent is, by definition, deviant. If, however, the designation "problem drinking" is reserved for that use of alcohol which is regarded as deviant by the adolescent's parents and age peers and which results in social complications for the drinker, problem drinking among adolescents in our society does not appear to be common. This designation is probably applicable to 2 to 5 per cent of the adolescents who drink. In perhaps the most careful study yet made on this point, Straus and Bacon (12) found that among college students only 1 in 3 males, and 1 in 5 females, reported ever having experienced social complications as a result of their drinking. The most commonly experienced complications were failure to meet obligations and damage to friendships. The more serious complications—accident or injury and formal punishment or discipline—had been experienced by only 1 in 16 males and 1 in 100 females. Studies of the drinking experience of adolescents in high school also indicate that repeated drunkenness is the experience of a small minority only (for a summary of recent research, see 18).

To emphasize that problem drinking, as it has been defined here, is the experience of a small minority of adolescents is not to dismiss this behavior as unimportant. Adults have a legitimate right to hope that adolescents will exhibit more responsibility in various areas of experience than they themselves exhibit. Nevertheless, insofar as drinking remains a culturally defined and institutionalized aspect of adult behavior, the adolescent who is learning what it means to be an adult is likely to continue to drink in spite of any risks which may be potentially involved, just as the adults he observes do. The adolescent, like the adult, is typically aware not only of what alcohol may do to him but also of what it may do for him, and he behaves accordingly.

N B

REFERENCES

1. McCarthy, R. G., and E. M. Douglass. "Instruction in Alcohol Problems in Public Schools," *Quarterly Journal of Studies on Alcohol,* 8: 609-635, 1948.
2. Slater, A. B. "A Study of the Use of Alcoholic Beverages among High School Students in Utah," *Quarterly Journal of Studies on Alcohol,* 13: 78-86, 1952.
3. Hofstra Research Bureau, Psychological Division, Hofstra College. *Use of Alcoholic Beverages among High School Students.* New York: The Mrs. John S. Sheppard Foundation, 1953.
4. University of Wisconsin. *Attitudes of High School Students toward Beverage Alcohol.* New York: The Mrs. John S. Sheppard Foundation, 1956.
5. University of Kansas, Department of Sociology and Anthropology. *Attitudes toward the Use of Alcoholic Beverages.* New York: The Mrs. John S. Sheppard Foundation, 1956.
6. Maddox, G. "High-School Student Drinking Behavior: Incidental Information from Two National Surveys," *Quarterly Journal of Studies on Alcohol,* 25: 339-347, 1964.
7. Maddox, G. L., and B. C. McCall. *Drinking among Teen-*

Agers: A Sociological Interpretation of Alcohol Use in a High School. New Brunswick: Rutgers Center of Alcohol Studies, 1964.

8. GLOBETTI, G. "A Survey of Teenage Drinking in Two Mississippi Communities." Preliminary Report No. 3. Social Science Research Center, Mississippi State University. State College, Mississippi (October, 1964).

9. MANDELL, W. et al. Youthful Drinking: New York State, 1962. New York: Wakoff Research Center, Staten Island, 1964.

10. BLACKER, E., H. DAMONE, and H. FREEMAN. "Drinking Behavior of Delinquent Boys," Quarterly Journal of Studies on Alcohol, 26: 223-237, 1965.

11. CAMPBELL, E. "The Internalization of Moral Norms," Sociometry, 27: 391-412, 1965.

12. STRAUS, R., and S. D. BACON. Drinking in College. New Haven, Conn.: Yale University Press, 1953.

13. PARK, P. "Problem Drinking and Role Deviation: A Study of Incipient Alcoholism," in D. PITTMAN and C. SNYDER (eds.), Society, Culture and Drinking Patterns. New York: John Wiley & Sons, Inc., 1962.

14. MADDOX, G., and E. BORINSKI. "Drinking Behavior of Negro Collegians," Quarterly Journal of Studies on Alcohol, 25: 651-668, 1964.

15. HOLLINGSHEAD, A. Elmtown's Youth. New York: Wiley, 1949.

16. LAZARSFELD, P., and E. KATZ. Personal Influence: The Part Played by People in the Flow of Mass Communications. New York: Free Press, 1955.

17. LEVANTHAL, HOWARD. "An Analysis of the Influence of Alcoholic Beverage Advertising on Drinking Customs," in RAYMOND G. MCCARTHY (ed.), Alcohol Education for Classroom and Community. New York: McGraw-Hill, 1964.

18. MADDOX, G. L. "Teenagers and Alcohol: Recent Research," Annals of the New York Academy of Sciences, 133: 856-865, 1966.

Chapter 5

THE INTERNALIZATION OF MORAL NORMS*

ERNEST Q. CAMPBELL
Vanderbilt University

A CENTRAL CONTINUING CONCERN of sociology and social psychology is the explanation of social order and conformity. At the macro level it is the issue of how societies maintain themselves in a state of relative equilibrium, order, and continuity. At the micro level it is the issue of how and why the individual becomes a socialized being.

It is somewhere within these complex issues that the concept of internalization enters the literature. Its importance in our explanatory efforts is difficult to determine, since the concept seems simultaneously to occupy a basic and a trivial position.[1] For it is a word of many meanings. Most writers who use it do not define it, and most writers who define it do not measure it.[2]

* Reprinted from *Sociometry*, 27 (December, 1964). Prepared under grant M-4302 to the author from the National Institute of Mental Health. As graduate research assistants, Nancy Gates, James F. Keith, Norman Alexander, Mary Ann Lamanna, and Joe Lella were invaluable, as were the facilities of the Institute for Research in Social Science, University of North Carolina. The late David M. Shaw of Duke University made substantial contributions to the initial formulation of the research problem and design, and I cannot express how much I have missed him in its execution. Harry J. Crockett helped write the story-completion items and, with Nancy Gates, devised the scoring scheme and scored the protocols.

[1] Winch, reacting to the general confusion surrounding the term's usage, has suggested that it be dropped from the vocabulary of the behavioral sciences. See Robert F. Winch, *Identification and its Familial Determinants: Exposition of Theory and Results of Pilot Studies* (Indianapolis: The Bobbs-Merrill Co., Inc., 1962), p. 28.

[2] Kelley and Volkart, who make substantial use of the term, and Blau, who uses it incidentally, are illustrative. Harold H. Kelley and Edmund H. Volkart, "The Resistance to Change of Group-Anchored Attitudes," *American Sociological Review*, 17 (August, 1952), 453-465; Peter Blau, "Structural Effects," *American Sociological Review*, 25 (April, 1960), 178-191.

What seems most common is the casual, incidental use of the term, without definition, for explanatory purposes. It is used often in conjunction with the related concept of identification. If there is any central tendency in the literature, it is to define internalization (or interiorization or introjection) as a condition of incorporation of norms and/or roles into one's own personality, with a corresponding obligation to act accordingly or suffer guilt. Identification, which usually means an emotional attachment to an object or person and a desire to please and/or imitate it, is then the major process which leads to internalization. This we may term the classical concept of internalization and of its relation to identification.[3]

Contrary to the "classical" meaning, Parsons generally treats internalization as a process leading to identification. Internalization of an object means "role-taking," that is, discriminating the other and understanding his behavior, values, and expectations. The end result of this is identification, in which there is a we-feeling, a feeling of group solidarity, and a commonality of values between ego and alter, hence a stable role relationship. The conceptual emphasis is on interpersonal reciprocity rather than normative commitment.[4]

Many who attempt to specify and distinguish internalization

[3] There is a special variant of this definition, often implicit though rarely explicit. As above, identification is the mechanism by which internalization occurs, but the theme that identification and internalization are different points along a continuum of commitment to a norm or role also appears. That is, one who supports or conforms to a norm because of identification is not as "deeply" committed to the norm as is another who supports or conforms to it because of internalization. Thus Bredemeier and Stephenson, describing the process of conscience development, observe that, "There is nothing inevitable about this development. In the first place, the socializee may or may not acquire a need for others' approval. In the second place, even if he does, he may or may not internalize their standards of approval." (Henry C. Bredemeier and Richard M. Stephenson, The Analysis of Social Systems [New York; Holt, Rinehart, and Winston, Inc., 1962], p. 68.) In other words, the actor internalizes norms (or roles) because he identifies with norm-senders (role-players), but he may identify with others without necessarily incorporating the norms or roles they represent into himself.

[4] See, for example, Talcott Parsons, "Family Structure and the Socialization of the Child," pp. 35-131 in Talcott Parsons and Robert F. Bales (eds.), Family, Socialization and Interaction Process (Glencoe, Ill.: The Free Press, 1955), pp. 56-57, 91-94; Talcott Parsons and James Olds, "The Mechanisms of Personality Functioning with Special Reference to Socialization," pp. 187-257, Parsons and Bales, op. cit., p. 229.

empirically require that conformity to a norm[5] occur in the absence of external pressures or even in the face of contrary external pressures.[6] Thus Rommetveit, having described internalization as "the subtle change occurring when an enduring social pressure exerted by a norm-sender gradually is felt or experienced by the norm-receiver as an obligation toward himself," then suggests that a criterion for the degree of internalization is whether or not the norm is carried out even when the norm-sender is physically and symbolically absent.[7] Similarly, Davis observes that "A norm is said to be internalized when it is a part of the person, not regarded objectively or understood or felt as a rule, but simply as a part of himself, automatically expressed in behavior."[8] Likewise, Miller and Swanson observe in discussing the internalization of moral rules that "Once a child has com-

[5] The "thing" that is internalized, or the object of internalization, is variously norms or values, roles, and objects or persons. Most commonly it seems to be norms or values, especially in literature reporting measurement efforts. Less commonly it is roles, and this usage tends to be more typical of the socialization literature that summarizes broad processes. Least commonly in the sociological literature (the notable exception being Talcott Parsons), but very common at least by implication in the psychoanalytic literature, it is persons or objects, especially punitive parent figures, that are internalized.

[6] It must be noted that a considerable literature on conformity and social pressures ignores the values and commitments that an actor brings to an immediate situation, and by treating outcome determinants as within the immediate field is entirely situational and ahistorical. An appropriate example of this is Hans L. Zetterberg, "Compliant Actions," *Acta Sociologica*, 2 (1957), 179-201. Campbell and Pettigrew have reviewed this tendency in some detail and urge the importance of considering the actor's self-commitment in the explanatory system. See Ernest Q. Campbell and Thomas F. Pettigrew, "Racial and Moral Crisis: The Role of Little Rock Ministers," *American Journal of Sociology*, 64 (March, 1959), 509-516.

[7] Ragnar Rommetveit, *Social Norms and Roles: Explorations in the Psychology of Enduring Social Pressures* (Minneapolis: University of Minnesota Press, 1954), pp. 56-57. Conformity that occurs when the norm-sender is present presumably might occur with or without an affectionate bond between ego and alter. If such a bond exists, the conformity base is identification; if it does not, the base is superior power. Here, again, implicitly there is the idea that internalization is "deeper" than identification. On another point, we should note that to Rommetveit the very definition of norm implies a sender and a receiver; it seems to follow that a norm which has been completely internalized is no longer a norm.

[8] Kingsley Davis, *Human Society* (New York: The Macmillan Co., 1949), p. 55.

pleted the process of patterning himself after important adults, the external observer is replaced by an inner voice."[9]

We may pause to note that a theoretically clear distinction—that drawn between conformity determined by norm-senders and conformity determined by valuing the norm itself—is full of empirical pitfalls. Not only is it that instances with significant others (i.e., norm-senders) *symbolically* absent are difficult to find (and demonstrate) empirically, but they are difficult to create even in the imagination. This is so in large part because the human actor has the ability to *imagine* the presence (and/or evaluative response) of absent significant others[10] and to adapt his behavior so as to avoid the pain of knowing he has not done what they would have wished.[11] It is true also because he has the capacity to generalize the expectations of significant others into religious representation and to believe, for example, that "God is watching," i.e., to create the presence of a surveillance figure.[12] The tantalizing difficulty of determining whether conformity that occurs when significant observers are absent truly results because of internalized norms probably accounts for much of the considerable ambiguity in the literature.[13]

An extensive literature in psychology supports the perspectives that we have drawn primarily from the sociological literature. Allinsmith, for example, having noted that developmentally there are at first two major forces influencing behavior—external reality and one's own impulses—observes that there develops in

[9] Daniel R. Miller and Guy E. Swanson, *Inner Conflict and Defense* (New York: Henry Holt, 1958), p. 136.

[10] Charles H. Cooley called attention to this many years ago in his famous discussion of the looking-glass self. See his *Human Nature and the Social Order* (New York: C. Scribner's Sons, 1902).

[11] We do not mean to imply that all actors would do this in the same degree. In the extreme instance, there is what Fenichel has termed the heteronomous person, one who has only one internalized standard, that of doing what is demanded. See Otto Fenichel, *Psychoanalytic Theory of Neuroses* (New York: W. W. Norton Co., 1945), pp. 520-521.

[12] For an empirical study, see Clyde Z. Nunn, "Child Control Through a Coalition with God," *Child Development*, 35 (1964), 417-432.

[13] To draw but one example, we may ask whether Mead's "generalized other" refers to a set of internalized norms or to the imagined responses of possibly absent others. For relevant statements, see Anselm Strauss (ed.), *The Social Psychology of George Herbert Mead* (Chicago: University of Chicago Press, 1956), pp. 231-233.

time a third force, social demands that originally were part of external reality but which became internalized. He then defines internalization as "that learning in which reinforcements became internal; the individual experiences *internal* reward or punishment for actions which, for him, have moral connotations. Through internalization a person becomes motivated to live up to a moral standard even if this means resisting temptation when no one else could know to censure him; he becomes motivated to go against the crowd, if necessary, in order to maintain his standard."[14] And Festinger, after postulating that there is no private acceptance of a norm if the compliant behavior disappears on removal of the source of induction or influence, then suggests that the appropriate mechanism for internalization ("private acceptance") is identification: "Public compliance with private acceptance will occur if there is a desire on the part of the person to remain in the existing relationship with those attempting to influence him."[15] Yet in the psychological no less

[14] Wesley Allinsmith, "The Learning of Moral Standards" (unpublished doctoral dissertation, University of Michigan, 1954), pp. 17-18.

[15] Leon Festinger, "An Analysis of Complaint Behavior," in Muzafer Sherif and M. O. Wilson, *Group Relations at the Crossroads* (New York: Harper and Bros., 1953), p. 234. The same general perspective appears in Ausubel's two major works: David P. Ausubel, *Theory and Problems of Adolescent Development* (New York: Grune and Stratton, 1954); and *Theory and Problems of Child Development* (New York: Grune and Stratton, 1958). Bandura and Walters see the development of internal controls as accomplished largely through the process of identification: Albert Bandura and Richard H. Walters, *Adolescent Aggression* (New York: The Ronald Press Company, 1959), p. 252. Bronfenbrenner observes that although Freud uses the word identification in many ways, it is always based on an emotional tie with an object: Urie Bronfenbrenner, "Freudian Theories of Identification and Their Derivatives," *Child Development*, 31 (1960), 15-16. Miller and Hutt see identification as a "significant and ubiquitous process for interiorizing social norms": Daniel R. Miller and Max L. Hutt, "Value Interiorization and Personality Development," *Journal of Social Issues*, 4 (1949), 22. And French, in distinguishing between "induced force" and "own force," observes that "An induced force which is accepted to a high degree produces in the person additional own forces in the same direction, so that the behavior instigated by induction becomes relatively independent of the inducing agent and will occur even if his power field is removed": J. R. P. French, Jr., "Organized and Unorganized Groups Under Fear and Frustration," *Studies in Topological and Vector Psychology, III. Studies in Child Welfare* (Iowa City: University of Iowa, 1944).

than with the sociological literature there are prominent problems of clarity and consistency.[16]

Careful review of the literature suggests the conclusion that there are four major issues in conceptualizing internalization. There is, first, the issue or dimension of *depth:* may internalization be thought of as a polar position on a continuum of degrees of self-control (i.e., internal control) over behavior? If so, may it be seen as representing a higher probability of conforming behavior under given conditions of deviance pressure, and as representing a higher probability of a self-punitive response to deviance, than other conformity bases, identification being a prime example? The second is the issue or dimension of *content:* what is it that the actor internalizes? The literature suggests, as we have seen, that this may be roles, or norms and values, or persons and objects, or simply the community and society, as with Mead's generalized other. The third issue is the *extensity* dimension: does internalization refer to all standards of conduct or merely to a subset which may be defined as moral? And is it extensive enough to be virtually coterminous with learning (i.e., anything that becomes a part of the behavioral repertoire is "internalized"), or does it refer to some particular form, type, structure, or content of learning? Finally, the fourth major issue is the *development* dimension: how does internalization come about? Is it the condition or product, with identification its process or mechanism, or is identification also a condition or product and may internalization occur via other routes than identification?

Definitions and Assumptions

The position assumed in this paper is that internalization does represent a deeper norm-orientation condition and should result in less frequent deviance than other conformity-bases; that as

[16] There is, for example, a smaller literature, initiated by Herbert Kelman ("Compliance, Identification, and Internalization," unpublished manuscript, 1956) and developed by Thibaut and Kelley, which is quite idiosyncratic in comparison to the literature reviewed here. These authors say that internalization occurs when the norm-sender has credibility and the norm is seen by the actor as having a practical utility for him: "Internalization exists if by virtue of his 'credibility' A can provide the means to B's acquiring 'useful content,' that is, right, true, valid, or meaningful outcomes." (John Thibaut and Harold Kelley, *Social Psychology of Groups* [New York: John Wiley and Sons, 1959], p. 245.)

a concept its most appropriate referents are norms and values; that its use should be restricted to a subset of standards called moral;[17] and that identification is both a process and a condition, and that as process it is the major means by which internalization occurs.

We will define internalization as a commitment to a norm[18] or standard, such that the actor would be expected to commit energy to its defense and maintenance even when external supports or pressures are not available. We will distinguish this from conformity based on identification by indicating that the conscious recall or construction of the responses and expectations of significant others is not an element.

Behavior tends to be consonant with the normative atmosphere in which action occurs. Although everyone in the actor's circle of contacts may be said to emit normative expectations relevant to the actor's decisions, it is clear from reference group theory that not all such expectations have an equal impact on the actor. Specifically, the more important the message-sender is to the actor, the greater the impact of his expectations on the actor's decisions and ultimate behavior. But it must be noted as well that decision-making is not ahistorical; or, in other words, some portion of the normative atmosphere affecting the actor's decision is "carried" by the actor as his personal norm and value

---

[17] One learns how to shift gears in an automobile and he learns that failure to shift them at appropriate speeds and road conditions is foolish, i.e., it causes damage and expensive garage bills. He learns also that if he wants to arrive somewhere in a hurry, he doesn't drive in second gear. These certainly are standards of conduct and they clearly are "internalized" if by this we mean simply acquiring a (any) response mode. But these standards are those of efficiency and performance, and any teacher who helps one learn such technical norms assists basically because as an expert he can save one the costs of "learning for himself." No emotional bond between alter and ego is required; the outcome is intrinsically linked to the act; and while one who strips his gears may call himself foolish, he will hardly call himself wicked, or be so called. It is when the linkage between act and outcome is not apparent except as defined or created by the norm itself, when the emotional bond between sender and receiver becomes, then, essential, and when the evaluative standards are expressed in terms of moral superiority, that the concept of internalization seems most applicable and appropriate.

[18] For a good general discussion of norm commitment, see William J. Goode, "Norm Commitment and Conformity to Role-Status Obligations," *American Journal of Sociology*, 66 (November, 1960), 246-258.

system. He attempts to emit behaviors that are consistent with his self-image, that is, with which he can live comfortably; and behaviors inconsistent with these self-imposed demands create a discomfort generally called guilt.

We may assume further that the actor is motivated to behave consistently with the expectations of any immediate circle of contacts toward which he is positively oriented. He wishes to be well liked, to "get along," to "be a good Joe," to "go along with the crowd," to "belong." Whether in fact he so behaves is a hypothesized function of the relevant expectations of absent meaningful others and of the internalized standards that he carries around with him. Thus he may be unwilling to conform to the immediate group expectations because he remembers the preferences of an absent loved one, or he may not conform because "I couldn't live with myself if I did anything like that." We may add parenthetically that it is the goal of any value-coherent social system to teach its members to punish themselves internally if their behavior violates its norms; self-control and self-punishment are primary goals of the socialization process.

If, relevant to any given norm, the actor's conformity is a simple minimax function of rewards and costs controlled by the immediate environment, then over time and varied circumstances his behavior will seem normatively random except as we know the physically immediate normative pressures affecting him. This conformity-base may be called surveillance. If, however, certain norm-senders in his not-immediate environment are affectively positive and meaningful—such that he is motivated to imagine their expectations and wishes to please them and not to hurt them, and especially if he experiences pleasure when he imagines their approval of his decision and pain when he imagines their disapproval—then the weight of these imagined responses of absent others may well be greater than that of the immediate environment and he will resist pressures to behave contrary to these remembered agents. This conformity-base may be called identification. Likewise, if the norms these meaningful others have sent have been internalized by the actor, such that they operate independently of their source and the actor commits energy to their maintenance without reference to actual or imagined external supports, here too we may expect that his behavior may not conform to immediate pressures. This base is called internalization.[19]

Deviancy rates in response to changes in the normative environment should reflect the prior conformity base. Those who conform because they have been under surveillance should have relatively high rates of deviance. The rates should be considerably lower than this for identifiers and internalizers. As between these latter two, deviancy should be higher among the former. Whereas the imagined responses of primary group members almost certainly affect the actor's normative decisions even when he is separated from them, there is at least the possibility that the belief that they cannot possibly learn of his behavior, hence cannot be "hurt" by it, may be sufficient to permit the deviant act; but the actor cannot by definition hide the fact of his deviance from himself, hence the internalizer must be "hurt" by his deviant behavior.[20] Finally, deviance should be less among "true" internalizers than among those whose internal commitments are "rational," since the latter are presumably more "open" to discussion, persuasion, and changed perspectives.

[19] Actually, in the data analysis that follows and in keeping with our own conceptual biases, internalization is limited to moral rather than rational internal commitments. That is, we wish to maintain the distinction established by Durkheim when he observes that violation of a moral rule does not inherently contain subsequent blame or punishment as does violation of a rule of technique, and we wish to extend this distinction to the different conceivable orientations that two different actors may have to the same norm; one's conformity may be morally based, another's identical behavior due to a rational orientation. With Durkheim, we take the position that when one conforms for internalized moral reasons, consequence is linked to moral rule only synthetically, via sanctions: "A sanction is the consequence of an act that does not result from the content of that act, but from the violation by that act of a pre-established rule . . . Thus there are rules that present this particular characteristic: We refrain from performing the acts they forbid simply because they are forbidden." And again: "We find charm in the accomplishment of a moral act prescribed by a rule that has no other justification than that it is a rule. We feel a *sui generis* pleasure in performing our duty simply because it is our duty." (Emile Durkheim, *Sociology and Philosophy* [Glencoe: The Free Press, 1953], pp. 43 and 45.)

[20] In the interest of simplicity, we ignore the obvious possibility that the actor may be skilled in the use of ego defense mechanisms such that he can in fact protect himself from the "hurt" of his own deviancy.

Design, Data, and Measures

Questionnaires were secured from seniors in 61 high schools in 10 counties in North Carolina in the spring of 1961. Those who continued their education into college were re-contacted one year later; approximately 1,575 were located. Data were secured from the parents of these students by mailed questionnaires. The substantive focus of most of the questions was drinking behavior of respondents, their attitudes toward alcohol as a social object, and the expectations of peers and parents. Theirs is a culture in which strong adult-based socialization practices encourage abstinence.[21] Mixed drinks cannot be sold in the state, for example, and of 100 counties more than half are dry. The Methodists and Southern Baptists, the two dominant religious groups of the state, are staunch advocates of complete abstinence. Ninety-two per cent of the mothers who returned questionnaires prefer that their high school senior child not drink; the corresponding figure for fathers is 87 per cent. The figures are exactly the same for both parents a year later. Nearly 91 per cent of the high school seniors report that both parents prefer that they not drink. Only 22 per cent of the 5,115 students had consumed any alcoholic beverages at any time during their senior year in high school.[22]

As part of the questionnaire, two paragraph-length stories were given to the college-bound students, each concerned with drinking by someone their ages. The stories and their accompanying questions were designed to elicit material relevant to internalization and identification.[23] The first of these two stories

[21] Of a sample of 1,466 Southern Appalachian households, 76.3 per cent regarded drinking as "always wrong." By residential groups, this characterized 61.2 per cent of metropolitan, 71.7 per cent of urban, and 87.8 per cent of rural respondents. See Thomas R. Ford, "Status, Residence, and Fundamentalist Religious Beliefs in The Southern Appalachians," *Social Forces*, 39 (October, 1960), 47, Table 4. Although many North Carolina counties are included in the Appalachian region, this is not true of any of the counties used in the present study and hence there is not a strict comparability.

[22] The form of the question: "Do you now (since the beginning of this school year) drink alcoholic beverages in any form? .... Yes .... No."

[23] The analogous form for females reads as follows: "Jane and her date were out with several other couples one Saturday evening. Someone suggested that they all ought to see what it's like to take a drink. Everyone

reads as follows (male form): "Mike went out one Friday evening with his buddies with nothing special to do. They drove around for a while and someone suggested that they see what it's like to take a drink. Each had several drinks, and they seemed to have a real good time. A little before midnight, Mike went home and went to bed. When he woke up next morning, what were his feelings about the evening? Give the reasons why he felt this way."[24] It is the results from this story (and its counterpart form for females) that are the data for our analysis in this paper.[25]

Briefly, a respondent was scored as having internalized a nondrinking norm if he affirmed that drinking is wrong as a matter of principle, on the basis of his own moral standards, not because others define drinking as wrong, illogical, dangerous, unnecessary, etc. It was required that there be a definite, explicit statement to the effect that drinking is wrong, evil, bad, etc., and that it be clear that the source of this anti-drinking norm was within the respondent, not outside him, anchored in parents, peers, situational pressures, etc. A statement that "he felt that he had done the wrong thing" was scored as internalization, while a statement that "he felt that he did wrong in going

---

got just a little high, and seemed to have a real good time. Jane got home before midnight and went to bed. When she woke up next morning, what were her feelings about the evening? Give the reasons why she felt this way." The reason for having Jane "get a little high" while Mike "had several drinks" is, frankly, lost to memory. The difference appears on the form for the first pre-test and—obviously—it was never changed.

[24] A second part of the story reads as follows: "Suppose that when Mike came up the walk to his home he noticed that his parents were sitting in the living room. How would he have felt then? What would he have done? Why would he have done it?" (with analogous form for Jane). We intended to score respondents "high" on identification if relevant materials appeared in the first story, before the introduction of parents as stimulus; "low" on identification if relevant themes of commitment, obligation, etc., appeared only in the second; and "negative" on identification if such themes appeared in neither story. However, so few cases were scored "negative" that they are combined with "lows" in analysis, making the criterion simply whether the respondent does or does not give identification materials in response to the first part of the story.

[25] The scoring scheme was developed as follows: guided by a general but not precisely established intention to distinguish conformity based on the wishes of parents from conformity based on internal standards, the author and his colleague, Harry J. Crockett, drafted a set of story-com-

against his parents' wishes" was not. Likewise, unequivocal statements such as "He would have felt like a criminal. He knew it was wrong," or "He would be disappointed in himself because he had done something he knows he shouldn't have," were scored as internalization, but equivocal statements such as "He might have wished he had done something else," or "She might feel bad about what she did" were not.

A respondent was scored as positive on identification if his protocol contained any statement of love, trust, admiration, or

---

pletion items and pretested them with juniors and seniors in a small city and consolidated rural high school. We did not check inter-rater reliability in analyzing the results. Rather, we asked this question of all protocols: is the student telling us anything significant about why he doesn't drink? What? The impressions we formed were checked informally against responses to numerous closed-end questions, to see if they "made sense." We also, again informally, tried to determine what parts of the stimulus story produced either minimal or ambiguous materials; and we made hopefully appropriate modifications.

Time pressures did not permit a third pre-test with high school students. About 60 college sophomores completed the revised story-items and the two of us again checked them to determine whether we were forming meaningful impressions from the protocols. Interviews were held with 12 of these students, focused on their orientations toward alcohol and their reasons for abstinence; all were male. We were interested in whether the six "internalizers" were more "deeply" committed to abstinence than were the six "non-internalizers," e.g. had they ever tasted intoxicating beverages, could they imagine being drinkers in the future, were they tolerant of drinking by others as a social convention? We also wanted to know whether they used different words and themes in explaining their abstinence. The small number of cases precluded meaningful quantification, but we felt encouraged to believe that we were observing an important qualitative distinction. Following final adjustment in the story-stems, the forms were made ready for field distribution.

When the field data came in, Crockett and the author independently scored a randomly selected 100 cases, and laid out scoring instructions for internalization and identification as well as for other themes (such as fear and autonomy) that occurred with some frequency. With dichotomized scores, we were in agreement on 88 cases on internalization and 85 on identification. Next, we instructed a research assistant, Nancy Gates, in the scoring routines and she scored 50 new cases which the three of us discussed. She and Crockett then scored 200 new cases, achieving agreement in 93 per cent of the internalization scores and 91 per cent of the identification scores. Following discussions among the three of us on points of difference, and minor modifications in conception and instructions, Miss Gates wrote a detailed description of the scoring routine and scored all remaining cases.

respect for parents and/or parents' wishes and expectations and rights, or any statement of the importance to the respondent of a favorable response from parents, of obligations to parents, or of a need to keep from hurting or disappointing them. A statement that he would feel guilty or ashamed because he has violated his parents' wishes or disappointed them was scored as identification, not internalization. Illustrative statements scored as positive identification are: "She knew her parents would be disappointed"; "He would have felt deep regret and remorse, because from all general indications parents are opposed to their children drinking and he went against his parents' wishes"; and "Unless his parents approved he felt guilty about last night."

Most college students drink. College for most people means living away from home, i.e., away from early primary norm-senders. The opportunity-structure for drinking increases. Our research question is, simply, can we predict who will become a drinker and who will not? More formally, these are the hypotheses:

1. Internalizers [of a non-drinking norm] are less likely than Identifiers [with parents who prefer abstinence] to become drinkers.
2. Internalizers are less likely than Non-Internalizers to become drinkers.
3. Internalizers who become drinkers are less likely than Non-Internalizers who become drinkers to develop positive attitudes toward alcohol as a social object.

The assumptions are simple ones. It is assumed that an actor who has internalized a norm will commit energy to its maintenance even in the face of contrary expectations; that college increases one's exposure to drinking-relevant pressures; and that, even when an actor who has internalized a norm succumbs to contrary pressures, a residue is left in the form of ambivalent attitudes toward the social object in question. We do not assume that the actor will commit energy indefinitely to the maintenance of an internalized norm without external reinforcement, nor that drinking-relevant pressures are constant across a series of collegiate institutions, nor that the attitude residues among deviants last forever. A drinker is defined as anyone who answers "yes" to the question, "Do you now, during this school year, use alcoholic beverages in any form?" An internalizer is one so

scored on the story-completion protocols as discussed above.
Identifiers are those so scored from protocols. Attitudes toward
alcohol as a social object are operationally defined at appropriate
points in the text below.

Certain results encourage the belief that the story-completion
scoring system has acceptable validity. We expect, for example,
that girls would be more likely than boys to internalize abstinence norms in American culture; 53.5 per cent of the girls in
the sample, compared to 36.9 per cent of the males, are scored
positive on internalization. Similarly, those who are active religious participants should show a higher incidence of internalization, since the numerically dominant religious bodies in the
area teach abstinence; 56.8 per cent of the most active church-
goers and only 40.1 per cent of the least active are scored as
internalizers.[26] The content of drinking-relevant communications
from parents should differ in predictable ways for those who
internalize the abstinence norm; specifically, they should more
frequently report communications defining abstinence as morally superior to imbibing. Relevant data are in Table 1. Internalizers are more likely to report that parents have told them
not to drink because the church opposes it, drinking is morally
wrong, and it signifies personal weakness; they are less likely to
say that parents have told them not to drink because of their
age, the health implications of drinking, and problems drinking
has caused in the kin group. Finally, we would expect that
within a population of abstainers the reasons given for not

[26] Several studies show a relation between religious participation and
drinking behavior. Goldsen shows that those scoring high on a religiousness
scale are less likely to drink, with the variable seemingly a stronger dis-
criminant among males than among females (Rose K. Goldsen *et al., What
College Students Think* [Princeton, N.J.: D. Van Nostrand, 1960], Table
8-1, p. 173). Skolnick observes that "The data illustrate, above all, the importance of religious belief and participation in supporting total abstinence
as a drinking pattern. Persons of abstinence affiliation, who actively support
and participate in church affairs, are more likely to remain abstinent than
persons less active. Most abstainers cite religious reasons for rejecting the
use of alcoholic beverages." (Jerome H. Skolnick, "The Stumbling Block:
A Sociological Study of the Relationship between Selected Religious Norms
and Drinking Behavior" [unpublished doctoral dissertation, Yale University,
1957], p. 375.) And Williams reports that members of religious sects drink
considerably less than either Protestant denominations or Roman Catholics
(Mary G. Williams, "Drinking Patterns among High School Students" [un-
published doctoral dissertation, University of Kansas, 1958], p. 23).

TABLE 1.—*Internalization Status and Parents' Communications on Drinking Norms: Parents Opposed Only*

Parents' Reasons for Preferring Abstinence	Internalizers Per Cent Ranking Item:				Non-Internalizers Per Cent Ranking Item:			
	1st	2nd	3rd	Not ranked	1st	2nd	3rd	Not ranked
Drinking sign of personal weakness	8.6	13.5	15.5	62.4	9.4	10.8	12.0	67.7
Church is opposed	20.1	16.2	6.6	57.1	14.9	13.9	6.8	64.4
Drinking morally wrong	35.8	21.5	5.5	37.2	22.6	12.0	4.4	61.1
Has caused problems in family	8.2	7.1	7.3	77.4	12.1	5.9	5.4	76.6
Child not old enough	2.7	2.9	3.8	90.7	6.1	5.0	5.0	84.4
Poor health practice	7.7	14.8	22.8	54.6	12.1	17.7	17.0	53.2

drinking would vary by internalization status. In Table 2 results are given from a question asking abstaining respondents to rank order, from among ten reasons, those four that are their most important personal reasons for not drinking. Two of the ten reasons are identificational: one abstains because significant others want him to. Four others are rational reasons: neither norm-senders nor the norm *per se*, but rather a sort of rational calculus of costs of risk-taking, is involved. The remaining four are termed internalized reasons; they suggest the moral superiority of abstinence. Non-internalizers are more likely to rate both identification and rational reasons high, whereas internalizers more often give internalization reasons. This is true without exception for the most important reason, and with only two exceptions (plus one tie) for the second reason. The collapsed data given at the bottom of Table 2 show these differences clearly. Our analysis thus gives us tentative confidence in the classificatory system.

Results

Drinking Behavior. The central concern of the research is to determine whether an empirical measure of the internalization of an abstinence norm at Time A can predict continued abstinence at Time B. Of those non-drinkers whose parents opposed drink-

TABLE 2.—*Internalization Status and Reasons for Abstinence: High School Senior Non-Drinkers, Parents Opposed Only*

	Internalizers Per Cent Ranking Item:			Non-Internalizers Per Cent Ranking Item:		
Reasons for Abstinence	1st	2nd	Not ranked*	1st	2nd	Not ranked*
Identification						
Would disappoint parents	7.1	17.4	75.5	9.9	17.3	72.8
Would disappoint loved ones	4.5	11.4	84.1	9.9	12.2	77.9
Internalization						
Church is opposed	7.7	9.7	82.6	3.5	9.7	86.8
Sign of personal weakness	12.9	11.2	75.9	10.4	9.9	79.7
Wrong in principle	41.2	13.9	44.9	29.3	7.4	63.3
Decent people don't	5.2	4.9	89.9	3.2	2.8	94.0
Rational						
Not old enough	1.7	0.9	97.4	5.5	4.2	90.3
Too many dangers	14.4	16.3	69.3	19.4	19.9	60.3
Poor health practice	4.9	12.9	82.2	9.0	11.1	79.9
Costs too much	0.6	1.3	98.1	0.7	4.8	94.5
Total identification	11.6	28.8	......	19.8	29.5	......
Total internalization	67.0	37.9	......	46.4	29.8	......
Total rational	21.6	31.4	......	34.6	40.0	......

* Question format calls for third and fourth most important reasons also. "Not Ranked" here means ranked third or fourth or not ranked at all.

ing[27] in 1961, fewer internalizers than non-internalizers became drinkers by the spring of their freshman year in college (21.6 per cent versus 32.6 per cent). If we control by sex and college, on 11 of the 14 campuses male internalizers are less likely than male non-internalizers to become drinkers; for females, 11 of 13. Overall, internalizers less frequently become drinkers in 22 of 27 campus comparisons. These results are consistent with self-prediction; of high school seniors who abstain and whose parents oppose drinking, 79.3 per cent of the internalizers and 62.7 per

[27] Of 1,499 classifiable respondents, 1,363 reported that *both* father and mother opposed their use of alcohol.

cent of the non-internalizers predicted that they would "definitely not" drink during their freshman year in college.

Given parental opposition to drinking, more dormitory students than those who attend college while living at home would be expected to begin drinking. This expectation is confirmed. But whether living at home or in a dormitory, fewer internalizers become drinkers. In fact, more non-internalizers living at home than internalizers living on campus began the use of alcohol during the freshman year (24.6 per cent versus 21.4 per cent). Internalizers living at home are least likely (13.2 per cent), non-internalizers living on campus most likely (32.4 per cent) to become drinkers.

A quite modest positive association between internalization and identification scores permits us to treat the two variables as substantially independent. We may inquire, then, as to their relative predictive value. If we assume an equal and adequate validity for the two measures, it would appear that internalization clearly is a better predictor. Within homogeneous residential categories (home or dormitory) the difference by internalization is greater than the (almost non-existent) difference between identifiers and non-identifiers. Table 3 supports the same observation: those who are internalizers but not identifiers are hardly more likely to become drinkers than are those who both

TABLE 3.—*Internalization/Identification Status and Drinking Behavior by Residential Status in College: High School Non-Drinkers, Parents Opposed Only*

Internalization/ Identification Status	College Drinking Behavior		
	Drinks	Doesn't Drink	Total
Internalizer and Identifier			
Lives at home	11.5%	88.5%	(26)
Lives on campus	21.4	78.6	(173)
Internalizer Only			
Lives at home	14.0	86.0	(50)
Lives on campus	21.1	78.9	(228)
Identifier Only			
Lives at home	23.5	76.5	(17)
Lives on campus	30.8	69.2	(159)
Neither			
Lives at home	25.0	75.0	(40)
Lives on campus	33.6	66.4	(229)

internalize and identify; and those who identify but are not internalizers are almost as likely as those who are neither to become drinkers.

Values, Attitudes and Self-Image. If a person internalizes a norm, this fact should have a significant effect on his perceptions of the objects or behaviors to which the norm is relevant, and an effect on his perceptions of himself in relation to the relevant objects and behaviors. We assume further that the fact of norm-violation in one's behavior is not in itself proof that the effect of the internalized norm no longer appears in the deviant's values and attitudes. That is, among a population of those characterized by identical behavior, we would expect variation in evaluative response to this behavior as a function of their orientation to the relevant norm.

All respondents were asked whether they had ever tasted beer and hard liquor, and if so, whether they liked the taste. Data in Table 4 show that within each of the three drinking groups (here referred to as Old Drinker, New Drinker, and Non-Drinker) internalizers are less likely to have tasted beer and whiskey, and that among those acquainted with the taste, internalizers

TABLE 4.—*Per Cent Who Do Not Like Taste of Beer and Whiskey (among Those Who Have Tasted) and Per Cent Who Have Never Tasted Beer and Whiskey, by Drinking Behavior and Internalization Status*

Drinking Status	Do Not Like Taste of:		Have Never Tasted:	
	Beer	Whiskey	Beer	Whiskey
Non-Drinkers				
Internalizers	91.9%	94.0%	70.9%	73.9%
	(111)	(100)	(382)	(383)
Non-Internalizers	91.3	83.4	59.7	70.0
	(122)	(91)	(303)	(303)
Drinkers 1961 (Old Drinkers)				
Internalizers	79.0	50.0	5.1	20.0
	(62)	(32)	(39)	(40)
Non-Internalizers	73.5	42.9	2.1	2.8
	(98)	(140)	(144)	(144)
Drinkers 1962 (New Drinkers)				
Internalizers	64.9	88.5	35.4	45.3
	(37)	(52)	(96)	(95)
Non-Internalizers	32.9	81.1	30.5	32.6
	(143)	(95)	(141)	(141)

are less likely to like it. Several of the differences are very small, but there are no exceptions. The differences do not disappear when drinking experience (estimated amount consumed) is introduced as a control.

Table 5 reports differences between internalizers and non-internalizers in each of the three drinking groups on a series of items relating to the self in relation to alcohol as a social object.

TABLE 5.—*The Effect of Internalization Status on Perceptions of Self-Alcohol Relations, Two Measurement Dates, with Control for Drinking Status*

Drinking Status	1961	1962

I. As the person you would be if all your dreams could come true would you. . . . (per cent "not drink at all").

	1961	1962
Old Drinkers		
Internalizers	33.3% (48)	29.2% (48)
Non-Internalizers	13.0 (193)	12.5 (192)
New Drinkers		
Internalizers	70.9 (110)	34.3 (108)
Non-Internalizers	56.0 (159)	23.1 (156)
Non-Drinkers		
Internalizers	93.0 (400)	86.7 (398)
Non-Internalizers	85.4 (328)	83.6 (323)

II. Drinking is wrong as a matter of principle; people ought not to drink. (Per cent agree)

	1961	1962
Old Drinkers		
Internalizers	47.9 (48)	16.6 (48)
Non-Internalizers	28.4 (194)	6.2 (194)
New Drinkers		
Internalizers	66.7 (108)	20.2 (109)
Non-Internalizers	59.5 (158)	15.7 (159)
Non-Drinkers		
Internalizers	87.3 (400)	63.4 (399)
Non-Internalizers	73.5 (328)	53.6 (328)

III. Do you now believe that God will punish you if you drink alcohol? (Per cent saying "yes")

	1961	1962
Old Drinkers		
Internalizers	18.8 (48)	12.8 (47)
Non-Internalizers	14.7 (191)	9.0 (189)
New Drinkers		
Internalizers	29.9 (107)	18.5 (108)
Non-Internalizers	28.0 (157)	11.6 (155)
Non-Drinkers		
Internalizers	56.6 (391)	41.6 (387)
Non-Internalizers	41.4 (326)	27.9 (323)

Each of the three items was administered in 1961 and again in 1962, and results are shown separately. Again without exception, the differences are in the expected direction; internalizers are more likely to define the ideal self in abstinence terms, to see the use of alcohol as wrong in principle, and to believe that God punishes those who drink. Generally, internalizers are somewhat less subject to *change* in perceptions over the year's time, although many of the differences are small and the conclusion seems not to apply to non-drinkers (computations not given).

Finally, whether we deal with the close intimacy of the roommate relationship, the primary relationship with friends, or the more remote character of the college community, internalizers in each drinking category are more likely to say that it is important that their roommate not drink; to prefer strongly that their friends not drink; and to insist that "drinking reputation" is an important consideration in their selection of a college. Data are in Table 6.

TABLE 6.—*Associational Preferences by Internalization Status and Drinking Behavior: Parents Opposed Only*

Associational Preference Item	Internalizers			Non-Internalizers		
	Old Drinkers (1961)	New Drinkers (1962)	Non-Drinkers	Old Drinkers (1961)	New Drinkers (1962)	Non-Drinkers
1. Preferred drinking behavior of roommate (1961):						
Definitely not drink	22.0%	70.5%	89.2%	9.0%	47.9%	74.2%
Preferably not drink	43.9	17.9	8.5	25.0	34.3	21.4
Tolerant of drinking	34.1	11.6	2.4	66.0	17.9	4.3
	(41)	(95)	(378)	(144)	(140)	(299)
2. Preferred drinking behavior of friends (1962):						
Definitely not drink	14.6	6.3	66.8	1.4	4.3	51.3
Preferably not drink	24.4	45.8	26.9	15.9	34.8	37.3
Tolerant of drinking	61.0	47.9	6.3	82.7	61.0	11.4
	(41)	(96)	(383)	(145)	(141)	(306)
3. Would drinking reputation of college affect decision to go there? (1961):						
No drinking is important	12.2	17.9	43.7	2.8	10.1	27.2
No drinking is preferred	24.4	52.6	41.8	17.2	39.6	48.8
Drinking is accepted	63.4	29.5	14.6	80.0	50.4	23.9
	(41)	(95)	(378)	(145)	(139)	(301)

Associational Patterns. As with preferences so with actions: independent of drinking behavior, internalizers are more likely to form peer associations that encourage personal abstinence. Pertinent data are in Table 7, which reports the respondent's estimate of the proportion of his friends who prefer that he not drink. Within each of the three drinking categories, those who score positive on internalization are less likely to report a strong peer pressure to drink.[28]

The relationship of drinking behavior and norm internalization to fraternity/sorority membership and orientation constitutes one of the most interesting aspects of the study. Drinkers '61 are most likely, non-drinkers least likely, to have pledged a fraternity or sorority. (See Table 8; we exclude those who report that their college does not have these social clubs.[29]) Among those who did not pledge, however, Drinkers '62 are especially likely to wish they could join, while non-drinkers are least likely. The relationship between drinking status and pledge status holds for high, middle, and low socio-economic groups separately (data not given).

TABLE 7.—*"Thinking again of the people you enjoy being with, how many of them prefer that you not drink?"* Parents Opposed Only

Per Cent of Friends Who Prefer that Respondent Not Drink	Internalizers			Non-Internalizers		
	Drink-ers (1961)	Drink-ers (1962)	Non-Drink-ers	Drink-ers (1961)	Drink-ers (1962)	Non-Drink-ers
Less than 20% (high drinking pressure)	51.2	41.5	11.2	57.4	47.5	26.8
20-49%	12.2	22.3	9.6	28.4	27.7	11.7
50-79%	7.3	21.3	23.5	9.2	15.3	20.7
80% or more (low drinking pressure)	22.0	14.9	55.6	5.0	9.5	40.8
	(41)	(94)	(374)	(141)	(137)	(299)

[28] Generally, the same conclusion is supported by analysis of a question that asks the respondent to report the number of non-drinkers among his five closest friends. However, an exception appears among the new drinkers, with internalizers less likely to have large numbers of abstinent friends.

[29] Results for Cornell men are similar. See Goldsen *et al., op. cit.,* Table 3-3 and pages 70-73. Gusfield, too, finds that within religious groups fraternity affiliates are more likely to drink, and that overall, 60 per cent of the fraternity members and only 32 per cent of the non-fraternity members drink. Joseph R. Gusfield, "The Structural Context of College Drinking," *Quarterly Journal of Studies on Alcohol,* 22 (September, 1961), 428-443.

TABLE 8.—*Drinking Behavior, Fraternity Affiliation, and Fraternity Orientation of Students Whose Colleges Have Social Fraternities*

| Drinking Status | All Respondents | | | | Those Who Did Not Pledge Only | | |
	Pledged	Would Like to Pledge	Don't Want to Pledge	(N)	Would Like to Pledge	Don't Want to Pledge	(N)
Old Drinkers	36.4%	37.2%	26.4%	(121)	58.4%	41.6%	(77)
New Drinkers	30.1	45.2	24.7	(146)	64.7	35.3	(102)
Non-Drinkers	16.0	36.7	47.2	(362)	43.8	56.2	(304)

When drinking status is disregarded, internalizers are less likely than non-internalizers to have pledged a fraternity, and, among those who did not pledge, they are less likely to wish they could (see Table 9). But if an internalizer does pledge a fraternity, he is less likely to be or to become a drinker than is his counterpart among the non-internalizers. Similarly for those who would like to pledge but didn't: internalizers are less likely to drink (see Table 10). Generally, these observations hold for each of several socio-economic groups.

One final aspect of these data should be noted. Among those who pledged, the proportion who are non-drinkers is substantially higher among the internalizers (55.8 per cent to 30.8 per cent). There is a similarly large difference among those who would like to pledge: 68.2 per cent to 43.8 per cent. (We assume that the fraternity system is a positive reference group for these who would like to pledge even though they did not.) But among those who do not wish to affiliate, the difference (76.9 per cent to 66.1 per cent) is not as great. These comparisons

TABLE 9.—*Internalization Status, Fraternity Affiliation, and Fraternity Orientation of Students Whose Colleges Have Social Fraternities*

| Internalizers Status | All Respondents | | | | Those Who Did Not Pledge Only | | |
	Pledged	Would Like to Pledge	Don't Want to Pledge	(N)	Would Like to Pledge	Don't Want to Pledge	(N)
Internalizer	18.6%	38.2%	43.2%	(280)	46.9%	53.1%	(228)
Non-Internalizers	26.9	39.3	33.8	(349)	53.7	46.3	(255)

TABLE 10.—*Fraternity Affiliation and Orientation, Drinking Behavior, and Internalization Status Among Students Whose Colleges Have Fraternities*

Fraternity and Internalizer Status	All Respondents				Non-Drinkers 1961 Only		
	Old Drinker	New Drinker	Non-Drinker	(N)	Drinker 1962	Non-Drinker 1962	(N)
Pledged Fraternity							
Internalizer	19.2%	25.0%	55.8%	(52)	31.0%	69.0%	(42)
Non-Internalizer	36.2	33.0	30.8	(94)	51.7	48.3	(60)
Would Like to Pledge							
Internalizer	6.5	25.2	68.2	(107)	27.0	73.0	(100)
Non-Internalizer	27.7	28.5	43.8	(137)	39.4	60.6	(99)
Don't Want to Pledge							
Internalizer	8.3	14.9	76.9	(121)	16.2	83.8	(111)
Non-Internalizer	18.6	15.3	66.1	(118)	18.8	81.2	(96)

suggest the hypothesis that the magnitude of the difference in behavioral outcomes between internalizers and non-internalizers is a function of the degree of deviance pressure encountered. When deviance pressures and opportunities are low, whether a norm has been internalized is of relatively little moment as a determinant of the behavioral outcome. But when they are high, those who have internalized the norm should be significantly less likely to violate it. Thus for those students who orient themselves toward the fraternity system, we might expect that the opportunity-structure for deviance is high and that within such a group the orientation of the actor toward the abstinence norm would be a significant determinant of whether or not he drinks. Among students not positively oriented toward this system, however, encouragements to imbibe are less sustained and intense, with the consequence that norm-internalization plays a reduced part in determining outcomes. Moreover, another finding seems consistent with the present interpretation. In "wet" communities (those in which both whiskey and beer are sold), the incidence of drinkers among high school seniors is considerably higher among non-internalizers than among internalizers. In "damp" communities (where beer is sold locally in an otherwise dry county or throughout the rural areas of a county which permits the sale of whiskey as an exception in a major city) the difference is reduced but is still substantial. But in "dry" communities (no beer sold locally and no whiskey sold in the county) the difference virtually disappears. Again, as in the prior case, when the opportunity or pressure to drink is not presented within the social system (as in "dry" communities), norm internalization should have little if any differentiating power; but as opportunities for deviance increase, difference in its incidence between internalizers and others widens substantially.

Summary and Discussion

Typically, the concept of internalization is used in the literature either to explain a behavior after it has happened or as commentary upon behavior without an effort at measurement. This paper reports certain of the results of one effort to measure norm-internalization with the use of the semi-projective technique of story-completion, and then to use these measures to predict certain behavior outcomes in a panel design. The normative issue has been the use of alcohol among high school seniors and college freshmen.

The data are encouraging if one heeds the consistency of the results, but less encouraging if he notes the often meager magnitude of the category differences. It is easy to develop a perspective on internalization that leads us to expect it to make much *more* difference than it seems to make here. Does our failure to observe more striking differences, then, result from an invalid measure or from a trivial predictor?

There are several signs to indicate that the measure itself can be improved. On many items answered by high school seniors, internalizers (by our classificatory procedure) who become drinkers during their freshman year in college behave quite differently from those internalizers who remain abstinent over this period. That is, we use knowledge obtained at Time B to subdivide what seemed at Time A to be a homogeneous group, only to discover from other data secured at Time A that the group was not homogeneous to begin with. Perhaps some subjects were classified as internalizers through coding errors or because of imperfect stimulus materials. Or, perhaps, some respondents so classified are internalizers in fact but they are also something else—that is, perhaps we made fallible and incomplete use of available data. Clearly, to reduce to attribute data a phenomenon so complex is the grossest over-simplification, and one can hope that future efforts will permit a range of scores from strong to moderate to weak to no internalization. Also, both Goode[30] and Rosen,[31] as well as the present author,[32] have pointed to certain basic dangers involved whenever analysis of behavior focuses on a single norm or on a specialized sub-set of norm-senders.

Even so, present results would seem to encourage the conclusion that survey research efforts to determine empirically whether or not given norms are internalized, and to use these measures to predict future behavior, can even now enjoy at least a modest success. Those whom we scored as having internalized an abstinence norm were less likely to drink; less likely to become drinkers; less likely to have tasted intoxicating beverages and more likely to dislike the taste if they had; more likely to believe in abstinence as part of the ideal self; more likely to wish to associate with non-drinkers; and they were less likely to join a fraternity or sorority and more likely to remain abstinent if they did join. Each of these results is consistent with expectation and encourages the belief that more refined survey measures will yield more exact predictions.

[30] Goode, *op. cit.*, p. 252.

[31] Bernard C. Rosen, "The Reference Group Approach to the Parental Factor in Attitude and Behavior Formation," *Social Forces,* 34 (December, 1955), 143.

[32] Ernest Q. Campbell, "Moral Discomfort and Racial Segregation: An Examination of the Myrdal Hypothesis," *Social Forces,* 40 (March, 1961), 233-234.

Chapter 6

DRINKING AND ABSTINENCE: EMERGENT PATTERNS AMONG SELECTED NEGRO FRESHMEN*

GEORGE L. MADDOX
Duke University

THE CULTURE of a social group outlines its shared strategy for living. Group members, by virtue of their association with each other, share some common notions about goals to be pursued; tasks to be accomplished and how to accomplish them; ways to think about and evaluate themselves and others. They also share some notions about the meaning of words and things and how to use these words and things in their interaction with each other. New members of a group need not, and typically are not encouraged to, invent their own strategy for living; they learn more or less willingly and well the existing shared culture of their group.

Applied to drinking behavior, such an explanation of why group members tend to behave alike and why new members of a group become increasingly like their peers would lead one to conclude that individuals rarely have to invent notions about drinking and abstinence. Shared definitions of drinking are available for learning in interaction with others. In groups in which drinking is a culturally defined and socially structured way of

* This research was supported in part by a grant from the National Institute of Mental Health (MH-2185). Support was also provided by the Scientific Advisory Committee, Licensed Beverage Industries, and the Duke University Research Council. Michael Sherman, a research assistant, was supported by a grant from the Board of Christian Social Concern of the Methodist Church. Parts of this chapter are reproduced with the permission of the *Social Science Quarterly*.

relating to others, one would expect most members to drink and most new members to learn to drink. In a group in which drinking is not a shared or approved way of relating oneself to others, most members would be abstinent and new members would learn to be abstinent. If such unambiguous situations existed, one would expect deviant behavior only if the socialization of new members were inadequate or incomplete. The individual's development as a drinker or as abstainer would, for the most part, follow a predictable course and his career as a drinker or as an abstainer would present few surprises. The fact is, however, that ambiguous social situations in which a shared cultural strategy is not evident or does not exist are common. Drinking behavior in the United States, especially among youth, is a case in point.

Two aspects of the American experience are especially relevant in understanding why ambivalence about drinking is common and why drinking careers are often erratic in the United States. First, Americans are a hard-drinking people who have, nonetheless, experimented with prohibition. The prohibition experiment polarized feeling about drinking and abstinence and the proponents of abstinence continue even now to represent a persistent, substantial, and occasionally a politically effective minority in the population. If we recognize that an individual is never exposed to culture in general but to culture as it is lived and transmitted by particular groups to which he is exposed, then a substantial number of persons are continually exposed to groups attached to a culture of abstinence within the cultural mainstream in which drinking is accepted behavior. In a geographically and socially mobile society, both drinkers and abstainers have many opportunities to be aware of contradictory ways of thinking about and behaving in relation to beverage alcohol. Second, there is the matter of age. In the American experience, children are typically expected to be abstinent even if their parents drink. Adults may drink if they prefer, and most in fact do. Young people in the process of becoming adults —literally, adolescents—negotiate this transitional period with increasing experimental drinking and, by the time they are graduated from high school, have become drinkers. For most the transition appears to be negotiated with no special difficulty and their career lines as drinkers seem to be unproblematic (1). Some tentativeness about this description of learning to drink is necessary since, in fact, very little is known about the emergent drinking careers of younger people, especially those who have no identifiable or socially visible difficulty associated with their drinking. Even in the case of older problem drinkers about whose drinking patterns and histories something is known, little reliable information about their drinking careers as youth is available (2).

The research reported here focuses on emergent patterns of drinking and abstinence among selected Negro youth. Specifically, the objectives are to describe their behavior, to explore the stability and change in this behavior during their first year in college, and, insofar as possible, identify the factors which underlie the observed patterns. Negro males in college were selected for both practical and theoretical reasons. Practically, little is known about the drinking behavior of Negroes, although such literature as there is suggests that Negro males drink heavily and have considerable trouble associated with their drinking (3, 4, 5). This gap in the literature warrants attention. But there is also a theoretical justification for focusing on Negro men in college. It appears, again on the basis of the available literature, that middle-status Negro men are exposed to substantial ambivalence toward drinking. On the one hand, alcohol seems to be an obvious and accessible drug for use in narcotizing and in reality transformation within a highly constraining and frustrating environment. On the other hand, a desire for respectability, stereotypically defined in terms of the virtues of the white middle class, occasions serious questions about the propriety of drinking. Thus there are reasons to believe that Negro youth who, by being in college may be presumed to have middle-status parents or middle-status aspirations, would be maximally exposed to ambiguity in regard to drinking. More than this, the fact that they are young provides an opportunity both to observe the emergence of their careers as drinkers or abstainers in the face of cultural and social ambiguity and to explore the negotiations involved in their emergence or continuation as drinkers and abstainers during the first year in college.

In the presentation which follows, the impossibility of using the information reported as a basis for generalizing about Negro collegians or Negro youth should be obvious. This limitation is explicitly recognized by the author. Moreover, at this time, there is neither the basis nor the inclination to conjecture with any conviction or in any detail about the future careers of these young men as drinkers or abstainers on the basis of their behavior as freshmen. In time such conjecture will be appropriate and possible, but at this time the objectives are more modest.

Role theory (6) and balance theory (7) provide useful theoretical perspectives for understanding the emergent careers of drinkers which are our immediate concern. Individuals know about social roles. In social interaction they act "as if" there were a script which informs their interaction with others. They act as if behavior can be grouped into consistent units which are appropriate for types of actors in given situations and that the role models implied are useful in interaction with others who also may be expected to be informed in a similar way about these models. Role models are one of the ingredients of culture and, to the extent that an individual is informed about the culture as lived in his groups, his behavior may be described in terms of the roles he takes and the degree to which his role playing conforms to the role model. However, role taking and role playing can be complex tasks. When role models are contradictory or ambiguous, as may very well be the case for a young male who is no longer a child but not clearly a man living in an environment in which both drinking and abstinence can be variously rewarding and punishing, the individual cannot simply take a role. Rather, he may have to make a role which allows him to operate effectively in the midst of conflicting demands from others who are in a position to reward and punish him. He may know, for example, that a man drinks. But he may recognize that, while he thinks he is a man, and his peers think he is a man, his parents, the police, and school authorities may think otherwise. The situation would be made even more complex if, for any reason, he has middle-class aspirations and feels that drinking is inappropriate for respectable, middle-class men. In the ambiguous or contradictory situation, an individual must negotiate the conflicting expectations of people who are important to him. Balance theory is helpful in understanding the problem posed by conflicting or ambiguous expectations and the processes involved in negotiating resolutions in such situations.

Briefly, balance theory postulates the necessity of achieving some degree of perceptual constancy in adapting to the potentially contradictory demands of complex social environments. The socialized human individual depends heavily on agreement with others in establishing and maintaining a stable orientation to himself, others, and the non-human objects in his social environment. Thus balance theory also postulates an uncomfortable psychological condition (tension, strain, stress) which results when there is a perceived disparity between one's attitudes and behavior and those of significant others. This discomfort underlies an individual's attempts in the typical cases to minimize the perceived discrepancy by changing his behavior, his groups, or perhaps both.

The data which follow are introduced as an illustration of role taking and role making of male Negro youth during their first year in college. If the descriptions of drinking behavior among Negro men commonly presented in the literature are accurate, one would expect most of these young collegians to be drinkers and, in fact, relatively heavy drinkers. To the extent that this is found to be the case, these collegians will illustrate role taking behavior. But it has also been emphasized that a single role model for Negro males with middle-class backgrounds or aspirations in regard to drinking is improbable and, moreover, that these collegians are older adolescent, or at most, only marginally adults. These considerations would lead one to expect, and look for, indications of instability and change in drinking behavior among those students who must negotiate conflicting or discrepant role models. Hence, one would expect their behavior to illustrate role-making as well as role-taking. The ratio of these two processes is a matter for empirical determination in the absence of evidence. However, to the extent that the hypothesized ambiguity about and ambivalence toward drinking among young Negro males in college exist in fact, indications of instability in patterns of drinking and abstinence should be prominent. The choice at any point in time to drink or not to drink would not necessarily be a decision once and for all.

Methodology

The initial sample consisted of 262 young Negro men, 91 per cent of the males entering a state-supported institution in a southern state as freshmen in the Fall of 1963. Median age in the sample was 18.7 years, and 9 of 10 were residents of the state in which the study was done. Although the socioeconomic status of Negroes is difficult to assess, the average status of parental families among these students is best described as middle to lower middle class.[1] Eighty-eight per cent of the students identified themselves as Protestants, a majority specifically as Baptists; 9 per cent identified as Catholics and the remaining 3 per cent had no religious preference.

The initial sample has subsequently been treated as a panel for purposes of studying stability and change in drinking behavior and in 1967, as seniors, those who were still in school were interviewed for the fourth and last time. However, at this point, only the 188 panelists (72 per cent of the initial panel) interviewed early in their freshman year and again one year later as sophomores are under consideration.[2]

Negro upperclassmen in the college in which the research was done were specifically trained to use a pre-tested interview schedule which required about one hour and a half to administer. In addition to items which permitted the social placement and description of panelists, the schedule was designed to elicit information about drinking patterns and experiences; estimates of self-esteem; descriptions of relationship with parents; and social interaction with fellow students. The interview schedule, while not identical both years, did include a common core of questions about drinking behavior.

The extent of an individual's drinking was measured by a Quantity-Frequency Index based on his report of the number of drinks, converted to absolute alcohol, he ordinarily consumed at a sitting, combined with the reported frequency of such sittings in a given period. Drinkers are classified into one of five

[1] There are no clearly established procedures for deriving interchangeable measures of status for non-whites and whites. As a rule of thumb, one may generally assume that measures of status which are useful in the study of whites tend to underestimate the status of non-whites. For example, the Hollingshead two-factor Index of Status Placement (8, Appendix Two) applied to the parental family of the students indicates that, on the average, they are just below middle class. However, in terms of education and income, the parental families of panelists are above average for non-whites both in the state and nationally and also compare favorably, on the average, with the white families in the state.

[2] The 74 panelists not available in 1964 were, almost without exception, dropouts. The dropouts were not significantly different from available panelists in any relevant characteristic except their definition of alcohol. Dropouts were more likely than others to define alcohol in terms of its reality-modifying rather than its social functions. They also tended, in contrast to others, to be somewhat heavier drinkers and to be preoccupied with their drinking but these tendencies were not statistically significant.

types following the procedure described in detail by Mulford and Miller (9) with two modifications. First, at the suggestion of Jessor and Grossman (10), attention was given to the specification of the individual's typical "sitting." Each student was asked initially to think of all the times he had had wine recently; if he had used wine, he was then asked to recall how often he drank it and how often on recent drinking occasions he had drunk five or more glasses. If he had drunk this much on fewer than half the occasions recalled, he was asked how often he had drunk about three or four glasses. If he had drunk this much wine on fewer than half the occasions, he was asked how often he had drunk only one or two glasses. This type of inquiry was then repeated separately for beer and liquor, substituting respectively "bottles" and "drinks" for "glasses." Jessor and Grossman have devised an absolute alcohol conversion table which permits an estimate of the total quantity of each beverage consumed during the sittings a respondent describes. While it is possible with this procedure to estimate the average daily consumption of absolute alcohol for an individual, it was used in this research primarily to determine the most used beverage and to estimate more accurately the amount of that beverage consumed at a typical sitting. An individual's quantity and frequency estimates of the beverage most commonly drunk were used to classify him in one or another of the five types outlined by Mulford and Miller. Second, the justification for the common practices of collapsing the five drinking categories into three (9, 11) was re-evaluated. For purposes of analysis Type 1 (infrequent drinking/small amounts) and Type 2 (infrequent drinking/medium or large amounts) drinkers have usually been classified as *light* drinkers. Type 3 (moderate frequency/small amounts) and Type 4 (moderate frequency/medium or large amounts) have constituted the *moderate* drinkers; and Type 5 drinkers (frequent use/medium) have constituted the *heavy* drinkers.[3] Although these categories have generally proved useful in or-

[3] Definitions of frequency and quantity of use are as follows:

Frequency: Infrequent = once a month at most
             Moderate frequency = two to four times a month
             Frequent = more than once a week

Amount: Small = less than 1.6 ounces of absolute alcohol
             Moderate = 1.6 to less than 2.88 ounces of absolute alcohol
             Heavy = 2.88 ounces of absolute alcohol or more

ganizing data, Type 2 drinkers have always been troublesome. For example, in an analysis which cannot be reported in detail here, the correlates of the drinking patterns associated with each type of drinking consistently suggested that Type 2 drinkers are more similar to Type 4 and 5 drinkers than to either Type 1 or 3 drinkers. The most recent work of Mulford (11, p. 20) indicates that he has reached the same conclusion; he now combines Types 1 and 3 ("lighter") and then Types 2, 4, and 5 ("heavier"). In the report of findings which follows, students will be classified as abstainers, *lighter* drinkers, and *heavier* drinkers as suggested by our own research experience and that of Mulford.

Two attitudinal dimensions of drinking behavior—the definition of alcohol and the imputation of beneficial changes in self-esteem for the drinker—were explored. Determination of definitions of alcohol emphasizing use for narcotizing effect as distinct from social use followed the procedures described by Mulford and Miller (12).[4] The imputation of beneficial changes in self-esteem for the drinker was assessed by an adaptation of semantic differential procedures. Students were asked, for example, to describe themselves "as I really am," "as I would most like to be," and "as I am when I am drinking" in terms of nine pairs of descriptive terms, with each pair constituting a seven-point scale. A positive score was assigned if a student indicated that, when drinking, his self-evaluation moved in the direction of his ideal evaluation and a negative score was assigned if that evaluation was away from the ideal evaluation and less than the evaluation of actual self. When the evaluation of actual self and of the self when drinking coincided, an item was evaluated as neutral. A student was asked to impute beneficial changes in self-esteem to drinking when he scored positively on at least five of the nine items.[5]

Self-esteem was measured by acceptance or rejection of 15

---

[4] The coefficient of reproducibility for the Definition of Alcohol scale is well above the minimum .90.

[5] The specific scales used were happy-sad, fast-slow, hard-soft, successful-unsuccessful, active-passive, strong-weak, nice-awful, sharp-dull, and large-small. Since the procedure of analysis could produce an artificially low number of positive or negative responses if evaluations of actual self concentrated at the extremes of the item scales, the distribution of responses by item was checked. The number of extreme (1 or 7) responses constituted only 16 per cent of the total and in no case constituted the majority of responses by any given student.

essentially derogatory descriptive statements which an individual might apply to himself and of 6 similar statements which significant others (e.g., family and friends) might use to describe him. In the absence of established standards against which the mean response of panelists on these items may be compared, high and low self-esteem must be understood as internal comparisons only.[6]

Assessment of problems associated with drinking, in addition to the measurement of self-esteem, includes Straus and Bacon's Social Complication items and Warning Signs (13, Chapter 12), Park's Index of Problem Drinking (14), and Mulford and Miller's Preoccupation with Alcohol Scale (15).[7]

Findings

The panel of students fulfills the expectation that, in any collectivity of Negro males, a large proportion will not only be drinkers but will also drink heavily (Table 1). Both as beginning freshmen and as students with a year of college experience, eight of ten panelists drank; and, of these drinkers, half of them were heavier drinkers. Compared with college students generally, the proportion of drinkers among panelists is not strikingly high. It is probable, however, that if comparable groups of college freshmen were available, the proportions of drinkers and of heavy drinkers would be found to be quite high. The basis for this conclusion is that the proportions of drinkers and

TABLE 1.—*The Quantity-Frequency of Drinking among Panelists as Freshmen and as Sophomores*

| Q-F Type | College Year | | | |
| | Freshman | | Sophomore | |
	%	N	%	N
Abstainer	22.3	42	20.2	38
Lighter drinker	38.3	72	40.4	76
Heavier drinker	39.4	74	39.4	74
Total	100.0	188	100.0	188

[6] For a description of the items and their previous use, see Maddox and Borinski (3).

[7] The coefficient of reproducibility for the Preoccupation with Alcohol Scale is well above the minimum .90.

of heavy drinkers in a college population might be expected to increase over time. The observed proportion of panelists who drink in their first year in college matches the distributions found in the most nearly comparable samples of older collegians and college educated males in this country which have been studied. The proportion of panelists who drink heavily exceeds that of any population yet studied (4). The panelists, therefore, are precocious drinkers.

The Quantity-Frequency distribution among panelists as freshmen and as sophomores is quite similar. This similarity, however, masks several important changes. During the year under consideration, for example, the quantity of alcohol consumed increased from a standardized daily average of .43 to .84 ounces of absolute alcohol. Moreover, the proportion of panelists who defined alcohol in terms of narcotizing and reality-modifying effects increased from 44 per cent to 56 per cent. Similarly, preoccupation with drinking increased. For example, 18 per cent of the panelists fell initially into categories I-III on Mulford and Miller Preoccupation with Alcohol Scale, a rating which Mulford feels is indicative of probable trouble with drinking (11). A year later 32 per cent were preoccupied, while panelists with no indication of preoccupation decreased from 64 per cent to 39 per cent. A more optimistic view of changes in drinking behavior which are masked by the format of the data in Table 1 is suggested by the fact that the prevalence of problem drinking as measured by Park's Problem Drinking Index, shows a slight decrease (from a mean of 2.0 to 1.90).[8] Also on the optimistic side, the probability that panelists who drank would experience one or more of the Warning Signs or Social Complications discussed by Straus and Bacon (13) increased only slightly during the freshman year.

[8] Comparable data which provide a basis for evaluating observed levels on the Park index are scarce. Park, in private correspondence, indicates that the mean index score found in a 10 per cent sample of collegians used by Straus and Bacon in their Drinking Survey was 3.2. Park found a mean score of 2.2 in a random sample of Yale undergraduates. Alan Williams, in private correspondence, reports that, in a sample of 289 junior and senior male undergraduates, the mean score on the Park index was 2.5. Thus, comparatively, the mean index score of the panelists under consideration is only slightly below the mean scores of older collegians. Extrapolating, one might consider the observed score of panelists to be high when their age is considered.

The apparent stability in drinking behavior suggested by the data in Table 1 masks another significant kind of change among panelists, i.e., change in patterns of use. For example, while the proportion of abstainers remains essentially the same among panelists, the abstainers are not always the same individuals in both years (Table 2). Sixty-seven per cent of the abstaining freshmen reported behavior which classified them as either *lighter* (24 per cent) or *heavier* (43 per cent) drinkers a year later. Conversely, 16 per cent of the drinkers initially were classifiable as abstainers a year later (14 per cent of the *lighter* and 19 per cent of the *heavier* drinkers). Over-all, panelists were more likely to change (56 per cent) than to remain in their initial Q-F category.

The credibility and significance of these changes cannot simply be taken for granted. In the first place, the reliability of reports about abstinence and drinking behavior cannot be determined without the kind of detective work subject by subject which would have been prohibitive in this investigation. Second, data on the natural history of the careers of abstainers and drinkers with which the reported change among panelists might be compared are simply not available currently. Third, in all longitudinal research, the assessment of reliability of observations is always confounded by the possibility if not the probability of some actual change in behavior. As noted previously, there are substantial reasons for expecting the middle-status Negro youth to have important issues to negotiate and resolve in regard to drinking. Such considerations make caution necessary in the subsequent discussion of stability and change in patterns of abstinence and drinking among panelists.

TABLE 2.—*Stability and Change in Q-F Category among Panelists during the First Year in College*

Q-F as Sophomore	Q-F as Freshmen						Total
	Abstainer		Lighter Drinker		Heavier Drinker		
	%	N	%	N	%	N	N
Abstainer	33	14	14	10	19	14	38
Lighter drinker	24	10	51	37	39	29	76
Heavier drinker	43	18	35	25	42	31	74
Total	100	42	100	72	100	74	188

No special claim is made for the reliability of the initial or later classification of panelists as abstainers, lighter drinkers or heavier drinkers. However, reasonable confidence in the data does seem warranted. A technique was used in eliciting information about drinking behavior which, taken at face value, was sensitive to differences in that behavior. The interviews were conducted by Negro upperclassmen specifically trained in the use of the pre-tested interview schedule; the interviews were private; almost without exception, the panelists were cooperative; and the drinking behavior of panelists was uncorrelated with the reported drinking behavior of their interviewers. Of greater significance is the fact that stability and change in patterns of abstinence and drinking are not random, as will be illustrated subsequently. Therefore, with the need for caution duly emphasized, consideration now turns to the characteristics and experiences of panelists during their first year in college which might suggest an explanation for changes in their drinking behavior. Attention will be given first to some of the *background factors* (e.g., social class, religious preference and behavior, parental attitudes toward use of alcohol) associated with stability and change in patterns of abstinence and drinking among these young Negro males. Then, *social-psychological* factors (e.g., the meaning of alcohol and self-esteem); *experiential* factors (e.g., preoccupation, warning signs, and social complications); and *sociometric* factors (e.g., group cohesion, social integration) will be considered.

Background factors. A direct relationship between the quantity-frequency of drinking and socioeconomic status was found; the higher the status of a panelist as compared with other panelists, the more likely he was to drink and to drink heavily. Among those panelists whose Q-F category did not change during the year, for example, abstainers had the lowest status and *heavier* drinkers the highest. Moreover, among those who changed Q-F category, social status was associated with the direction of change. Abstainers who became *lighter* drinkers were of lower status than those who became *heavier* drinkers. Similarly, among drinkers, lower status was associated with a shift to abstention or to *lighter* drinking. The meaning of *lower status,* as it is used here, is important in interpreting this finding. A *lower status* panelist, in comparison with other panelists, was one whose Index of Status Placement (Hollingshead's two-factor index [8]) was in the lowest quartile of the distribution of index scores. Compared with his peers, a lower status panelist is thus most probably middle class in terms of his aspirations or identification but not in terms of parental status. This marginality might be associated with a cautious attachment to a norm of middle-class respectability among Negroes which is imputed to value abstinence. At any rate, the status marginals in the panel tend to negotiate their behavior in the direction of abstinence.

Among the panelists, religious orientation was also associated with social status, and, in turn, with drinking behavior. The lower the status of a student's parental family, the more likely he was to be religiously involved as a Protestant, indicating preference for a religious orientation which, in the region, has been historically identified with abstinence and prohibition.[9] Among students who did not change Q-F category, those with no or little Protestant involvement were most likely to be drinkers (93 per cent) and those with most involvement were least likely (75 per cent). Those marginally involved were intermediate (80 per cent). The *involved* Protestants who were abstainers initially were least likely to become drinkers (50 per cent) and the *non-involved* most likely (75 per cent). However, the *involved* Protestants who were initially drinkers were less likely than others to become abstainers and more likely to increase the quantity and frequency of their drinking. A plausible interpretation of this finding is suggested by an analysis of the relationship between the parental family's perceived preference for abstinence[10] and reported drinking behavior of panelists. This interpretation focuses attention on the extent to which the *in-*

[9] Lenski's measures of association, orthodoxy, and devotionalism (16, pp. 22ff.) were used to develop an index of Protestant involvement and panelists were categorized as *non-involved* (including non-Protestants as well as Protestants who were low on association, orthodoxy, and devotional measures); *involved* (those high on all three measures); and *marginally involved* (a residual category).

[10] An index of the parental family's preference for abstinence was constructed on the basis of the father and mother's reported use or non-use of alcohol and the advice given the panelist about drinking. A high score was given when both father and mother were reported to be abstinent and both advised the panelist to abstain. A low score was assigned when the opposite situation obtained. An intermediate category was formed by those with combinations of parental behavior and advice. This information was available for only 146 panelists; of these, 40 had low scores, 30 had high scores, and 76 had intermediate scores.

volved Protestant as an abstainer is clearly in a tenuous position in relation to most of his peers and presumably perceives pressure to behave like his peers. There are also indications that some of the changes are in reaction to perceived pressures to remain abstinent.

Among the stable panelists, those with a low index of parental preference for abstinence were in fact least likely to be abstinent (9 per cent). Those with intermediate scores were more likely to abstain (24 per cent); but, unexpectedly, panelists who perceived parents as most opposed to drinking were not the most likely to abstain (17 per cent). Moreover, among panelists who were initially drinkers, those who perceived their parents as abstainers were much less likely (11 per cent) to become abstainers during the year than panelists who perceived their parents to be more positive toward drinking (42 per cent). This suggests that in environments and in families in which drinking is perceived most negatively, drinking assumes a special significance. That is, drinking may be a way for expressing disaffection with or hostility toward parents, as well as an obvious means for identifying with the perceived cultural mainstream exhibited by a majority of one's peers. For youth who are exposed to a family or a religious tradition which opposes behavior typically observed among their peers, negotiations involving their own behavior take on a special significance. Such youth must literally make a role rather than simply take a role. Among panelists, exploration of abstinence on the part of a drinker whose family and religious tradition does not discourage drinking appears to be a more attractive option than it is for the drinker whose behavior is in violation of his family or religious tradition. Balance theory would suggest that, among the latter type of drinkers, there would be strain to resolve the contradiction by reevaluating religious involvement, the importance of parental vis-à-vis peer approval, or both. The data currently available on the panel do not permit an adequate test of specific hypotheses derived from balance theory, although, in time, such data will be available. Some data on the relationship of perceived closeness of panelists to fathers and of peer group integration to changes in Q-F category do suggest, however, the importance of family and peer group identification, particularly the latter. These relationships will be discussed below.

Social Psychological Factors. Panelists were asked to conceive and indicate their perceived closeness to mother and to father in terms of five concentric circles with maximum closeness designated by the center circle. Perceived closeness to mother did not differentiate among panelists since 9 of 10 indicated the maximum degree of closeness. However, perceived closeness to father did vary among panelists (60 per cent were maximally close) and was related to reported patterns of drinking and abstinence (Table 3). Although a majority of panelists drank, regardless of the degree of closeness to the father and regardless of whether the father was perceived to be a drinker, closeness to the father did increase the probability initially that the reported behavior would correspond to that of the father. Initially, for example, 90 per cent of those who were maximally close to a drinking father were drinkers themselves; 82 per cent of those who were less close to a drinking father drank. In contrast, 62 per cent of those close to a non-drinking father were drinkers as compared with 73 per cent of those who were less close. During the first year in college, however, some adaptations were made. At the beginning of the sophomore year, differences in the probability of drinking based on perceived closeness to the father and the perceived behavior of the father have decreased. The sons of non-drinking fathers were more likely to be drinkers than were the sons of drinking fathers, regardless of closeness. The panelists who were maximally close to the father were more likely to change their behavior, with some drinking sons of drinking fathers experimenting with abstinence and some abstaining sons of abstaining fathers experimenting with drinking. In order to understand these changes, it would be necessary to know more than is, in fact, known about both the drinking behavior of the father and the father-son relationship. Two relevant factors

TABLE 3.—*Percentage of Drinkers among Panelists as Freshmen and as Sophomores, by Perceived Closeness to Father and by Reported Drinking Behavior of Father*

Relation to father is	% of drinking panelists as	
	Freshmen	Sophomores
Close and father is described as a		
Drinker	90	76
Non-drinker	62	87
Not close and father is described as a		
Drinker	82	77
Non-drinker	73	83

in understanding the observed changes, in addition to the father's reported behavior, suggest themselves, however. First, although the social climate to which the panelists are exposed in college generally recommends drinking, drinking is not uniformly rewarding behavior. The particular peers with whom an individual finds himself repeatedly as a freshman may and, as will be indicated below, sometimes may not, prefer abstinence. If these peers are preferred comparisons, balance theory suggests that the individual who drinks has the option of changing his behavior instead of his group. Also, drinking in itself is not necessarily socially integrative and may, if it results in disturbing personal or social experiences, provide an occasion for the drinker to try abstinence. The data presented later also suggest this factor as relevant in understanding why some panelists became ex-drinkers during the year. Thus, it can be said at this point that closeness to father is associated with changes in drinking behavior. Whether these changes reflect a greater sense of security which promotes experimentation, a greater sense of responsibility which promotes caution, or a combination of both remains to be determined. Second, the probability of changes in Q-F categories may also reflect personality differences such as field dependence or independence. This possibility is noted but the data available are insufficient for systematic exploration.[11]

[11] Although personality differences were not systematically explored in the research reported here, one personality measure, a flexibility of closure test developed by the Educational Testing Service (17), was given to 100 of the panelists by another investigator, Michael Sherman. Flexibility of closure is a concept generally related to field dependence and independence in the tradition of Witkin (18). The expectation is that, following Witkin, the capacity to distinguish figures within a complex background is related to an analytic, as distinct from a global, orientation to the environment and indicates relative independence of environmental cues in giving meaning to stimuli. Hence, persons who display a marked analytic capacity (field independent) are also expected to depend less on drugs such as alcohol for reality modification and to present more stable patterns of behavior than others. The limited data available support these expectations. One hundred per cent of the 24 selected panelists exhibiting the lowest (4th quartile) Flexibility of Closure scores (field dependent) were drinkers as compared with 89 per cent of the 52 panelists in the middle range and 65 per cent of the 24 "field independent" panelists exhibiting the highest (1st quartile) scores. Moreover, 71 per cent of those with lowest scores changed drinking categories during their first year in college in contrast to 50 per cent of those in the middle range and 29 per cent of those with the highest scores.

The extent to which religious involvement, perceived closeness to father, and family tradition interact and the relative importance of these factors in explaining the observed patterns of drinking and abstinence among the panelists remains to be explored. However, it is clear from preliminary analysis that these factors do interact in complex ways. This complexity is further illustrated by an analysis of the relationship between self-esteem and patterns of abstinence and drinking.

Two aspects of self-esteem were considered: self-evaluation and the evaluation of self attributed to others. While these two estimates of self can be different, what is known of the origins of self-concepts leads one to expect that how an individual views himself is, to an important degree, correlated with the concept and evaluation of himself he imputes to others who are important to him.[12] Among students whose drinking pattern remained stable, initially both a negative self-evaluation and the imputation of a negative evaluation of self by others were more likely among drinkers than among abstainers and, among drinkers, was higher among *heavier* drinkers (Table 4). At the end of a year in college, the evaluation of self among abstainers and *lighter* drinkers was quite similar and both had a more positive image of themselves than did *heavier* drinkers. Although evaluations of the self generally became more negative during the year, suggesting that factors other than drinking *per se* were involved, the observed changes were apparently not independent of drinking behavior. Of particular interest are the *lighter* drinkers, who

TABLE 4.—*Mean Number of Negative Items Applied to Self, by Self and, by Imputation to Others, among Panelists with Persistent Q-F Patterns as Freshmen and Sophomores*

| | Mean Number of Negative Items | | | |
| | Applied by Self as | | Imputed to Others as | |
Persistent Q-F Pattern	Freshman	Sophomore	Freshman	Sophomore
Abstainers (N=14)	2.5	4.3	0.5	1.9
Lighter drinker (N=37)	3.7	4.2	1.1	1.7
Heavier drinker (N=31)	4.4	6.1	1.7	2.3
Total	3.5	5.1	1.6	2.1

[12] In an analysis not shown, there is a significant positive correlation between self-evaluation and the evaluation of self imputed to others by panelists.

showed the least changes in self-evaluation during the year and who as sophomores had the most favorable image of themselves. The *lighter* drinker is interesting precisely because he may represent the optimum solution in regard to drinking for the panelist. On the one hand, he meets the modal peer group expectation by drinking; on the other hand, he drinks in a way which has some chance of being personally and socially justified as respectable. The persistent abstainers, in contrast, exhibited a substantial decline in self-esteem. Thus, while the *heavier* drinkers among panelists had consistently the most negative image of themselves, the abstainer exhibited a pronounced loss in self-esteem during the year, particularly in his imputation of evaluation by others. Additional evidence that patterns of drinking and abstinence are related to self-esteem is provided by those whose Q-F category changed during the year.

A change from drinking to abstinence or a reduction in drinking was associated with an improvement in self-esteem, while a change from abstinence to drinking or an increase in drinking was associated with an increase in negative self-evaluation (Table 5). The effects of Q-F changes on self-evaluation are more clear-cut than on the evaluation imputed to others. Among drinkers who changed from *lighter* to *heavier* drinking, and vice versa, the perceived change in evaluation by others is minimal. Otherwise, the observed relationship between drinking and a negative evaluation of the self holds.

Again it should be emphasized that multiple factors are probably involved in changes of Q-F category among some panelists

TABLE 5.—*Mean Changes in Acceptance of Negative Items Applied to Self by Self and Imputedly by Others among Panelists Who Change Q-F Category during the First Year of College*

| Patterns of Q-F change | Mean Change in Negative Items | |
	Applied by Self	Applied by Others
Lighter drinker/abstainer (N=10)	−0.6	−0.4
Heavier drinker/abstainer (N=14)	+0.7	−1.1
Abstainer/*lighter* drinker (N=10)	+0.5	+1.1
Heavier drinker/*lighter* drinker (N=29)	+1.6	+0.2
Lighter drinker/*heavier* drinker (N=25)	+3.1	+0.4
Abstainer/*heavier* drinker (N=18)	+4.0	+1.6
Total	+1.6	+0.5

during their first year in college. However, it seems clear that, among panelists, drinking, and particularly heavy drinking, tends to have a negative effect on self-esteem. Role-making exacts a price, and the more extreme the changes negotiated, the greater the price.

Another illustration of the negotiations in which many of the panelists are involved is provided by changes in the preference for self-description in terms of the use or non-use of alcohol. In previous research (3, 4) some young people who do not drink have been found to reject the label *abstainer* and to prefer the designation *non-drinker*. Those who drink usually prefer to label themselves as a *social drinker* rather than as a *drinker;* and some drinkers even prefer to designate themselves as *non-drinker.* The designation *abstainer* apparently connotes not only avoidance of alcohol but also total avoidance based on moral conviction. The designation *non-drinker,* on the other hand, apparently connoted minimal use, perhaps even non-use, related to situational factors rather than to moral conviction. For example, almost four times as many panelists ($N=77$) label themselves as *abstainers* or *non-drinkers* as are in fact abstainers in terms of Q-F classification. *Drinker* without the adjective *social* is rarely accepted as a self-designation even by those who, in terms of their Q-F classification, drink heavily. The avoidance of this label appears to reflect an association of *drinker* with excessive or deviant drinking behavior.

Balance theory would lead one to expect increasing congruence between drinking behavior and the self-description. This is in fact the case among panelists. Among those whose Q-F classification remained constant, all abstainers (no alcohol reportedly consumed) labeled themselves as *abstainers* or *non-drinkers* both initially and a year later. Similarly, almost all *heavier* drinkers (97 per cent) initially, and all of them a year later, designated themselves as *social drinkers* or as *drinkers.* As might be expected, while the *lighter* drinkers were less in agreement about an appropriate designation for themselves initially (54 per cent preferred a label recognizing their drinking), a year later 95 per cent of them accepted the designation *social drinker* or *drinker.* Correspondingly, while those who changed Q-F category, like the *lighter* drinkers, initially had a substantial number of incongruous self-designations, a year later approximately 9 of

10 of them presented a self-designation which was congruous with their reported behavior.

Alcohol may be perceived and used primarily as a drug for modifying reality or as a social beverage for relating oneself to others in a conventional way. A reliable, valid procedure for measuring such a distinction, a Definition of Alcohol scale, has been proposed by Mulford and Miller (15; see also 11). One would expect that drinking for reality-modifying effects (Types I-III on the Definition of Alcohol Scale) would be associated with amount of drinking and this was found to be the case among panelists. Forty per cent of the persistent *lighter* drinkers initially associated their drinking with reality modification and 74 per cent of the *heavier* drinkers did also. A year later these percentages had increased, respectively, to 57 per cent and 94 per cent. Among panelists who changed Q-F classification, the perception of drinking primarily in terms of reality-modifying effects was related to the changes in drinking behavior reported. More simply, those who initially perceived alcohol as a social beverage were slightly less likely to decrease their use of alcohol during the year than were those who perceived alcohol as a reality-modifying drug. If one can assume that some panelists perceive drinking for reality-modifying effect as potentially dangerous and suspect, the observed pattern of changes could be explained in part. The *lighter* drinkers who increased their drinking in the direction of an environmental norm which tolerates fairly heavy drinking were more likely than others to define drinking in social terms. The *heavier* drinkers who decreased or gave up drinking were more likely than others to think of drinking primarily in terms of reality modification. It is as though those *lighter* drinkers who describe their motivation in socially acceptable terms feel justified in increasing their consumption while those *heavier* drinkers whose motivation is socially suspect feel compelled to reduce consumption. In both cases, however, these maneuvers, if that is what they are, are unsuccessful. A year later, among panelists who had increased their drinking, 72 per cent of them perceived drinking in terms of reality modification, an increase of 30 per cent. Among panelists who were initially *heavier* drinkers, reduction of drinking during the year had very little effect on their perception of the reality-modifying function of alcohol. Moreover, 79 per cent of the abstainers who initially were *heavier* drinkers still perceived drinking in reality-modifying terms even though momentarily they were not drinking. The perception of alcohol as a social beverage, therefore, did not protect the panelists from the discovery of its potential as a drug if they drank heavily; and once having made this discovery, they continued to associate drinking with its reality-modifying potential.

The relevance of reality modification as an orientation to drinking for understanding observed changes in Q-F categories among panelists receives additional support from another measure of differential perceptions of what alcohol can do for or to the drinker. This semantic differential measure focuses specifically on the perceived positive or negative modifications in self-evaluation associated with drinking. Drinkers in the panel, for example, were asked to describe themselves "when I drink," while abstainers were asked to describe themselves hypothetically "if I drank." Thus with information about how a given individual described "myself as I really am" and "myself as I would most like to be," it was possible to identify individuals for whom drinking was perceived to modify the actual self in a positive, that is, the ideal, direction as well as those for whom the reverse was true.

Twenty-six per cent of the panelists indicated that drinking modified their self-evaluation positively; 63 per cent reported the effect to be negative; and 11 per cent reported no effect. Given the high percentage of drinkers and of *heavier* drinkers in the panel, the proportion who perceived drinking in negative terms is interesting but not surprising in the light of a literature which usually predicts such an evaluation of drinking among middle-status Negroes. Nor is it surprising that, among panelists who did not change Q-F category, the proportion of drinkers is highest (100 per cent) among those who report that drinking is a means of manipulating their self-perception positively; lowest (74 per cent) among those who report the opposite effect; and intermediate (86 per cent) for those for whom alcohol makes no contribution to self-evaluation one way or the other. But another finding is less obvious although anticipated by the association between the perceived function of drinking and changes in drinking behavior noted above. Panelists who perceived alcohol primarily as a social beverage, it was noted above, tended to reduce their drinking. A similar relationship was found in the association between the perceived potential of alcohol for modifying the self concept and changes in drinking behavior.

Among panelists who were drinkers initially, those who associated drinking with positive modifications of self-evaluation were most likely to become abstainers (45 per cent); those with the opposite association least likely (19 per cent); and, again, those who made neither association were intermediate (29 per cent). This suggests that a negative association between drinking and self-realization may provide reassurance to the drinker that he is not inordinately dependent on a potentially dangerous type of behavior. Recognition that drinking is being used to modify self-evaluations apparently leads some panelists to a radical modification of drinking behavior. Whether such adaptations are temporary remains to be determined.

Experiential factors. How an individual drinks, when he drinks, why he drinks, and where he drinks, and not simply how much he drinks, are associated with the kinds of troubles he has with his drinking if, in fact, he has such troubles. In fact, however, the more one drinks, the greater the probability of experiencing trouble, all other things considered. This is illustrated by the data in Table 6 which summarize the experience during the freshman year of those panelists who presented a persistent drinking pattern. In general, a similar relationship between patterns of drinking and trouble experienced held for these panelists also as sophomores, although, in the case of preoccupation with alcohol, *heavier* drinkers were more likely (+16 per cent) and the *lighter* drinkers were less likely (—8 per cent) to be preoccupied with drinking. Among those whose Q-F category changed during the year, a pattern is clear and increasingly familiar: the

TABLE 6.—*Trouble with Drinking Initially Reported by Panelists with Stable Drinking Patterns during the First Year in College*

	Indicators of Trouble			
Q-F Category	Preoccupied with Drinking	Warning Signs	Social Complications	Problem Drinking Index
	%	$\overline{X}$	$\overline{X}$	$\overline{X}$
Lighter drinker (N=37)	21	0.8	0.3	1.2
Heavier drinker (N=31)	42	2.0	1.5	3.0

absence of trouble with drinking appeared to encourage heavier drinking while trouble appeared to encourage reduction in use. Panelists who increased their drinking reported initially fewer indications of trouble than those whose drinking remained constant or whose drinking decreased. For example, among *lighter* drinkers who became *heavier* drinkers, only 13 per cent were preoccupied with their drinking initially. On the other hand, drinkers who during the year reduced their drinking most radically were those who were having the most trouble. For example, the *heavier* drinkers who became abstinent during the year had the highest index of problem drinking ($\overline{X}=3.4$) found among the panelists.

The results of such maneuvers cannot be evaluated adequately over a short period of time. But there are indications that, even in the short run, increased drinking by panelists who had not experienced much trouble with their drinking initially increases the probability of trouble. Moreover, the *heavier* drinker who reduced his consumption, in part in response to the trouble he experienced presumably, did not reduce the trouble he experiences very much if he stopped short of abstinence. For instance, 33 per cent of the *heavier* drinkers who during the year became *lighter* drinkers were preoccupied with drinking. A year later 27 per cent of them were still preoccupied, which is twice the proportion among panelists who were persistently *lighter* drinkers.

Sociometric factors. Drinking behavior is potentially important in social interaction in several ways. It follows that, in an environment in which drinking is encouraged, socially active and integrated people will have many occasions to drink and drinking people will have at least one interest in common with many other people in a variety of social situations. The abstainer, especially the abstainer whose behavior reflects moral conviction about not drinking, will experience constraints in such an environment. Most simply, the abstainer surrounded by drinkers has only a limited number of people whose behavior matches his own and a limited number of social situations in which drinking is not a common activity. The experience of the panelists illustrates the problems of the abstainer and his attempts to deal with them as well as the problems of the drinker whose drinking does not prove to be socially integrating.

The panelists were asked to list the fellows with whom they

were spending as much time as possible at the beginning of the freshman year. They were then asked, "How close do you fellows feel to each other?" and "How close are you personally to the center of things that go on in this group?" In each instance the panelists were shown five concentric circles with 1 in the center and 5 at the outer circle and asked to indicate the degree of perceived closeness and peer group integration. They were also asked to estimate the number of hours spent with this group during an average week. Only four panelists indicated they spent no time regularly with at least one other person. Among those that did spend time with a group of peers and who had stable Q-F patterns, drinking was found to be positively related to perceived closeness, integration in group activities, and in the number of hours spent with the group (Table 7). The patterns presented in Table 7 hold also for the report a year later with a single modification; as sophomores the abstainers had increased the average time per week they spent with peers, although they still spent less time with their peers in group activity than did either category of drinkers.

Among panelists who reported a change in drinking behavior, changes in their group relationships may be characterized as follows. In general, during the year perceived closeness to preferred groups increased. In four of the six types of Q-F changes (e.g., abstainer/*lighter* drinker, *lighter* drinker/abstainer, etc.) the mean closeness score improved and, in the remaining two categories, remained unchanged. The perception of being at the center of things in group activity also improved for five of the six change-categories. Only the abstainers turned *heavier* drinkers felt less at the center of things. In regard to the average number of hours per week spent with the preferred group, the

TABLE 7.—*Perceived Closeness, Integration, and Hours per Week in Peer Groups, by Q-F Category, among Panelists with Stable Drinking Patterns*

Q-F Category	SOCIOMETRIC INDICATOR		
	Closeness $\overline{X}$	Integration $\overline{X}$	HPW $\overline{X}$
Heavier drinker (N=31)	1.6	1.6	26.5
Lighter drinker (N=37)	2.0	2.1	26.9
Abstainer (N=14)	2.2	2.2	16.5

more socially active abstainers became drinkers and the less active drinkers reduced their drinking or became abstainers. These changes in drinking pattern increased the number of hours spent with the preferred peer groups in the sophomore year with a single exception. The abstainer turned *heavier* drinker was less active but still, on the average, was more active than the persistent abstainer.

Individuals continually negotiate with their peers for social acceptance. In these negotiations there is a strong tendency for groups to develop in which there is some consensus about appropriate behavior or for group affiliations to be unstable in the absence of some degree of consensus. Since drinking is a common, and presumably important, activity for most panelists, the observations that perceived closeness within groups of peers and integration in group activities were most likely among those for whom drinking is a frequent activity are consistent with the expectation. The probability that a panelist would be a member of a stable group was also found to be related to drinking behavior and to the similarity of drinking behavior within a group. Among panelists who did not change their Q-F category during the year, for example, the persistently *heavier* drinkers were most likely to list the same persons as belonging to their preferred peer group both years $(\overline{X}=2.4)$, the abstainers were least likely to report continuity of group membership $(\overline{X}=1.6)$, and the *lighter* drinkers were intermediate $(\overline{X}=1.9)$. The negotiative aspect of the peer relationship can be best illustrated briefly by focusing the analysis on the behavior of those panelists who represented initially or later the minority position, abstinence.

The persistent abstainers consistently reported small groups, composed predominantly of abstainers who also labeled themselves as abstainers. As noted previously, the number of hours spent per week in these groups was small. All the persistent abstainers imagined that drinking would, if they drank, be deleterious to their self-evaluation, which was uniformly high. Significantly, however, the generally positive evaluation of themselves imputed to others initially disappeared during the year.

The abstaining panelists who became drinkers during the year present a different picture. Whether the ex-abstainer became a *lighter* or a *heavier* drinker, initially he listed a preferred group composed predominantly of drinkers. The single exception, who initially described participation in a group of abstainers, reported a year later that he and his best friend both became drinkers. With few exceptions, the ex-abstainers had initially and maintained an above-average number of hours per week in their preferred groups and maintained a high level of perceived closeness to and integration with them. The ex-abstainers who became *lighter* drinkers and those who became *heavier* drinkers were different in some ways, however. These differences provide a basis for speculating about the probable stability in drinking patterns of each type of drinker in the later years of college.

Among the ex-abstainers, the *lighter* drinker was more likely to impute a positive evaluation of himself to others initially than was the *heavier* drinker and was also more likely to make this imputation a year later. The new *heavier* drinker was also more likely to experience a loss of self-esteem and to experience problems with drinking. No new *heavier* drinker was free of indications of problem drinking (a zero score on Park's Problem Drinking Index) while half of the *lighter* drinkers presented no indications of drinking problems. The ex-abstainer who moved to make his drinking behavior consistent with that of his group, therefore, was only partially successful in minimizing the costs of his change and was more successful if his drinking was *lighter* rather than *heavier*.

If the ex-abstainer is conceived as an individual attempting to bring his behavior to conform with that of his preferred peers, the ex-drinker may be similarly described. It has already been noted that the experience of drinking problems and the perception of alcohol as a reality-modifying drug were related to a decrease in drinking; this maneuver, however, did not appear usually to be very successful. The same conclusion is suggested by the sociometric data. For example, half of the sophomore ex-drinkers, whether initially *lighter* or *heavier* drinkers, described preferred groups composed primarily of abstainers in the freshman year and were below average in the number of hours per week spent with their groups. In general, they perceived their closeness to and their integration with their groups to be low. The *heavier* drinkers, in contrast to *lighter* drinkers, were more likely to have had trouble with their drinking. All the *heavier* drinkers had experienced trouble and their mean score on the

Problem Drinking Index was 4.0, twice the average of all drinkers. Half of them had experienced social complications associated with their drinking, and the same proportion expected to improve their evaluations of self when drinking. The *lighter* drinker who became an abstainer, on the other hand, had not had unusual trouble with drinking. They were distinguished from others by the very positive evaluation of themselves which they imputed to others and the improvement in self-evaluation which followed their termination of drinking. These data suggest that the ex-drinker whose drinking has been moderate or minimal experiences some positive rewards from his abstinence and hence has some reasons for maintaining the new pattern. No such rewards are apparent for the new abstainer who has been a *heavier* drinker. In addition to the description of this situation already given, it should be added that not a single panelist who was a *heavier* drinker turned abstainer had a reciprocal choice within his preferred peer group either initially or a year later.

The sociometric data provide insights into the role of drinking in the negotiations through which stable peer groups are created and maintained. Although the full complexity of the data presented here can only be hinted, the negotiations in which drinking figures among these young collegians are clearly complex; these negotiations involve attitudes toward drinking which reflect family background, self-esteem, and the initial composition of peer groups. For a student beginning his freshman year in a new environment, the panelists illustrate pressure to bring their drinking into conformity with that of their peers. Those who are most active, whose preferred peers are drinkers, and who perceive themselves as most integrated in groups either drink or become drinkers. Drinkers who are least active, whose preferred peers are abstainers, and who are least integrated in groups are most likely to become abstainers, especially if they have had trouble with drinking. The probability that the panelists who changed Q-F category during the year, especially those who changed radically, will continue their new pattern is problematic. In the case of the abstainer turned *heavier* drinker and the *heavier* drinker turned abstainer, the probability seems small since there were indications that the negotiations suggested by these changes were not experienced as rewarding by the panelists involved.

Conclusions

The complex factors which underlie the variable patterns of abstinence and drinking found among youth are illustrated by this panel of Negro collegians followed through their first year in college. As young Negro males with middle-status backgrounds or aspirations, they are exposed to the acute ambivalence toward drinking which has characterized the American tradition. Most youth are exposed to ambiguous messages about the legitimacy of their drinking, and the problem is intensified by the precarious legitimacy of drinking among *respectable* Negroes at any age. One result of this ambivalence and ambiguity is that being an abstainer or becoming a drinker involves more than simply taking a predetermined social role. Literally, many, if not most, youths must make a role for themselves; they must negotiate potentially contradictory expectations about their behavior as they explore what it means to be a male, a collegian, and a young adult. Choosing to drink is clearly not simple and is not done once and for all, if the experience of the panelists in this study is at all typical of Negro youth in college. For most of these young men, drinking is a common, important activity and their college environment is more tolerant of heavy drinking than it is supportive of abstention. Some panelists did maintain their abstinence into the sophomore year but they seem to have done so by constricting their social activity and by finding friends who were also abstinent, which is not an easy task in an environment in which most of one's potential friends drink. The persistent drinkers were also likely to have found like-minded friends; but, in contrast to the abstainers, the drinkers were socially active and felt themselves esteemed. The majority of panelists modified their abstinence or their drinking in some way during the freshman year. Socially active abstainers whose friends drank tended to give drinking a try. Panelists whose drinking did not secure for them group acceptance or personal satisfaction tended to give abstinence a try. Among lighter drinkers, the quantity and frequency of use tended to increase if they had had no trouble with their drinking and did not associate drinking with reality modification. Heavier drinkers, on the other hand, tended to reduce their drinking if they perceived their use of alcohol to modify reality and experienced trouble. Thus, the marginal people—whether in terms of their patterns of abstinence or drinking, their social characteristics, their experiences with drinking, or their social integration—had the most to negotiate during their first year of college and were the most likely to change their behavior. The success of their negotiations remain in doubt. From the limited data in hand, some of the resolutions attempted by the panelists seemed inadequate even to the panelists. The abstainer turned heavy drinker and the heavy drinker turned abstainer are cases in point. But only subsequent study can provide insight into when and how satisfying and stable patterns of drinking and abstinence are achieved among youths in the process of growing into adulthood. Among the panelists, the maintenance or achievement of social integration and self-esteem were most likely for those who drank, moderately and socially.

REFERENCES

1. MADDOX, GEORGE L. "Teenagers and Alcohol: Recent Research," Annals of the New York Academy of Sciences, 133: 856-65, 1966.
2. JELLINEK, E. M. "Phases of Alcohol Addiction," in D. PITTMAN and C. SNYDER (eds.), Society, Culture, and Drinking Patterns. New York: John Wiley & Sons, 1962.
3. MADDOX, G. L., and E. BORINSKI. "Drinking Behavior of Negro Collegians: A Study of Selected Men," Quarterly Journal of Studies on Alcohol, 25: 651-658, 1964.
4. MADDOX, G. L., and J. R. WILLIAMS. "Drinking Behavior of Negro Collegians: A Comparison of Selected Men," Quarterly Journal of Studies on Alcohol, 29: 117-129, 1968.
5. STERNE, M. W. "Drinking Patterns and Alcoholism among American Negroes." Occasional Paper #7, Social Science Institute, Washington University, October, 1966.
6. TURNER, RALPH. "Role-Taking: Process or Conformity," in ARNOLD M. ROSE (ed.), Human Behavior and Social Processes. Boston: Houghton Mifflin Company, 1962.
7. ALEXANDER, C. NORMAN. "Consensus and Mutual Attraction in Natural Cliques: A Study of Adolescent Drinkers," American Journal of Sociology, 69: 395-403, 1964.
8. HOLLINGSHEAD, A. B., and F. C. REDLICH. Social Class and Mental Illness. New York: John Wiley, 1958.
9. MULFORD, HAROLD A., and D. E. MILLER. "Drinking in Iowa, II. The Extent of Drinking and Selected Sociological Categories," Quarterly Journal of Studies on Alcohol, 21: 26-39, 1960.

10. JESSOR, R., and P. GROSSMAN. Unpublished manuscript from the Tri-Ethnic Research Project, University of Colorado.
11. MULFORD, H. A. "Identifying Problem Drinkers in a Household Survey." National Center for Health Statistics. Series 2:16, May, 1966.
12. MULFORD, H. A., and D. E. MILLER. "Drinking in Iowa, III. A Scale of Definitions of Alcohol Related to Drinking Behavior," *Quarterly Journal of Studies on Alcohol*, 21: 267-78, 1960.
13. STRAUS, R., and S. D. BACON. *Drinking in College*. New Haven: Yale University Press, 1953.
14. PARK, P. "Problem Drinking and Role Deviation," in D. PITTMAN and C. SNYDER (eds.), *Society, Culture, and Drinking Behavior*. New York: Wiley, 1962.
15. MULFORD, H. A., and D. E. MILLER. "Drinking in Iowa, IV. Preoccupation with Alcohol and Definitions of Alcohol, Heavy Drinking and Trouble Due to Drinking," *Quarterly Journal of Studies on Alcohol*, 21: 279-91, 1960.
16. LENSKI, G. *The Religious Factor*. Garden City: Doubleday Anchor Books, 1963.
17. JACKSON, D. N., S. MESSICK, and C. T. MEYERS. "Evaluation of Group and Individual Forms of Embedded Figures Measures of Field-Independence," *Educational and Psychological Measurement*, 24: 177-192, 1964.
18. WITKIN, H. A. "Psychological Differentiation and Forms of Pathology," *Journal of Abnormal Psychology*, 70: 317-336, 1965.

Chapter 7

COLLEGE DRINKING: STUDENTS SEE IT MANY WAYS

ROBERT D. RUSSELL
Southern Illinois University

FACETS of the answer to the question "What is drinking among collegians?" are discovered or derived in a number of ways—surveys of a range of students, surveys of smaller groups, observation, in-depth interviews, and so on. As these become part of the literature, however, they achieve a certain similarity in that most of the writing is non-student, adult writing. Professors, researchers, journalists, and others put their findings together and write about collegians and the way they drink, usually interspersing a short quote or two to establish credibility. The following pages will effect a reversal of the typical ratio and will present primarily words of students with a minimum of adult commentary.

In no sense is this presented as *the* answer to the opening question. The student-written words contained herein are from papers submitted to the author by senior students in a colloquium entitled "Beverage Alcohol and Society," at Stanford University during the 1960-65 period. These are not presented as "typical college students" (though some of them might be, in certain ways). They are male and female, but mostly male. They are all over 21, and most are drinkers and have been through their college years. Most are second or third generation college students—or at least grew up "knowing" they would be going to a "good" college, possibly Stanford. In general they were not visible student leaders nor distinguished scholars, but just a self-selected (the course was elective but enrollment was limited to eighteen) group of students over a six-year period who were soon to graduate and who, for some combination of motives, wrote papers and did not balk when the professor refused to return them.

The papers were not written for publication, so to avoid predictable and unpredictable complications they are presented anonymously, with an occasional detail changed to maintain the anonymity.

Since the author is a non-student adult, and he has selected the papers and the excerpts to fit some conceived frame of reference, the question certainly can be posed: "How is this really any different—except that it is a bit less scholarly?" Simply, in the balance of this chapter, student-written words tell the story rather than add a trimming. This does not make it superior to other papers in this volume—nor is it necessarily inferior. It is just different—and therefore may add another dimension to our understanding of this life phenomenon.

Drinking before College

The studies of youth drinking behavior present a fairly consistent picture of alcohol use beginning to be evident in the mid-teens, with a larger portion of the age group becoming at least occasional drinkers with each subsequent year. Thus, a sizeable number of those who drink as collegians had drinking experiences before entering college. The nature of some of these experiences follows.

This young man's narrative begins with his sophomore year in high school:

Prior to this time drinking had been a subject only very remotely related to me. None of my friends or acquaintances drank at all, to my knowledge, and the topic of drinking was something for movies, television and senseless adults. I realized I was "too young to drink" and was perfectly happy, unable to understand why any sane person would ever submit to the unpleasant taste and unhappy consequences of drinking such awful stuff. Then Ed Ferguson, a senior whom I admired very much and looked up to, came up to me in a drive-in restaurant and was obviously drunk. I went over to a car with him and saw several others sitting in the car drinking beer in short, concealed gulps.

Suddenly, alcohol was no longer a remote stranger, but had moved in on my life without my being aware of its approach: in the shock of one incident, drinking became both a threat and a challenge. My first reaction was repulsion—both in relation to alcohol and to those who used it. I did not openly express my feelings, but merely sought the company of those who didn't drink and avoided those who did. This reaction lasted, roughly, through my junior year, but I was slowly beginning to be swayed by social pressure and the attraction of the adventure in drinking.

During this period, I was just beginning to feel a desire to drink, and combatted this feeling mostly by an unfounded fear of some sort of drastic consequences. I was genuinely afraid of drinking, but had nothing to satisfy the secret desire for the adventure of doing something "wrong." Only my fear and a sense of religious morality held me back, and when autumn sports and their necessary training came along, I was very relieved to have a justifiable reason for abstaining. Football was followed by basketball in the winter and most of the guys I went around with who were considered "good athletes" did not drink during this time.

Thus, substitution involved not finding something to take the place of alcohol, but finding something to use as an acceptable barrier to keep the temptation sublimated. This barrier was keeping training. During the six-month period of football and basketball in my senior year, I made many new friends, and I suppose was considered to be "one of the boys," and when basketball season was over and my ostensible reason for not drinking gone, the temptation mounted in new and larger dimensions.

Drinking became the means of identification with the group, and there were simply no substitutes that would allow one to keep his identification and "respectability" as a BMOC, one step ahead of the rest of the student body who looked to this group to supply strong leadership and backbone to the campus. Drinking being inconsistent with my religion, one or the other had to go. The religion took the rumble seat. When most of my friends were drinking, the fear that I formerly had of the consequences seemed very small. When girls were drinking, my pride and sense of male superiority were so inflamed that there was not a moment's hesitation regarding the direction of my action.

I discovered that it was easy to drink and have a good time and was welcomed to the group as a full-fledged, finally sensible member.

Another young man's description includes these observations:

> In the early years (13-16) drinking, at least in my case, was
> a very furtive thing. Because of this and the fact that we had no
> access to cars, our rare drinking occasions occurred mainly in
> some hide-out or while walking through the city alleys. During
> this time drinking was not so much for the sake of enjoyment or
> intoxication as it was a case of kids seeking a thrill in something
> forbidden (not even indulged in by my parents).
>
> With the advent of the car in my later high school days, a
> place to drink was no problem. All we had to do was drive to
> the beach along a deserted road, or to a drive-in movie . . . By
> far the most popular place to drink, especially in mixed company,
> was the drive-in theater. . . . During the summer the next most
> popular place . . . was the beach, especially during night-
> time beach parties . . . out of metropolitan areas and free from
> adult interference. Much of the worst kind of alcoholic abuse by
> minors occurs at such parties.

He goes on to describe a beach party at which he and a friend,
both seventeen, drank vodka rather rapidly, passed out, and were
picked up by the police. His conclusion provides his transition
to college.

> Our parents were phoned and when they arrived to carry us
> home, I was as scared as I've ever been in my life. My home
> punishment was severe, but the police did nothing and actually
> joked with me about getting drunk enough to get picked up.
> Naturally this event greatly affected me, and I drank very rarely
> and then very cautiously until I came to Stanford.

Another male student, writing on the transition from high
school to college, described pre-college drinking in these ways:

> During the high school years, the teen-ager is under the direct
> influence of his parents; he still lives with them, and their rules
> are, in general, the rules he must abide by. In regard to liquor,
> it has been my experience that most parents do not give absolute
> rules which forbid their teen-agers to drink, but rather the par-
> ents do let their opinions on the subject become known in such
> a way that the teen-ager formulates some absolute rules for him-
> self from these opinions. My own ideas were formed by such
> statements as "your mother and I would rather give you a drink

here at home if you want one than have you running off somewhere to drink. . . . I have found that most teen-agers in high
school either are convinced they should not drink, decide they
will not drink, or are afraid to drink for fear of what their parents
will say or do.

He goes on to expound on two other deterrents to pre-college
drinking.

Many boys refrain from drinking in high school because they
are participating in athletics. Not only do coaches' rules forbid
drinking, but most athletes realize their ability in a sport is reduced to some extent by alcohol. Very few high school athletes
participate in collegiate sports, however; this eliminates their
former excuse for not drinking. And it seems almost paradoxical
that quite often these former athletes become the heaviest drinkers in college. Whether this is because the athletes are seeking
some sort of substitute for athletics or whether this is because
athletes often congregate together in social groups because of
their common interest in athletics, and alcohol becomes more of
an excuse for socializing, I do not know.

Another factor is the availability of alcohol. While attending
high school, the teen-ager has few means by which he can obtain
liquor. Parents usually will not purchase beverage alcohol for
their teen-agers, and very seldom will the teen-ager have close
friends who are old enough to buy liquor for him. Therefore,
unless the high school student can obtain false identification or
unless there is an unusually lenient tavern owner in the community, the student will be unable to acquire the liquor.

His summation:

The student upon entering college changes directly from an environment which acts to prohibit his drinking to an environment
which, in its own way, encourages the student to drink.

Finally, a young lady from an upper-class suburban town
where the vast majority of young people are expected to and,
in fact, do go on to college, describes her community and its
youth drinking mores:

High school boys usually begin drinking somewhere around
the age of fifteen and drink approximately two or three times
a month in the early stages. The frequency of drinking increases

gradually until they are drinking at least twice a week (usually Friday and Saturday nights only) by the end of their junior year, or age sixteen. Degree of intoxication shows little increase, for it seems that moderate drinking is a stage that these students rarely go through. Drunkenness is common from the very outset, and the philosophy behind high school drinking is, "If there isn't enough alcohol around to get you sufficiently drunk, don't bother to drink at all."

The female population of our town do not usually commence social drinking until the early part of the senior year. More frequently than as is the case with boys, the girls are given their first drink by the parents in their own home along with a perfunctory lecture on the evils of alcohol for sweet young things. Somewhere around sixteen, a slumber party or a casual "Friday-night-with-the-girls" brings the first occasion of drinking with peers. This first ritualistic introduction is done very secretively and the average girl would "just die" if any of the boys at school ever discovered that she drank. As is the case with the young males of her peer group, she never reports "mild intoxication," only complete abstinence or complete intoxication, operating on the same philosophy: That it's not worth the effort unless you get "good and drunk."

Our town has an unwritten tradition that New Year's Eve of the senior year is more or less a "coming-out" party of the wildest nature . . . completely lacking in the social refinements of moderate social drinking. At this time in the young girl's life she makes her debut to the drinking world. At last she can drink in front of the boys and taste the unknown pleasures of a vodka and lemonade "heat." The use of hard liquor is infrequent, though there is little problem in obtaining it. Beer is almost universally the first choice, vodka and gin second, and never wine.

Drinking parties almost always take place in the private home of the student—never in bars or public places. . . . The students are clean, well-dressed, and generally well-behaved. Even after intoxication pervades the atmosphere the only real manifestations are louder music, louder laughter, more strenuous dancing, and an occasional surreptitious dirty joke. . . . The really bad manifestations . . . take place in aggressive destructive behavior —after the party. Never (in any of my experience) did any destruction take place in a home.

Thus, the student who comes to college has had some experience with drinking, but it is not the same for all youngsters or for all communities. Some seek drinking experiences, others just "fall into them," and others feel bothered enough by the restrictions to drink very little, if at all.

And do adults—parents and teachers—give any guidance on the development of this behavior? A bright but lazy male student summarizes his observations in this way:

It is my impression from experience and from taking a senior's view of freshmen that most parents do not offer any education in the field of drinking. Most of what they say is in the way of orders, or warnings of what will happen as a result of drinking. I have not made the acquaintance of anyone who has come from a home where there has been any attempt to educate the sons by giving them some of the known and accredited facts about the consumption of alcoholic beverages. It seems that the most understanding parents merely offer to give the son a drink when he decides he wants one, and this in order to take some of the adventure out of taking that first illegal drink. Usually this or any other mention of alcohol comes too late and is of insufficient content to do any good towards giving an understanding of what alcohol is and what the accepted behavior norms are concerning its use. There is the feeling that the parents who say nothing are relying on the high schools to furnish this training, but few of these do this and those who do cannot devote adequate facilities to this part of education. In reality, the only valuable guides and understanding that we can get from our parents is from their actions, and even these may not be the best to follow, especially since we do not get the reasons behind the behavior or the facts supporting the reasoning. It simply becomes a matter of blind following the blind in many cases.

If there has been a genuine attempt in the home to give advice to the son, statistics show that most of it is toward abstinence. If there is not a conflict created from parental actions, there certainly is one from those of society. And it is further shown that many of these sons who have been advised to abstain do go on to drink, whereupon they develop an anxiety over doing so against the will of their parents, and therefore, they have no conception of how they should react to drink except from what they have heard, namely get drunk, which is exactly what they do!

Drinking in College

Two senior students, one male and one female, developed and conducted a survey of 56 randomly selected freshman women during the spring quarter. One of their concluding paragraphs reads:

> Of the 77 per cent who drink now at Stanford, 55 per cent drank in high school and continue to drink in college; 22 per cent began drinking at Stanford. The former group continues to drink for the following reasons which are listed in order of their importance: Feel happier and relaxed, like the taste, feel you are a better date, and forget about your problems. There is a general trend of the freshmen girls to drink more now than when they first began drinking. The majority of the latter group began drinking by the end of the fall quarter. They considered college the first opportunity to drink acceptably. The majority wanted to please their date and satisfy a curiosity. Some saw no reason not to drink. A few wanted to appear older. However, 32 per cent of all the drinkers are reluctant to drink. The following reasons for reluctance are listed in order of their importance: Fears she may do something under the influence of alcohol of which she would not be proud, feels reluctant to break the law, fears she may be caught for underage drinking, is afraid of what other people will say and family doesn't know.

They commented later on 16 per cent of the sample whose "attitudes and actions toward alcohol and its use were characterized by indecisiveness" by predicting:

> Because of the Stanford environmental influence which is favorable rather than unfavorable to the consumption of alcohol, one may expect that the majority of this indecisive group will become drinkers who show little reluctance and indecisiveness in their future habits.

A senior woman student surveyed the girls in her residence and came up with these observations on the drinking of upperclass women.

> . . . Of the 34 respondents, 32 of them replied "yes" to the question, "Do you drink alcoholic beverages of any kind?" . . . Almost 90 per cent of the drinkers drink at least once a week, half of whom are under the legal drinking age. . . . The increase in frequency of drinking from freshman to sophomore year is the most marked trend. . . . Not one woman stated that she felt she would be looked down upon by her living group if she chose to abstain completely. . . . The great majority of the

girls in the house do drink, so they *expect* everybody to drink but do not try to directly pressure anyone into doing so . . . while the majority of the respondents condone getting drunk at a social function there is a significant minority (⅓) who would condemn this type of behavior.

The drinking habits of college women are more apt to vary with the type of men they date than with their place of residence or any other single factor. . . . All senior women respondents had gone out drinking on the night before an exam . . . seniors do not seem to worry nearly as much about the possible effects of this drinking as do the younger women.

The majority of women feel that their drinking habits are about the same at Stanford as they are at home, with a slight tendency to drink more at school than at home.

A young man who lived in one of the "houses" at the University (comparable to a dormitory at most institutions, but organized into groups of less than 100 students—non-fraternity men) surveyed his living group and reported, in part:

Abstainers numbered 13 out of 59 returned questionnaires, a 22 per cent abstention rate in the house, which is 14 per cent above the national statistics for men at a private coeducational, nonsectarian university (according to Straus and Bacon) . . . [however] the total group living in the house tend to be light to moderate drinkers, no matter what class (age group) they are in . . . In answer to the question on the desirability of on-campus drinking all seem to agree that men and women should be treated equally . . . the moderate and light drinkers favor lowering the drinking age to 18 while the abstainers, who possibly fear drink's evils, favor 21. The moderate heavy drinkers who possibly realize what excessive drinking can do, are not strongly in favor of the 18 age. In relation to the administration's present stand, abstainers perceived it to represent a liberal attitude while more frequent users perceived a more disapproving attitude.

We can say that, disregarding abstainers, grade point tends to decrease with increased drinking habits . . . the more one drinks the less he tends to study . . . lower grades, higher drinking and lower study hours can be correlated. A curious conclusion is that light drinkers study the most and have the best grade point average. (Light drinkers were those who called themselves moderate drinkers but drank no more than one ounce of whiskey [pro rata] per week, were high a few times, seldom drunk, and never had passed out.)

Generalizing from these returns, I speculate that men in the Stanford House system are lighter drinkers than those in fraternities or eating clubs. And because of this they study more and maintain a higher grade point average.

Finally, a senior member of a "hard-drinking" fraternity, a young man with a personally established place in this group, surveyed and analyzed the drinking habits of what he called the "drink-oriented" segment of the Stanford student body. His conclusions follow:

. . . drinking plays a definite, in fact almost primary, role in the social life of some of the students in college.

The tempo and amount of drinking has been greatly increased from high school, and the concern for drinking under age has greatly decreased. Only seventeen drank at least once a week during high school, whereas in college, 53 drank at least once a week. This, of course, represents the growth in maturity and the assumption of the adult role; whether it is deserved or not is of no concern—a college student has his role and he plays it.

The important position that drinking holds in campus life can be seen from the fact that one-third of those questioned drink on school nights, and 72 per cent were willing to drink before noon. In other words, most of the students sampled were willing to drink any place, any time—in the morning, afternoon, or late evening.

Often, many in the sample do not exhibit a well-developed sense of responsibility. Many do not leave the bar after an afternoon drinking bout to go home and eat; they either eat at the bar or fail to eat at all. The dating pattern reflects a trend of irresponsibility; week nights are typically "stag nights." Male college students behave far more responsibly with dates than without. With a date, the boys often close down the bar and continue the party elsewhere with a "couple for the road"; this to the obvious detriment of their class attendance. The tendency to drink in the afternoon with its aftereffects is also not good for one's academic pursuits. It is observed that beer frequently wins over books, even to the extent that mid-terms and papers are "forgotten."

I think that an obvious trend has been discovered which concerns the compulsive nature of much of the drinking that is carried on. It often is the case of a student having one or two beers and, then feeling, "what the hell, I'll stay." The fact that extra beer is purchased when the bars close is definitely a compulsive act; the fact that 22 out of 67 admit to going on "binges" conclusively illustrates this compulsive trend. From observation, this investigator is led to conclude that these binges take place during "free" stretches of the academic quarter—between series of midterms, etc. It appears that there are always enough drinkers around so that anyone going on a "binge" will have company— even though this company is continually changing.

Two trends, one a minimization of responsibility and the other a proneness to compulsive drinking, have been observed during this analysis of the sample. It appears to be dangerous, having such tendencies displayed at such an early age, but some ex- tenuating circumstances may be noted. First of all, those ques- tioned were asked to exaggerate. Secondly, this drinking involves beer primarily. Although bad habits can be formed with beer, this hardly is as serious as if it involved the same amount of hard liquor. Finally, the need for responsibility and the type of responsibility involved is over-magnified. Most of those inter- viewed come from successful families to whom the expense of their child's education does not appear as a great sacrifice. Their children, on the other hand, reflect by their actions the "com- fortable" social life enjoyed by their parents. They do not have the drive or need for behavior with the same amount of respon- sibility as one working his way through school does.

For the most part, the trends observed are still compatible with controlled drinking—this college-level drinking is controlled. The difficulties of the uncontrolled phase of drinking, which might arise from a continuation of these habits, would happen when the switch or "graduation" to hard liquor occurs. Those in the "drinking-oriented" segment of the student body would be the most prone to any such difficulty.

Drinking Means Many Things

The college community is like the larger adult community to the extent that drinking means different things to different peo- ple. A sample of these meanings spring forth from the selections which follow.

A senior fraternity man presents three arguments for drinking that represent its meaning to at least some Greeks; two of these arguments are fairly well known, but sandwiched between is a relatively new meaning, albeit overstated.

Many college students have led relatively sheltered lives at home. College represents a breaking away from rigid controls.

In breaking away, there is a great temptation to experiment with all previously forbidden forms of pleasure. Similarly, there is a tendency to overindulge. One such new activity is, commonly, drinking. Experimentation is a good and necessary part of learning; however, the "newly liberated" student too often knows no limits or control. Consequently the experiment often runs rampant and assumes control of the experimenter. In this manner a fertile soil for problem drinking is developed.

A corollary factor is not quite so obvious. Many college students (Stanford in particular) have come from schools where they were looked upon as eggheads and teacher's pets. They were greatly chastised by their peers and unjustly left out of many activities. College provides these people with a new start. They can establish themselves as okay guys and thus include themselves in the fun. Part of the image building which many of these students seem to consider necessary is to be a good drinker. Again, too many of these people know of no control for their drinking and are prime prospects for problem drinking.

A third contributing factor to the rise of a drinking problem among fraternity men (and indeed people of that age in general) is the attraction of the forbidden fruit. Fraternity men are given the responsibility of deciding their course of study, their choice of career, the duty of military obligation, and in general of their behavior. They are told that they are being regarded as adults and are expected to behave as such. Yet they are forbidden to make the choice of whether or not to drink. The denial of this privilege and responsibility represents a contradiction of all else that they are told. This contradiction is very keenly felt, and the response to it is the creation of an "artificial" desire to drink. To my mind this desire is *not* simply one to defy authority, as is often suggested, but rather it is an expression of confusion at the inconsistency of the denial. This reaction is a very real one whether consciously considered or not.

Meaning can be personal or it can be situational (within the college environment) but it also must, at some points, take the "outside world" from which students come and to which they finally go as a referent. A transition observation, indicating that college students may well possess this awareness, is offered by a senior man.

One of the hardest decisions that a young man entering college has to make, and one of the earliest, is whether he should drink or not, and in what quantity, presuming of course, that his drinking habits (as opposed to attitudes) have not already been formed in his pre-college excursions into the realm of high school beer blasts. Even if he has become a social drinker of the brewer's art he will have to decide his limits. These two segments of the over-all question seem to be the most important ones concerning college drinking, but there are other divisions which arise when he stops to evaluate the initial decision. He must decide whether he is right or wrong; whether to agree with his parents, his school, and the existing liquor law, and whether his decision is worth the conflict it causes within him, if he recognizes any. Our modern American culture has not yet geared itself for minors' drinking, which a majority of college men who drink are, and such archaic phrases as "liquor will ruin your body" are only erroneous reminders to us young people that outside society has not yet condoned drinking in college, and it will preach anything it seems to think will keep us from it.

Later in the same paper this answer to the question of reason for drinking is offered.

One may rightly ask if there is any reason for drinking in college. In other words, should college men drink? The answer is yes, if they so decide. College is a maturing place for many students. We enter college not knowing what we want out of life, or even what it is for. One might say that college is a "fenced-in proving ground" wherein all of the students' values are questioned and tested by the individual himself. We are more excessive drinkers because we are testing, and the exuberance shown even after one beer comes from this. The basic question to us becomes one of how far society will let us let down our inhibitions, given the rationalizing element of alcohol. We can test in this surrounding, whereas if we were placed directly in society we would be restricted to follow doggedly what it proclaims. In college we have the friends who will put us to bed if we go too far, whereas if we were in society we would only receive the disdain of our friends and probably a night in jail. College is also a time when there are very few responsibilities placed on us, and so we can afford to experiment, as it were, without the risk of hurting family or friends. It is while in college that the most can be accomplished toward gaining an understanding of the outside world without hurting or being hurt.

Another student says essentially the same thing, putting it in the words of a hypothetical student he is describing:

"If I'm going to drink, my college days are the time to get most of it out of my system, because after I get out of school I'm going to have too many responsibilities to carry on like this. Now all I have to do is keep my grades at an adequate level which gives me all the time I need to drink."

These expressions seem to be within the realm of responsible behavior, though perhaps with somewhat of a future orientation. A fraternity man, quoted earlier, pictures the senior drinker with less of a hopeful future than the immediately previous writers.

The senior student has commonly reached the "magic age," twenty-one. He can now drink legally and seizes every opportunity to do so. He has convinced himself that he no longer cares about school; it is too late to really improve over-all gradepoints, and he is tired of the whole ratrace. His lack of concern for school leaves our senior with plenty of free time. This time generally is put to good use in pursuing some leisure activity, such as drinking: So he can watch color TV at the local bar . . . be sociable, relax after a hard day, etc. The problem of excessive drinking is now fully evident. Without even realizing it the senior has come to use alcohol as the medium through which he has all his fun and spends his idle hours. Alcohol is now an integral and basic part of his life.

At this point I might mention that many people I know who would fit the pattern which I have described have continued to lean on alcohol after graduation. The cruel world has offered even new reasons to drink. They now find it necessary in order to escape from the tension of the business world. Many of these people directly attribute their drinking habits to their college days.

Now that it is established, on the basis of student reporting which this paper assumes to be credible, that there are heavy, "hard" drinkers on the campus, what are these like and why are they as they are? The literature on alcoholism immediately replies that they are likely to be diverse and heterogeneous. What, then, is one of them like? In a paper which he titled "Why Do I Drink Heavily?" a representative of this group relates his perceptions of the meanings alcohol has for him. An initial observation is provocative:

Most students seem to have drunk alcoholic beverages before they came to college. This puts me in a minority, for I never

had so much as one beer until Easter vacation of my freshman
year here at school. It wasn't so much that I was against it as
that I had never been exposed to it. None of my peer group
drank. All this changed when I joined a fraternity.

He goes on to make a good case for the "heavy" quality of his
drinking and then asks himself some questions about his feelings while sober and while drunk.

There are a few occasions when I know absolutely why I
drink, for I admit it to myself and make no rationalizations. A
couple of these occasions are before meeting a good blind date
or before going out with a girl whom I am not really interested
in. In both cases I get extremely upset, and know that when I
do first see them, I'll be very unsuccessful in making a good impression because of my nervousness. Thus with no pretext, I
drink enough to get "high" so that I will be relaxed and be able
to converse smoothly with them. There are no hidden reasons
here, for I simply drink to gain the confidence I know alcoholic
beverages give me. I contend that this is basically always the
reason I drink heavily, but it is harder to see this when I just go
beer drinking with a lot of my fraternity brothers.

Only a short amount of space will be devoted to questions
concerned with getting at my expectations towards getting intoxicated. I ask myself if I like loud gatherings and I have to
answer that I do very much, but usually only if I know a lot
of people involved in the gatherings. I associate loud gatherings
with drinking and because I like these loud groups I can conclude that my expectation for drinking is that it is something I
like. The rest of the questions I can explain similarly but will wait
and draw one conclusion at the end of this section. I next ask
myself if I like conventional behavior or do I like to rebel. The
answer is that I like to rebel but do not have the nerve unless
intoxicated. Another question concerns what I think of when I
see a drunk. Do I think he is repulsive or funny? I almost in-
variably derive a great amount of enjoyment out of seeing a
person really drunk. What is my opinion of the fraternities on
campus that have a big reputation as being "big drinkers"? I
admire them far more than any of the other "typed" houses and
I often regret that I am not in one of those houses. Another
question is what do I think of "big drinkers" as individuals. Here
again I admire them and wish I had the reputation they have.
There are many more questions of this nature that could be asked
to derive my expectations but this sampling is all that this paper

has room for. My answers to these questions and similar ones seem to show I like heavy drinking and heavy drinkers. When I go drinking I expect to get drunk and thus get happy and loud. This is not enough of an explanation of why I drink because I often get really intoxicated by myself or with just one or two other people. There has to be some other reason than to get loud.

As I have previously mentioned, to get to the reason I drink heavily, I feel I have to ask some personal questions. I must answer them normally and then while under the influence of alcohol or answer them as I would normally while intoxicated. Some of the questions are direct in that they ask if I like to do something. They then ask if it is easier to do when drunk. The first type of question will be asked now. I ask myself if I think I am attractive to most girls and then am I attractive to the "top" girls. While sober I am very negative on both of these. I feel very inferior to many of the men around me in this respect. When drunk I do not exactly think I am attractive to girls, but I think they like me a lot more. I also do not really care so much about this question when drunk. (This seems to be standard for many of these questions. They bother me a lot when I am sober, but I relegate them to relative insignificance when drunk.) Do I consider myself a good athlete? When sober, I think I am a good skier, surfer, and volleyball player at times, though in general I think I am a poor athlete. When intoxicated I answer that I am really good in this respect and am usually willing, even in that state, to take any one on in any sport I know.

Another question I asked myself was do my old friends at home really like me. I do not think they really like me though they enjoy my company somewhat. When drunk I think they do really like me and even envy me. This is also proved because at a party with them when I get really drunk I become the "life of the party" for I feel I am among people who really like me. A similar question is, do my fraternity brothers like me? Again I do not believe so. Most of them like me but I only have one or two really good friends in the house. When drunk I believe they all really think of me as a lovable person. This is shown by when I get drunk and go up and turn beds over on the sleeping porch, and other such stunts. When drunk, I think they will not be mad at me at all when I do these things. Now we will go to the questions of the second type. Do I find it easy to talk to someone I barely know? Unless under the influence of alcohol, I have trouble talking to casual acquaintances because I am too nervous to carry on a conversation smoothly. When drunk, I can go up to complete strangers and get along with them easily, whereas when sober I find this impossible to do. I am afraid of any social event in which I am not fully aware of what is happening. I even fear taking a date to a fancy restaurant for the first time, simply because I am not sure what I am expected to do. When "high," these problems all disappear and I either do everything correctly and smoothly, or else I do not care if I do anything wrong.

His rather poignant closing statement indicates that he is one of the optimists who does not see college drinking as inevitably progressing into heavy adult drinking.

I sincerely believe I am nowhere near being an alcoholic, for I feel once I am out of school this pattern will change completely. I may be wrong, for this paper shows that I appear to be somewhat dependent on alcohol. . . . But this paper, on the whole, forced me to look deeply into my drinking patterns and made me try to analyze why I drink. I have come up with an answer that satisfies me. Simply because I understand the problem now I may be able to alleviate it.

It is well known that academic and intellectual ability does not necessarily correlate with personal and social adequacy. When the intelligent individual finds himself in a new environment in which he is inadequate he may suffer a good deal of "psychic pain." In general the university has to assume the bright student's personality is adequate for the total experience of a college education. In some cases it may not be.

This raises the further question of how individual college students, of the type making up the Stanford student body who have been raised to see themselves as excellent performers, to expect excellence of themselves, to judge this essentially in relation to the performance of others, and who, in fact, having performed well, do adjust to an academic, political and social situation where, although all were selected for excellence, half are, by definition of the grading curve, average or below. And for many of these students, as freshmen, a B is perceived as an unsatisfactory mark.

A male student, in describing drinking games, gives his answer to this dilemma as it applies to drinking.

At stag parties, games are concocted to determine how drinkers stand against one another. "Thumper," for example, is a round-robin type of game where the individual who makes a mistake must gulp a drink. Little more thinking goes into parties than what kinds of alternatives can be found to "thumper." Many parties dispense with any such ritual and "get directly to the matter at hand"; that is, they have "chugging" or "chug-a-lug" contests in which the goal is merely to discover who can drink the most the fastest. I maintain that those individuals who engage in this sort of activity the most eagerly are trying to excel in the area of drinking because they have no other area in which they feel that they can succeed. Such an individual would rather be known as the best drinker than just an average student or athlete.

The "double standard" in drinking behavior for men and women on campus indicates that the meaning of drinking is not the same for the two sexes, at the social group level, at least.

An attractive young woman, obviously a part of the campus drinking complex, describes the sex differences in these terms.

Whatever the reason, Stanford men do drink in all types of situations, and to varying degrees—and to them, there seems to be no unacceptable way. They drink socially at a party, or alone in their rooms; they drink champagne like a gentleman at a fancy affair—but more often they drink beer like a truck driver. In general, they are quite adaptable, sober when called for; drunk and speaking in four-letter words when called for also. One might say that there are probably few alcoholics at Stanford, but many drunks can be found (or heard) on a given night. There is no pressure or social control forcing one to contain himself when inebriated—it might restrict individuality and self-expression —and there is no guidance in acceptable modes of drinking given by those from whom it would be effective. Here, where the student is away from home influence, experience is not only the best teacher, it is the only teacher as far as the school goes—for it hesitates to give advice on a situation it wants to ignore.

Among the girls, the double standard again applies, and restricts their drinking, for the most part, to social affairs. They find that drinking alone, and getting drunk, while acceptable for their male counterparts, will result in loss, rather than a gain, in prestige for themselves. And group opinion seems to provide a fairly effective social control of their habits. That is not to say no girls drink alone, or get drunk, but if they do so, they do so on the whole with less frequency than the man, and do not tend to proudly "advertise the fact."

Most Stanford women do drink to some extent, and just as with the men, the exception is the one who does not drink. Social acceptability again is probably the chief reason for this, also, and with the females, as stated above, this implies not drinking alone or to get drunk, for this is not socially acceptable.

Each conforms to the pattern set, each knows their limits, and for the most part stays within them. And since the limit is so liberal for fellows, drunkenness is as acceptable to them as sobriety—and after five, almost as common.

Recognize that the two sexes on a college campus are not, finally, just biosocial categories, but live, often lusty human beings—with sexual drives and yet also certain inhibitions against sexual intimacy. A brief glimpse of this role or meaning for drinking is presented in a "handbook" prepared by a male student (as a paper but also for distribution to other male undergraduates), the purpose of which is capsuled in one sentence from the Preface: "The problem we now face is to make you a 'lover.'" After indicating proper standards for personal appearance, material possessions, fraternal and group associations, personality and attitude—a "beautiful role" a man can play, guaranteed to succeed in seduction—he observes:

> Drinking and smoking are something that you must learn to do with a quality of experienced rapport. The amount of actual participation will depend on the occasion and the girl. In no case is there an excuse for excess. Chain smokers, even to other chain smokers, are thought of as obnoxious. Getting completely bombed is void of purpose and benefit on a date, as it dulls the senses—quite the opposite of what girls are for! Drunkenness also endangers your control of the situation, the worst result of which is that you forget the beautiful role we have been creating.

Changes in Drinking Patterns

Since students are still human beings and human beings do change their behaviors, a student may not sustain a drinking pattern even after establishing it. The reasons for such changes are many and as varied as the individuals and circumstances involved, but this does not preclude a look at several, portrayed in the student's own words.

Though, in general on this campus, moving to an off-campus house or apartment is done in order to increase drinking activity, it did not have this effect in the case of this male student. It also is interesting to see the interplay of residence, companions, and dates (the effects of dating partners upon one another is obviously a two-way proposition) upon drinking behavior.

As a sophomore I became an active member of the fraternity but did not live in the house. Although no radical change took place, my exposure to liquor continued to increase. I dated a girl who drank very little but did not disapprove at all of drinking. However, as I dated her quite a bit I drank less as a result of her company. Thus although my frequency of drinking increased as a result of the fraternity influence, the amount I consumed upon each occasion remained small. At this point I still drank out of sociability and curiosity. The two most important points to bear in mind are that first I lived off campus with a small group of fellows, all of whom were light drinkers, and secondly that my frequency of drinking did increase due to attendance at the weekly fraternity parties.

My junior year was the year of big changes both in my drinking habits and my attitude towards drinking. For the first half of the year I lived in the fraternity house. This resulted in increased participation in the Friday night stag drinking parties which were held within the house itself. These were really the first occasions upon which I became quite high. Furthermore, living in the house made beer or liquor available constantly. Again my frequency of drinking increased, this time to two or three times a week. But, the majority of my drinking still occurred on weekends.

With this move into the fraternity house a gradual change of friends occurred. I became close friends with three or four fellows all of whom drank more than I did at the time. However, my drinking habits soon came to resemble theirs. I am still very close to these people, and our drinking habits are still much the same.

The second half of my junior year saw an important change in my social life which, interestingly enough, had little effect upon my attitude towards alcohol. I moved into an apartment with one other fellow and disaffiliated completely with the fraternity. With the move to apartment living began the first consistent drinking during the middle of the week. But, on the other hand, this was usually only one beer or cocktail, and the amount I consumed per occasion declined from its fraternity house level. With the shift to apartment living a coincidental shift to beer and away from hard liquor took place.

As a senior I am again living off campus, and the trend away from hard liquor to beer is now complete. Two factors bearing upon my drinking habits are significant. First, I am now twenty-one years old, and, secondly, I have dated one girl exclusively. This girl enjoys drinking and has much the same drinking habits as I do. The combination of these two factors resulted in a heavy trend towards the tavern circuit. I began to go to taverns as often as three nights a week, always with a date and usually with at least one other couple. On these occasions I often reached a stage of mild inebriation, and it was with this that I drank not out of enjoyment of taste or sociability, but because I liked the ensuing feeling of mild exhilaration.

Students, feeling restricted or at least "unfree" in regard to overt drinking, often muse about places like Europe where drinking is a "normal, natural part of life." Probably some who go to Europe do "tie one on" for a time, but for this young man who reports on himself and his experience, a self-defined "hard drinking fraternity man" in a "boozing house," the trip produced a different result.

At the end of my junior year, I went to Europe with three close friends, all Stanford students and all the same age. There, all restrictions were freed. No longer did I have to think about studies, the law or any of the things which might have restricted the amount of drinking I did in the past. Europe, with all its cheap beer, wine and local hard liquor was the ideal place to really break loose and see what real drinking was like.

After a short fascination, I was soon dissatisfied with "power drinking." With ample shoving to the back of my mind for four years, my conscience began to creep out and I had to face it and try to resolve the questions not only of drinking, but of the whole scope of my personal morality and integrity and to try to set some tangible goals for myself that would not be too idealistic to live by nor too contrary to the ideals which had somehow ingrained themselves in my mind. Alcohol was definitely one of the focal points of the knotty problem which I had dredged up.

With nothing but opportunity and convenience of drinking, it seemed to lose a great deal of the original fascination which was such a part of my taking my first drink several years before. The social pressure was, of course, still there, but it had changed direction. Instead of being from people I looked up to, in general, the pressure came laterally from friends I considered completely on my own level. Having developed a sense of independence and personal responsibility, the pressures toward drinking lost some of their magnitude and forcefulness.

Gradually, toward the end of the summer, I drank less and less, but never really made up my mind with regard to a concrete course of action or hard-fast rule for the future. I began savoring the nectars of European fruits as substitutes for the amber products of European grains. The scoffing of my friends only served to intensify my independence in the decision of what I was to drink on different occasions. With the threat of ostracism by those socially above now non-existent, and with an increase of independent thought on my part, my course was beginning to become more clearly defined.

A third student, a hard-drinking fraternity man and varsity athlete, was able to combine these two roles, but when marriage entered the picture, a change took place. Speaking of his every night, every weekend drinking pattern he says:

I enjoyed the frivolous life. It had become routine, a habit, and I was used to it. I liked this type of existence, and it would be hard to change to a more normal pattern of life. Nothing is static though, for suddenly I fell in love with a girl from my home town. We got married, and I brought her down to school ready to fit both of us down in that familiar niche. At first I blissfully thought I could successfully combine both existences— that of a drinking and carousing fraternity man and that of a mature and responsible married man. However, in my Jekyll and Hyde role, I was completely oblivious of the transition required when a person begins or attempts to settle down. At this time the individual has a new audience, not the raucous fraternity crowd, but a girl, a girl who looks to him for security, and for responsibility. In later marriages after college this transition is not so abrupt, but in my situation it was as different as night and day.

I found myself in this transitory position and at first I had serious doubts as to whether or not I could successfully make the necessary adjustment. During the first few months of my marriage my wife and I attended many fraternity functions. She found it hard to accept the riotous experiences, and I found it hard to reject them. My wife, after three years of college and two years of sorority life, did not appreciate the more carefree, impulsive, and immature Stanford fraternity type of existence. She felt that some of their actions were immature, destructive, and obscene. She felt so strongly about the subject that frequent quarrels would arise when we discussed the topic at home.

I defended the actions of my fraternity brothers rather hypocritically because I realized that her conclusions about the behavior of my fraternity brothers were valid. This posed another problem, however, for most of my close friends were my fraternity brothers. It was a choice between maintaining my friends while my marriage was suffering or to break my fraternal ties. Of course this was no real choice, but still I wanted to maintain the friendship and companionship of some of the fellows.

Finally I decided (with mutual consent) to attend only the parties which I believed would be of a less rowdy nature. My drinking had been lessened by the infrequency of our attendance at fraternity parties and by the concentration on a more balanced home life.

Soon I began to notice an even larger change in my drinking at the parties. I no longer made it a contest to see how much I could drink but instead drank slower and more conservatively. The less I drank the less I saw in the drinking parties, and soon I found myself avoiding them and attending only the smaller informal parties. I enjoyed these parties more because the emphasis was not upon heavy drinking and roughhousing but upon social drinking, primarily for enjoyment and companionship. I began to enjoy myself in a more mature fashion and my drinking began to lessen itself.

As I look back in recollection of my past fraternity-life type of existence I begin to realize the motivations for the heavy drinking type of parties. First of all there was the aspect of the possible seduction of a date; second, the desire to be with the group and to impress them; third, the desire to relieve yourself of tensions; and last, the desire to drink for drinking's sake. All of these aspects are nullified by marriage.

Marriage changed my whole pattern of drinking—for the better, as I see it, in my now-prejudiced view. I drink less now than I did before I was twenty-one. Even though alcohol is readily obtainable in our apartment I have no desire at all to drink heavily. My drinking now is primarily for the purpose of satiating my thirst or for purely social occasions.

In conclusion I would like to make this statement: The institution of matrimony, unless it is a marriage for economic convenience, establishes new goals, goals which provide alternate paths to the heavy and immature drinking. Marriage provides and bestows upon you responsibility and warm mutual love which negates any temptation to escape and impress via the vehicle of alcohol.

Expectations for Adult Life

Each colloquium group during the six-year period was asked, at the very beginning, to describe their own drinking pattern or patterns, how these matched with friends and living companions, and how these matched with parental patterns. The largest portion, over the six-year time span, could only be classified as moderate drinkers, both in amount and in frequency of drinking. The next largest category would be called erratic drinkers, mostly moderate, but sometimes heavy and sometimes light. Light drinkers followed and then heavy drinkers. Typically there was one abstainer in the group, usually a woman.

In general, over half the students classified their drinking as "about the same" as friends and living companions. Those who felt they drank less and those who felt they drank more were about equal, with a slight edge to the former. The most typical comparison of personal with parental drinking was the assertion that both were "about the same." A larger portion of students felt they drank more than their parents compared with those feeling they drank less.

The last question to which students were asked to respond was, "Do you think your present pattern will carry over pretty much 'as is' into your post-university, adult life? Why or why not?"

Again, following the pattern of previous answers the majority felt they would carry over the patterns now established as seniors into later life. A married male student epitomized this generalization with:

I believe my pattern will remain the same. My tastes for alcohol and my attitude toward it are well-established, and I do not foresee any radical changes in my life that should modify or increase the pressure on me to drink.

Another answered in this way.

Yes. After experiencing both positions of a heavy drinker and a non-drinker I have arrived at the position I believe to be the best.

One young woman predicted that her drinking

> Probably will be pretty much the same. It may taper off as young children come into the picture and with them fewer opportunities for social gatherings.

Another senior woman said:

> Pretty much. I enjoy drinking and I enjoy getting a little high once in a while. I feel my drinking patterns are acceptable for what will probably be my adult social and moral standards.

While yet a third, a very attractive young woman, stated her prediction in these terms:

> I'm sure my present pattern will carry over into adult life. I have no desire to learn to drink, and it certainly has been no handicap socially. I can have just as good a time without drinking, so what's the point when there are so many possible deleterious effects.

While generally predicting similarity, some students noted possible changes, such as:

> Pretty much yes. Perhaps I will cease to get good and plowed and be content with just feeling good. My wife to be deplores my being polluted—and she deplores herself in a like condition.

Another point made fairly often involved a change in beverage.

> Yes. I don't believe any great change will come over me. I enjoy drinking and see no reason to alter this simply because I am no longer a student. I do think the one change in my pattern will be to less beer and more hard liquor after college.

The most common prediction of change was from the "fraternity man" type, one representative individual stating the expected change as:

> After marriage I imagine I'll drop to a pattern comparable to my Dad's (a little less during the week and a little more at parties). I generally don't have one drink. If I drink, it's usually 3 or 4.

A change predicted by a young woman, destined to be a socialite, was:

I probably will drink more frequently, especially wine and lighter drinks, as an adult. Student life has never been very conducive to any established drinking pattern for me.

But the most typical Greek change probably is:

I expect that my drinking pattern will change—I imagine it will be less excessive and more regular. More intense, deliberately excessive drinking seems to be common behavior at college.

Put another way, the change envisioned is:

I think with marriage my alcoholic consumption will increase, but my drunken parties will be limited. I will settle for the mild, contented sensation and not aim for a drunken state. Cocktails each day, etc. will become the norm.

Finally, the responsible feelings of even the heavy drinking student shine through:

The heavy drinking will probably be reduced drastically when the "right girl" comes along, for there will be an understandable substitute of gratifications and more seriousness of purpose after marriage.

The Position of the Administration

The focus of this chapter is not on the administration position in relation to student drinking, but two written observations seem to present the best picture of "where the administration is when all this drinking is going on." In 1966 Stanford University liberalized campus drinking rules after eight years of an every-other-yearly effort to do so, but the generalizations here probably would hold for the majority of collegiate institutions in America today.[1]

In an article which put present college drinking practices in historical perspective, two deans of students at a state university concluded:

Colleges and universities bear more responsibility than any other social group for the behavior of the young men and women who are on their campuses. But most of the influences which

[1] For additional discussion, see chapter 19 in this volume.

mold and motivate these young people do not come from the colleges and universities. Like the public school, they provide the largest and least dangerous target. Many college officers throughout the country have developed a live-and-let-live attitude. They try to avoid problems, to strengthen student government, and, above all, to evade public notice. Their hope is that, like the chameleon, they will blend indistinguishably with the background. They have come to know that there is no formula, and that that policy is best which works at a given place, with given students, and at a given point in time. There is, of course, much which might be done in the way of education and instruction, but, except at the Yale Institute, there is very little evidence that anything is being accomplished. Perhaps the best policy was stated some one hundred and fifty years ago, when the authorities at William and Mary ordained "that the drinking of spirituous liquors (except in that moderation which becomes a prudent and industrious student) be prohibited."[2]

A senior woman student, researching the attempt for a change in rules at Stanford in 1962 captured the same spirit and hence indicates that the total situation is not misunderstood, but simply one in which, typically, "practice and policy cannot be brought closer together."

There are many sides and facets to the liquor problem on campus and to the liquor referendum itself. And although students and administrators agree that student drinking is a problem both on campus and off, the liquor problem will probably not be completely solved for a long time—if indeed it is ever solved.

Looking first at the administration's viewpoint, we find the administrators caught in a dilemma. They believe that it is their responsibility to preserve lawful, orderly conduct on campus, and therefore they oppose liquor on campus because it would probably tend to lead to disorder and also because it would lead to increased drinking by minors, implying an increased number of misdemeanors. However, the administration also seems to be hesitant in inviting outside authorities (the Alcoholic Beverage Control Commission) onto the campus, perhaps preferring to overlook the liquor problem as much as possible and hoping that by so doing they will avoid the criticism of parents, friends, alumni,

[2] Byron H. Atkinson and A. T. Brugger, "Do College Students Drink Too Much?", *Journal of Higher Education*, 30 (June, 1959), 305-312.

and would-be donors who might conceivably be upset by reports of student drinking.

The students, on the other hand, will undoubtedly continue to drink both on campus and off, disregarding the "authoritarian" University regulations, and wishing that a more lenient policy could be devised, bringing practice and policy closer together.

Chapter 8

THE FUTURE PROFESSOR: FUNCTIONS AND PATTERNS OF DRINKING AMONG GRADUATE STUDENTS*

PAUL M. ROMAN
University of Georgia

THE GROWING PROMINENCE of graduate education in the United States requires the inclusion of the graduate student body in the study of sociopsychological patterns and processes within the social system of the college and university (5, 10).[1] The attitudes and behavior of graduate students is a commentary on both their undergraduate educational experience and their perception of the life style to which they aspire. Moreover, their attitudes and behavior as graduate students is a prophecy about the models that they as teachers will present to future generations of students. The drinking behavior of graduate students is a case in point. This chapter presents some impressions of the functions of alcohol and patterns of alcohol use in the graduate student population of a large Eastern university and suggests some interpretations of the drinking behavior observed. These impressions are based on data gathered through partici-

* Support from the Christopher D. Smithers Foundation through the Program on Alcoholism and Occupational Health, Cornell University, is gratefully acknowledged. The critical comments of Dr. H. M. Trice are deeply appreciated.

[1] Few researchers have focused on the sociopsychological aspects of graduate education. Mechanic (14) studied the reactions of Ph.D. candidates to the stressful experience of final examinations. Hajda (11) analyzed the characteristics of graduate students exhibiting different degrees of alienation and intellectualism. Gottleib (9) has reported a study of career paths and factors related to career change in a large national sample of graduate students.

pant observation in selected graduate student and faculty-graduate student drinking groups over a three-year period.[2] We shall first consider the various functions of alcohol consumption in the socialization of graduate students and then examine factors which account for variations in drinking patterns.

Alcohol and Student-Faculty Interaction

There are a variety of social situations which include the consumption of alcohol at which both graduate students and faculty are present, particularly parties during the holiday season that are conducted under departmental auspices and private informal parties held at the homes of either faculty or graduate students. Observations at these occasions indicate the function of alcohol as a release for the tension that accumulates as a result of the social distance from students maintained by faculty and students' attempts to reduce this social distance, in addition to releasing the more general tensions arising from academic life. The consumption of alcohol introduces a camaraderie between faculty and students and there is a general relaxation of the boundary maintenance norms. Faculty members are apt to discuss aspects of professional life that are not brought out in day-to-day interactions with students, and students likewise feel free to express certain frustrations and dissatisfactions. In other words, the consumption of alcohol at social occasions involving graduate students and faculty reduces inhibition in such a way that the tensions surrounding boundary maintenance between faculty and students are released to a certain degree, and by this the system of boundary maintenance is maintained. The tension release of the social occasion that is accompanied by drinking serves to reduce the graduate student's feelings of marginality; but the separation of this tension release "ceremony" from the normal day-to-day interaction also actually serves to maintain the structure in which the student is by necessity marginal. Moreover, these occasions aid the socialization process by providing the

[2] There were approximately 75 students involved in the drinking occasions where the reported observations were made. Those engaged in graduate work in the social sciences were over-represented, although approximately 25 of the participants were from fields of the physical and biological sciences. Observations were well supplemented by open-ended interviews with ten students. The participants were primarily male Ph.D. candidates.

student with additional "facts" about the nature of his future professional life. Finally, student-faculty drinking occasions provide behavioral cues regarding appropriate professional behavior in social situations involving the consumption of alcohol.

Drinking that serves to release tension and to reduce temporarily feelings of marginality on the part of the student is not restricted to formal occasions. At certain times, following the completion of a project or paper or following an evening of work in the office, a faculty member or several faculty members may adjourn with students to a bar for an hour or two of drinking and conversation. Observation of such drinking groups indicates that processes occur which are highly similar to those observed on the more formal social occasions, namely the temporary "opening" of the student-faculty boundary and further socialization into the informal norms of academia.

Three additional observations should further illuminate this socialization process. First, the fact of having "gone drinking" with a faculty member is communicated within the student group as a mode of obtaining recognition and prestige for the drinking group participants. Indications of the close friendship relations implied are also apparently used to reduce feelings of marginality and to increase the student's identification with the faculty reference group.

Second, drinking groups that involve faculty and students do not persist over a period of time as they do in neighborhood drinking groups or in those that bring together a group of chronic heavy drinkers (18, pp. 49-61). Several insights may stem from this observation. For example, ceremonial tension release and the blurring of student-faculty boundaries cannot be carried out too frequently if boundary maintenance is to continue. Moreover, these informal drinking groupings of faculty and students tend to develop around a norm that drinking should be used as a reward for accomplishment rather than as an escape from work responsibilities or as a way of "killing time." In other words, faculty and students do not get together early in the evening and spend the night in a bar; rather they reserve the occasion of drinking for the completion of an activity. The absence of this former pattern may reflect a concern about damaging the boundary between faculty and students.

Third, it appears that faculty members may be stigmatized as being heavy drinkers and as having inadequate colleague relations, or both, if they are frequently observed in bars accompanied by students.

Finally, it should be noted that faculty-graduate student drinking groups almost always contain more students than faculty. This relates to the possibility that a drinking pair composed of a faculty member and a student may imply favoritism on the part of the professor and unfair advantage on the part of the student. To invite either inference would run counter to the universalistic norms governing graduate education and education in general.

To this point, it has been implied that, in order to understand the drinking behavior of graduate students, one must understand the social context in which they live and work. This implication warrants explicit development. Graduate education includes a variety of programs of preparation for entrance into a particular profession. The focus of this study is limited to the large segment of graduate students who are pursuing doctoral programs with the goal of obtaining teaching, research positions in colleges or universities, or both. It is recognized that other types of professional study such as business administration, medicine, law, pharmacy, theology, and dentistry are frequently included under the broad umbrella of graduate education. But the present effort is limited, for practical reasons, to the more "traditional" graduate career directed toward entrance into the academic profession.

Recently attention has been drawn to sociological frames of reference which view social processes longitudinally and which focus on the *life careers* of individuals (3, 4, 6, 7, 16). This orientation provides a conceptual scheme within which to consider one of the major functions of alcohol in graduate student life. It is hypothesized, on the basis of the exploratory observations made in this study, that drinking and drinking occasions provide a context for the *anticipatory socialization* of the graduate student into his future role as an academician. These occasions also serve to reduce his feelings of marginality. An examination of certain structural characteristics of graduate education specifies these notions more clearly.

Merton describes anticipatory socialization as a process by which actors "take on the values of the non-membership group to which they aspire" (5, p. 265). He points out that this process may serve the dual functions of improving one's chances for eventual membership in the respective reference group, and for rapid integration into the group once membership status is attained. Thus anticipatory socialization results in various degrees of "pre-programming" of appropriate behavioral responses and reduces the potential tension that may be associated with status transitions.

Behavior which is parallel to anticipatory socialization, but which serves different functions, is found among members of *marginal* occupations and professions. Marginality develops when the marginal individual is between two occupational subcultures and he conforms to certain of the norms of each group but is not accepted fully as a group member by either. Marginality is illustrated in the cases of engineering technicians, druggists, chiropractors and psychiatric attendants (8, 12, 17, 19). Marginality differs from anticipatory socialization in that the realistic possibility of attaining reference group membership is generally absent for marginal individuals because the basic credentials for membership are lacking. However, in both instances, formation of these "imitative" occupational identities appears to orient the actors in social space and to provide them with the reflected prestige that may accompany the imitated status.

The graduate student who aspires to the status of academician illustrates both anticipatory socialization and marginality. These two factors are intimately interrelated in his case. His status differs from some instances of anticipatory socialization and marginality in the sense that, in all probability, the anticipated status will be attained. Thus, in all probability, his marginality is temporary. In the university studied, for example, qualifying examinations for degree candidacy were taken shortly after entering Ph.D. work. Very few students who passed this examination failed final examinations. Thus, the case of the graduate student is different from situations in which failure to attain reference group membership is quite probable. Likewise, the graduate student is unlike some instances of occupational marginality in which mobility into the desired occupation is prevented by the lack of essential abilities, by a high degree of career commitment to the marginal position, or both.

The nature of the graduate student's marginality and the processes of anticipatory socialization are now examined more closely. Graduate status differs from that of the undergraduate in (1) the degree of commitment to educational goals; (2) the independence of the graduate student from parental financial support and the consequent "seriousness" of educational pursuit; and (3) the individualization of study which is an essential aspect of graduate work. Graduate students are frequently quasi-faculty members through assistantship appointments which involve them in teaching and research and which serve to further differentiate them from undergraduates. They do not, however, have full faculty status.[3] The residential and social organizations prominent in undergraduate systems are generally absent in graduate student life; the monetary cost of such involvements, the societal norms which ascribe such memberships to certain age segments, and the frequent involvement of graduate students in the formation of their own families are factors which reduce the probability of graduate student involvement in fraternities, sororities, and social organizations in dormitories.

These factors all contribute to the temporary marginality of the graduate student's status. He is a student in the sense of taking courses and being subject to faculty evaluation; but he is not involved in the social organization typical of undergraduate life. His marginality in relation to faculty status stems from the fact of his partial performance of the faculty role as an assistant while he lacks the credentials for fully obtaining this status. Structured social organizations among graduate students are not prominent, partly because of the individualization of graduate educational careers, and thus the lack of common goals which typify undergraduate systems, and partly because of the pressures of studies and work which prevent the allocation of time to extensive social activity. Thus, graduate students may be said to be both marginal as a group and marginal as individuals.

Anticipatory socialization among graduate students stems from (1) his marginality and the consequent need to establish an identity and (2) from the reality that he will be eventually as-

[3] Evan (8, pp. 86-87) differentiates between single group and dual group marginality, the former illustrated by those occupations which are on the border of a central institutionalized occupation while the latter is illustrated by those who are in an interstitial zone between two institutionalized occupational groups. In the studies of marginality, the druggist (12) is clearly in a dual-group marginal position while the engineering technician (8), psychiatric attendant (17), and chiropractor (19) are marginal to single groups.

suming a faculty role. The graduate student consequently tends to be highly perceptive of cues which provide information on the appropriate role behavior of the faculty member. He also generally has a much higher degree of interaction with faculty members than does the undergraduate and consequently has a greater opportunity for observing and possibly emulating faculty role behavior.

In the university where these observations were made, it is typical for the graduate student to obtain a high degree of professional and personal rapport with the chairman of his graduate committee or the supervisor of his work as an assistant, particularly if the assistantship is related to the development of his dissertation and if his assistantship supervisor is also his committee chairman. Through this interaction he may observe role behaviors such as faculty-faculty interaction and cooperation, the relation of the faculty member and the department chairman, the procedures involved in publication of articles and monographs, the subtleties of the art of "grantsmanship," and the patterns of obtaining consulting assignments. These interactions and the participation of the student in the faculty member's activities contribute a great deal to his professional socialization. However, these activities generally occur within a context of status differentiation in which it is clear that the power and prestige in the relationship reside in the position of the faculty member. Boundary maintenance between faculty and graduate students exists as an unwritten but very real code.

The marginality of the graduate student, together with his anticipation of eventual entrance into the faculty reference group, results in what appear to be definite efforts to override this boundary and close the gap between faculty and student as much as possible. On the other hand, faculty members strive to maintain the boundary or at least to control how, when, and by whom it is crossed. This is due to the fact that boundary maintenance serves to maintain the value of the graduate degree as the key to entrance into the reference group; consequently boundary maintenance may act to increase the motivation of graduate students to complete the degree requirements.

Drinking plays a part in the socialization process being described. Maddox and McCall (13) have argued, for example, that the status passage between adolescence and adulthood frequently involves drinking and such behavior often has the appearance of being a regularized part of the status transitions which are integral to the ongoing operation of social systems. They point out:

> If adult roles are perceived as having alcohol use as a normal component, in contrast to the abstinence perceived as normative for the teen-ager, then one might expect that the teen-ager's identification of himself primarily as an adult or primarily as an adolescent would be an important variable in determining patterns of drinking or abstinence. In fact, this is what was found (13, p. 99).

Although in the professional socialization of the future professor drinking does not play a direct role in determining identification, it does act as a catalyst for the learning of appropriate professional behavior.

In summary, it has been hypothesized on the basis of empirical observation that graduate education is a setting for anticipatory socialization and that the graduate students, both as a group and individually, are marginal to the undergraduate system and to the academic profession. Ongoing anticipatory socialization and the condition of marginality are both sustained by the boundary maintenance efforts of faculty members. Drinking serves as a catalyst for tension release and further socialization, and in several ways serves to reduce temporarily social distance between faculty and students. In the long run, however, drinking does not dissolve student-faculty boundaries and the social distance implied. Boundary maintenance appears to motivate the graduate student to complete his degree work and thereby attain membership in the reference group of professors.

Alcohol and Student-Student Interaction

Graduate students constitute a heterogeneous population in terms of the patterns of drinking to which they have been exposed as undergraduates. Although the specific social characteristics, in addition to drinking style, which differentiate graduate students from undergraduates can only be speculated, from this study, it appears that non-fraternity members are slightly overrepresented in the graduate population. This may reflect, among other factors, early commitment to serious pursuit of academic goals on the part of these students. In this sense, graduate students are a select and self-selected population.

Another characteristic common to graduate students is that their undergraduate performance was adequate for graduate school admission. Thus, it may be assumed that those who, for whatever reason, developed drinking patterns in undergraduate life which interfered with their studies had a low probability of entering graduate school. This is not to imply, however, that graduate students were never heavy drinkers as undergraduates; rather, it implies that those undergraduates who were heavy drinkers had a high degree of control over their drinking which minimized significant interference with their academic performance. Thus, the pre-graduate school patterns of drinking of the students who were observed may be said to include all types of drinkers except those whose undergraduate drinking seriously impaired academic performance.

The responsibility associated with the role of the graduate student definitely limits their drinking behavior in most cases and stands in contrast to the relative freedom from responsibility ascribed to undergraduates. First, there are the responsibilities of completing the courses and research included in the degree requirements in an environment in which performance is quite visible. Additionally, there is the responsibility of completing the work assigned to the student by the supervisor of his assistantship.[4] Second, a considerable proportion of graduate students are married and in many cases have children. The limited income provided by assistantships or fellowships requires a close budgeting of funds, and alcohol is seen by most as a definite luxury within this budget. Therefore, the need to spend long hours at work and support oneself or a family on a very limited income limits the kinds of drinking likely to be observed among graduate students.[5]

[4] It is recognized that a growing number of graduate students are supported by fellowships or traineeships which do not include work responsibilities. In this study, those with such arrangements were observed to be as highly involved in projects as those with assistantships. In a number of situations, students with fellowships had also undertaken part-assistantships to augment their incomes. It appears that the major difference between holders of assistantships and fellowships is that the latter group has more autonomy in choosing academic activities rather than having more free time for the pursuit of leisure.

[5] By contrast, Hajda (11, p. 763) characterizes graduate student life as "lacking the responsibilities and temptations of post-graduate life, its seriousness, and in many ways also its all-inclusive societal scope." The ap-

Related to these factors of responsibility which mediate against extensive and intensive drinking among successful graduate students is the over-all structure of graduate education. Currently, graduate education operates in a way designed to motivate the student to complete the degree requirements as rapidly as possible. As mentioned in the previous section, although the graduate student is in a marginal position, he is continually reminded that successful completion of his program will eliminate his marginality, greatly increase his prestige, and increase his autonomy. In addition, the economic rewards he receives enforce a considerably lower standard of living than that permitted by the income of faculty members. Thus, the completion of the degree is seen as distinctly rewarding in terms of identity, prestige, autonomy, and rewards, and thus most students are highly motivated to complete the degree.[6] These considerations limit the extent to which graduate students will engage in behavior, even routine drinking, in private, which is perceived as hampering progress toward the degree. It is noteworthy that several informants specifically mentioned their anticipation of enjoying cocktails before dinner when they eventually attained faculty status.

A factor which also restrained graduate students who were teaching assistants from engaging in routine drinking in public places was their quasi-faculty status in relation to their undergraduate students. Like their own mentors, they exhibited the need to maintain social distance in the interest of maintaining authority in graduate-undergraduate relations. This restraint is parallel to the reluctance of faculty members to be involved in regular drinking with graduate students, which was discussed in the previous section, and might be seen as another element of anticipatory socialization.

A final factor which sets limits on drinking among graduate students is the lack of informal social organizations, such as

---

parent increase in competition for graduate school admission in recent years as well as the possibility of graduate students' improving their chances for attractive faculty positions by displaying more auspicious pre-professional credentials appear to have changed the degree of "seriousness" in graduate student subcultures.

[6] The fact that there are few career alternatives outside the completion of the degree also serves to maintain motivation. The dynamics of this commitment process are outlined in (1, 2, 16, pp. 177-187).

fraternities and social clubs, which are conducive to the development of social drinking. This absence of organization is tied to graduate students' commitments to academic responsibilities, the presence of family life as a replacement for residential organizations, and to the lack of commonality in individual academic pursuits which might provide a basis for informal organization. In the very few cases where regular drinking groups were observed, they were each restricted to students in a particular academic department.

It can be seen, therefore, that there are a considerable number of structural restraints on drinking among graduate students. The drinking that does occur and that was observed is largely in the service of tension release and may occur on the completion of examinations or projects, or during vacation periods. This drinking is generally restricted to evening hours and may take place in bars or in graduate student apartments. In the case of the latter, parties are generally "B.Y.O.B." ("bring your own booze"). Such drinking appears to be more prevalent among single students than among those who are married. Drinking does occur, but it is compartmentalized from other activities and in general attempts are made to keep it from interfering with academic pursuits.

This was not a clinical study intended to derive patterns of developing alcoholism or problem drinking. Yet there is no doubt that some who pass through a graduate student career and become academicians will also become problem drinkers or alcoholics. There were certain students who regularly became "high" or intoxicated when they were in drinking groups, and there was some evidence that certain students regularly engaged in solitary drinking. No case was observed, however, in which the graduate career was visibly impaired or terminated by alcohol. It appears that undergraduates with drinking problems are unlikely to be in graduate school and that the vast majority of graduate students are highly cognizant of the structural restraints on drinking. Most of them also appear to be motivated toward completing degree requirements. Thus, heavy drinking, even when it is observed, is accompanied by internalized controls and social restraints.

Will the removal of restraints that accompany passage into faculty status result in problem drinking, that is, a drinking pattern which significantly impairs role performance (18, pp. 28-

30), and eventually, lead to alcoholism in some cases? Although almost nothing factual is known about the drinking behavior and problems of college faculty, a variety of factors affect possible outcomes of the styles of drinking behavior observed among graduate students. First, the entrance into faculty status may result in the removal of certain restraints peculiarly applicable to students but at the same time result in the imposition of new restraints. The necessity of adequate role performance in order to receive promotion, tenure, and prestige within the profession is a case in point. In such a case one might expect pressure for controlled drinking on the part of even heavy drinkers or a reduction in the amount of drinking. Second, entrance into a faculty group may involve the internalization of new norms regarding drinking. There appeared, for example, to be considerable tolerance of intoxication in graduate student groups studied. But this may not be the case in faculty groups, particularly in regard to a junior member of the faculty who has accumulated no social credits with which to trade with his new peers. Third, the faculty group that the individual enters may be one with few structural restraints and one which is congenial to heavy drinking. This may be the case if the individual enters a large organization and develops associations with an established deviant drinking group.

There is wide variability in the types of settings which the graduate student may enter as he obtains faculty status, and the combination of past behavior and learning with extant structural restraints and opportunities is probably unique in every case, thus preventing a simple prediction. It does seem reasonable to assume, however, that the graduate student who finds satisfaction and release in alcohol to the extent of routine dependence has a considerable chance of encountering problems stemming from alcohol use in the future in social situations which tolerate or encourage heavy drinking. Moreover, the autonomy associated with tenured positions within academic organizations makes it possible for drinking problems to be masked for long periods of time.

Summary

The results of this exploratory study indicate that drinking tends to reduce feelings of professional marginality among graduate students who aspire to academic positions. Drinking also is frequently a catalyst in the anticipatory socialization of the future professors. Various structural restraints inherent in graduate student status limit drinking by graduate students and will probably continue to do so in the early years of their subsequent careers as faculty members. The observed drinking behavior of graduate students is not, however, a sound basis for predicting their drinking behavior beyond their achievement of faculty status. The exploratory nature of the study is emphasized. Observations were made at one university only and only at one point in time. The limitation of generalizations from these impressions is explicitly recognized.

REFERENCES

1. BECKER, HOWARD S. "Notes on the Concept of Commitment," *American Journal of Sociology,* 66: 32-40, 1960.
2. BECKER, HOWARD S., and JAMES W. CARPER. "The Development of an Identification with an Occupation," *American Journal of Sociology,* 61: 289-298, 1956.
3. BECKER, HOWARD S., BLANCHE GEER, ANSELM STRAUSS and EVERETT C. HUGHES. *Boys in White.* Chicago: The University of Chicago Press, 1961.
4. BECKER, HOWARD S., and ANSELM STRAUSS. "Careers, Personality and Adult Socialization," *American Journal of Sociology,* 62: 253-263, 1956.
5. BERELSON, BERNARD. *Graduate Education in the United States.* New York: McGraw-Hill, 1960.
6. BRIM, ORVILLE G., JR., and STANTON WHEELER. *Socialization After Childhood.* New York: John Wiley and Sons, 1966.
7. CAIN, LEONARD, JR. "Life Course and the Social Structure," in ROBERT E. L. FARIS (ed.), *Handbook of Modern Sociology.* Chicago: Rand-McNally, 1964, pp. 272-309.
8. EVAN, WILLIAM. "On the Margin: The Engineering Technician," in PETER L. BERGER (ed.), *The Human Shape of Work.* New York: The Macmillan Company, 1964, pp. 83-110.
9. GOTTLIEB, DAVID. "Processes of Socialization in American Graduate Schools," *Social Forces,* 40: 124-131, 1961.
10. GRIGG, CHARLES M. *Graduate Education.* New York: The Center For Applied Research in Education, 1965.
11. HAJDA, JAN. "Alienation and Integration of Student Intellectuals," *American Sociological Review,* 26: 658-777, 1961.
12. McCORMACK, THELMA H. "The Druggists' Dilemma: Problems of a Marginal Occupation," *American Journal of Sociology,* 61: 308-315, 1956.

13. MADDOX, GEORGE L. and BEVODE C. McCALL. *Drinking among Teen-Agers: A Sociological Interpretation of Alcohol Use by High School Students.* New Brunswick, N.J.: Publications Division of the Rutgers Center of Alcohol Studies, 1964.

14. MECHANIC, DAVID. *Students Under Stress.* New York: The Free Press, 1964.

15. MERTON, ROBERT K. *Social Theory and Social Structure.* Glencoe, Ill.: The Free Press, 1957.

16. MERTON, ROBERT K., *et al. The Student Physician.* Cambridge, Mass.: Harvard University Press, 1957.

17. SIMPSON, RICHARD L. and IDA H. SIMPSON. "The Psychiatric Attendant: Development of and Occupational Self-Image in a Low Status Occupation," *American Sociological Review,* 24: 389-392, 1959.

18. TRICE, HARRISON M. *Alcoholism in America.* New York: McGraw-Hill, 1966.

19. WARDWELL, WALTER I. "A Marginal Professional Role: The Chiropractor," *Social Forces,* 30: 339-358, 1952.

Chapter 9

THE AGING COLLEGIAN: DRINKING PATHOLOGIES AMONG EXECUTIVE AND PROFESSIONAL ALUMNI

HARRISON M. TRICE, *Cornell University*
JAMES A. BELASCO, *State University of New York at Buffalo*

ONE OF THE MANY unanswered questions concerning the drinking patterns of alcoholic executive and professional alumni is the extent to which drinking behavior in college fore-shadows their later alcoholism. Data regarding the social complications of drinking behavior in college strongly suggest that specific signs and behaviors of developing alcoholism occur during the college period (1). It is reasonable to believe that these role impairment signs might continue to develop in such a way that they directly reflect in the career pattern of the young executive. In other words, the drinking pathologies of the college years might continue to develop and come to impair their performance as managers or professionals. On the other hand, many alcoholic executives may have shown few if any signs of developing alcoholism when in college, but as their careers developed the symptoms of alcoholism developed simultaneously.

This chapter addresses itself to two basic research questions: First, "What is the relationship between drinking behavior in college and the emergence of problem drinking in later life?" In essence, this question deals with the matter of continuities or discontinuities between college drinking and role impairment for executives. Simply, this question asks, "Is the college student who is in trouble with alcohol likely to be the same individual

as the executive who has drinking problems ten to twenty years
after graduation?"

The second basic research question poses the inevitable explanatory dilemma of "What factors are associated with the
emergence of problem drinking among executives?" One of
these factors may well be college drinking patterns. Other factors, however, of a more immediate and situational character
may also intervene.

The main thrust of this chapter is that historical and personal
factors such as college drinking patterns are overshadowed by
more "here and now" occupationally and organizationally oriented considerations. For years the alcoholic himself, as an individual, has been the major focus of research. Considerable
efforts have been, and continue to be, expended to find some
deep-seated psychological or physiological explanation for the
behaviors clinically defined as alcoholism. To this point, research has failed to isolate either an alcoholic personality or
significant physiological differences between alcoholics and non-
alcoholics before the onset of problem drinking. This leads us
to question the sufficiency of the individual as the primary
source of data. Rather individual personality and physical factors may establish the necessary condition for the emergence of
problem drinking. The sufficient conditions may well reside in
factors external to the individual, particularly those which
emerge from the pivotal societal institutions of the formal bureaucratic work organization and the family.

This conceptual approach shifts the major research emphasis
from the individual to the organization and the social systems
of which the individual is a part. It focuses our attention on the
relationship between the developing alcoholic and his social
situation, thus postulating the involvement of a wide range of
normals in an interdependent web of deviants (2). We suggest
that the informal power struggles which characterize the upper
echelons of many organizations may be one of the organizational
factors which can both precipitate and protect the putative
pathological behavior of alcoholics. This conceptual stance implies that certain organizational factors may actually encourage
the development of alcoholism and, furthermore, that alcoholism
may be functional in certain organizational settings. This more
sociological explanation of the etiology of alcoholism stands in
sharp contrast to the more traditional, psychiatric, clinically-

oriented explanations found in the literature. The data reported
in this article attempt to shed some light on the utility of this
possible explanation.

The reader should first be aware of the methodological pitfalls
which are present in the data which are available. In the first
place, our data are self-reported and retrospective and, moreover, subject to all of the serious biases of selective remember-
ing and forgetting which the passage of time can induce. Secondly, we really do not have a representative sample in any
sense. For example, membership in A.A., which was the point
of contact with the executives we will describe, is itself quite
selective. This prevents us from generalizing beyond the immediate responses. Thirdly, the case study material is subject
to all of the problems inherent in the more anthropological approach, particularly that of selective perception. In short, in
literal scientific terms we offer nothing more than a basic description of a highly selective and possibly unrepresentative
population. We offer only a suggestion and an hypothesis. Any
conclusion beyond this the reader reaches at his own risk.

Does College Drinking Carry Over?

In an effort to throw more light on the question of continuities in drinking pathologies as males move from college into
managerial careers, the data from a study on work behavior of
developing alcoholics were re-examined (3). The data consisted
of 552 questionnaire responses from members of Alcoholics
Anonymous from all regions of the United States plus 83 taped
interviews from the New York City and Syracuse, New York,
areas. Respondents described, in addition to work behaviors,
such as absenteeism and work performance, their drinking histories when various problems related to alcohol began, the
nature of these complications, and how early in their drinking
history they began. They were also asked to consider drinking
behaviors during adolescence, early adulthood, job entry and
developing career.

One quarter of the subjects were in the professional or managerial positions. Eighty-six per cent of the college graduates
in the population were also in these job categories. By examining
the drinking history of these 194 subjects, some suggestions should
emerge about the questions at hand. In addition, by looking at

the histories of the 14 per cent of the college graduates who were not in executive or professional positions, we may find some additional hypotheses.

The large majority, 82 per cent, of those in executive and professional jobs report few social complications from drinking while in college. Rather, they describe a drinking pattern that was incidental: fraternity and drinking cliques that were not disruptive but seemed to be relatively functional. They described drinking on dates, at dances, in taverns and in spontaneous friendship groups during the day and evening.

Nor was the period of immediate entry into labor market following graduation marked by the social complications described in Straus and Bacon (1). Here and there a subject described drinking behavior such as a hangover that temporarily impaired his performance. For most, however, there are no general trends or themes of this kind during the years immediately following graduation and entry into a career path.

In addition, this period seemed to be typical regarding job turnover for these future alcoholics. The subjects consistently described a period of searching and shifting during which they reconsidered job roles and future careers. Their concerns seemed to be far removed from alcohol dependency. Rather, it was with "settling in." Thus a future general manager of a large electronics firm described his career: "At that time I was looking around for the very best opportunity I could come by. I had more than the usual ambitions and was thrashing about to locate that company that looked the best." A partner in a Wall Street brokerage firm described the period "A time when I was drinking like a lot of my friends. I don't recall it as anything greatly unusual. What stands out in my mind was hopes to get with a 'going' outfit, one with a future for me."

The histories give the clear impression that drinking during this period was a rewarding experience. Practically none described fears or concerns about alcoholism. In contrast, their accounts emphasize the social role of alcohol: drinking at home with wife, either incidentally or during tension facing periods, such as problems in child rearing and company drinking either at cocktail parties or in business situations. None of the respondents emphasized bar or cocktail lounge drinking; rather, they underscored enjoyable drinking during ceremonials such as weddings, retirements and business conventions. The only definite symptom of alcoholism prominently mentioned for this period was an increase in tolerance to alcohol. Only in retrospect, however, did this seem to loom as having any significance. In contrast, they frequently noted that the drinking situations were relaxing, enjoyable and something to which they looked forward.

In short, these college graduates, who were later to become alcoholics, as well as executives, tended to describe a college career and the job entry period immediately following it, as relatively free from alcohol-related problems. Concern for securing advantageous jobs loomed large for them and they appeared to be involved in drinking group patterns that had more positive than negative sanctions.

Social complications from drinking and job impairment begin to enter the histories as the young manager or professional moved out of the period of searching for a favorable job location and into a competitive career effort. This trend is supported by one of the most consistent demographic findings in the study of alcoholism; namely, the concentration of distinctive symptoms in the ages of the mid-30's to the early 50's. Consistently these college-trained subjects linked the beginning of regular recurrence of alcohol-related social complications with the development of a commitment to their future, to a specific organization and to specific roles within it. Their descriptions suggest that the beginning of clear-cut alcoholism symptoms coincided with a career commitment.

For example, on-the-job absenteeism, i.e., going to work out of a strong sense of responsibility when in poor condition because of alcohol use, appears over and over as these college-trained executives and professionals began the ascent up the bureaucratic ladder. A motion picture director described in detail how as an assistant director he

> very seldom missed; I relied on the morning drinks to get me there, but because I wasn't a nine-to-five employee, I could often duck out and get enough to keep me going at a very poor pace, but going nonetheless. Then, too, I had a driving force that got me there. I know that if I couldn't get there I'd have to give up whiskey and I didn't want to do that.

Still others describe noon-time drinking as a definite "must" period for them, leading to clear-cut job and role impairment and to changed behavior that called for energy-consuming cover-up efforts. These pathologies began well before reaching a mature, high-status position and clearly appeared to accompany upward mobility in the organization during junior roles.

Interestingly enough, these role impairments of developing alcoholism apparently did not deter the subjects from originally getting ahead. Instead, they report a consistently even path upward despite early and middle-stage alcoholism symptoms. Apparently, executive careers in their formative stages are not unusually stymied by alcoholic symptoms that actually do impair specific role performance. Furthermore, as will be suggested in specific case studies later, their developing alcoholism may actually be functional for the organization.

Analysis of the responses of the 14 per cent of the college graduates in our population who were *not* in executive or professional positions throws some light on the validity of the process we have just sketched—a process in which there was no carry-over of college alcoholism symptoms but a development of alcoholic symptoms as the career developed. When the histories of college graduates who subsequently moved into clerical, service and semi-skilled occupations were examined, there was a definite increase in the number of alcohol-related social complications described during the college years. When the high-status (executive, professional) college graduates are compared with the lower status ones (clerical, service and semi-skilled) on the basis of the number of college-period impairments described in the interview data, there is a chi-square significant difference at the 5 per cent level. This difference holds up in the questionnaire responses but with the differences significant at the 10 per cent level.

Clearly suggested is the possibility of two types of career patterns among college graduates who develop drinking problems. One is the alcoholism pattern that develops simultaneously with the executive or professional career and which shows no symptomatology during the college period. The second is that type which develops definite social complications in the early adult years of college training and whose ability to move and compete in a career pattern is thereby damaged. Although the data are purely suggestive, it seems reasonable to hypothesize that the first type is more typical but far more difficult to identify, while the latter is sufficiently visible and impaired so that career development is stymied.

In short, there were few continuities between college drinking and alcoholism among executives. The answer to the first research question is, then, "The college student in trouble with alcohol during his college days is *not* the alcoholic executive who appears ten or twenty years later."

Probably more fundamental, however, is the implication that job and organizational factors may contribute to the career-related type of alcoholism, while this may not be true for the non-career related type whose role performances had already been damaged as early as college days.

The "Here and Now" Hypothesis

Insight into this "here and now" hypothesis can be gleaned by an intensive look at three case studies which involve the presidents of three large organizations—two in the electronics area and one in the service field. None of these executives reported any drinking problems at all during his college career. All three reported an increase in drinking and the appearance of role impairment before and during the tenure of their presidency. All three were relatively heavy drinkers previously but deny any major impairment until after they were near the top of the bureaucratic ladder.

By all traditional business standards, the three organizations which these alcoholic executives head are highly successful. For instance, Organization A—a major force in the electronics industry—owes its current prosperity largely to its president. The president joined the organization sixteen years ago when it was a small, largely regional company. Under his leadership the organization has increased ten-fold to the point where it is now the second largest company in the industry and is listed as one of the fifty largest companies in the country. As an indication of its success, its stock price has increased thirty-fold since his accession to the corporate throne. The dividend has been increased every year in the last decade and the stock is now listed as a leading growth stock by major brokerage houses. During the period of this phenomenal growth, the chief executive officer was a "wet" alcoholic.

Similarly, Organization B is a leader in one of the newly emerging consumer goods industry largely because its alcoholic president insisted that the organization stay with basic research in an area after other companies had written it off as commercially unfeasible. Earnings of the company, one of the fifty largest in the country, have doubled in the last few years and it ranks as a leading "glamour stock."

Organization C, a service industry organization, has experienced a similar, somewhat less spectacular growth pattern. The number of clients served by this organization has increased steadily during the president's tenure of office. The assets of the organization have doubled and it ranks today as one of the largest organizations of its kind in the world.

Thus, the three companies have risen dramatically under the leadership of alcoholic executives. The relevance of these studies for this article lies in a more intensive look at the relationship between these three alcoholic executives and their organizations.

Take the case of the president of Organization A, for instance. Obviously, the alcoholism of the chief executive is a closely guarded, well-kept secret; only a few key persons are aware of the president's drinking problem. Of the two dozen or so vice-presidents who report directly to the president, only three know of the president's condition. The others probably don't even suspect.

The president hides his problem from the public and members of his own organization with the cooperation of a small coterie of insiders. This group of insiders include his two executive assistants, three vice-presidents and his personal secretary. These six persons successfully insulate the president from the rest of the organization.

A typical day goes something like the following. One of the executive assistants picks up the president at his mid-town apartment at approximately 8:30 A.M. Normally by this time the president has had four or five drinks to overcome the bad hangover and shakes from yesterday's drinking. Several times, of course, after a particularly extended drinking session the night before, it takes an hour or so of working by the executive assistant to get the president in shape, though this is not usual. Since the early part of the morning usually is the president's most productive time of the day, he spends an hour or so reviewing yesterday's stock market transactions and preparing his trades for the coming day. The president is an ardent student of the stock market. He studies and knows hundred of stocks and actively trades both under his name and several pseudonyms. Over the past decade he has accumulated through trading almost a quarter of a million dollars—all done like Lord Keynes—in an hour or so in the morning.

To avoid the morning rush, the two leave for the office at about 9:15 A.M. in the company car. By now the president has had seven or eight drinks and is reasonably alert, if still somewhat testy and irritable.

Once in the office building, the president goes right from his car to his office via a specially constructed private elevator. The private elevator was an idea of one of the vice-presidents after the president's morning unsteadiness and irritability had resulted in an embarrassing situation in the public elevator. One morning the president came in in the middle of the 9 A.M. rush and managed to knock over an urn full of coffee being delivered to a group of secretaries. The hot coffee spilled all over him and several of the other elevator passengers. Besides losing his temper, he immediately banned all morning coffee for the corporate headquarters, thus causing considerable consternation throughout the organization. The private elevator was designed to avoid repetition of such an event.

Once upstairs in his office the president has a few more drinks and is ready to see the first of his appointments. From 10:30 to 12:30 or so, he sees individuals from both inside and outside the organization. In all of these interactions the president merely listens and takes things under advisement. He makes no decisions at all but concentrates rather on making general statements of approval or disapproval. By 12:30 he needs a few more drinks before attending a regularly scheduled executive luncheon. At these luncheons he rarely drinks more than one cocktail "in order to keep up appearances." At the conclusion of the luncheon, at 2:30 or so, the president is through working for the day. He normally leaves with one of the executive assistants who stays with him well into the evening until he is certain that the president is safe in his apartment.

It is apparent that the president has little or nothing to do with the actual administration of his company. While he serves as a figurehead, the actual authority in the organization has evolved to this small group of insiders. Orders are issued, authorizations signed and the corporation run by these people in the name of the president. The responsibility for the actual operation of the corporation is divided by functional areas with each of the vice-presidents responsible for a series of major product lines. Administrative decisions are handled by the executive assistant and the secretary. Conflicts between and among the members of the insider group are resolved in an informal meeting, usually after working hours or on weekends.

Of course, this has not always been so. At the beginning of his tenure, the president was an active, able administrator. He launched an expansion program which in a short space of time more than doubled the size of the organization. In an effort to handle the administrative burden, the president surrounded himself with a "kitchen cabinet" of young trusted advisors. While it is difficult to reconstruct the past from interview data, it seems that two events occurred reasonably simultaneously. First, the president's ability to make decisions and follow up on details was more and more impaired by his drinking. This created an organizational vacuum. Concurrent with this was a push on the part of several key insiders for more responsibility and authority. Sensing the authority vacuum, these ambitious persons moved in to fill it and the current *modus operandi* is the result.

Thus, the insiders cover up for the president largely because the current situation is in their best interests. They exercise a considerable amount of decision-making authority, are recognized in the organization as "men behind the throne" and receive handsome economic rewards. Should the status of the president change in any way, their positions might be impaired. So, these six people put up with, tolerate and exploit the president's drinking problem. From the president's point of view, the current arrangement is also beneficial. He retains his occupational label, his prestige and his material comforts. At the same time, he has a situation in which he can continue to drink with the prospect of few, if any, negative sanctions.

The case of the president of Organization B closely follows that of the president of Organization A. In both cases a small group of loyalists surround the president and insulate him from exposure to the outside world. In return for this protection, these insiders have stripped away a good deal of the authority vested in the president's office and have taken it for their own.

The experience of the president of Organization C is somewhat different. A similar protective clique pattern emerged in which the president was isolated from the balance of the organization and effectively stripped of his authority by the insiders. Only in this instance, the insiders decided to further add to their power at the expense of the regional vice-presidents. This generated an organizational rebellion on the part of the vice-presidents which precipitated into a major proxy fight. When confronted with the reality that he might lose his job, the president sobered up. During the campaign the president remained dry for almost three months. After the election, however, he reverted to his former habits.

There are five interesting implications of these briefly stated but intensively studied cases. First, in all of these instances, the emergence of pathological drinking behavior was accompanied by support and protection from a group of significant role definers. In fact, problem drinking clearly emerges as behavior which is encouraged and rewarded by powerful role definers—particularly those in the alcoholic's occupational role. This involvement of non-alcoholic normals in the precipitation and maintenance in the deviant behavior lends some support to the sociological explanation postulated in the beginning of this article. For instance, in all three cases a protective clique emerges which envelops the alcoholic executive in a cocoon which effectively isolates him from the rest of the organization. This relationship between the clique members and the alcoholic executive is a symbiotic one (4). The clique members satisfy personal ambitions for power and materialistic gains while the executive continues to drink without the threat of job or status loss. As a part of this protective clique pattern much of the power in the president's position is extracted and decentralized to the clique members. As an example, in Organization C, the alcoholic president easily becomes a pawn in the organizational struggle for power.

Second, the label of "alcoholic" is employed as a weapon in the organizational struggle over scarce power assets. The in-group clique members, for instance, were able to control the president of Company A by the simple, clearly understood, yet never voiced threat of exposure. For the president, exposure meant personal humiliation and probable loss of status and job. He often acceded to the group's wishes rather than run the risk of this exposure. Thus, the very process of labeling itself is employed as a weapon in the informal power struggle to control the president.

Third, by the control of the communication channels both to

and from the president, the inner clique is able to perpetuate a pattern of exclusiveness and exclusion. Since the president's interactions are limited to this group he is prohibited from any significant "testing of reality."

His circumscribed population of role definers constantly treats him differently—expecting him to behave like an alcoholic—with the result that, as with Lemert's paranoids, this reinforces the alcoholic behavior. By expecting the president to act like an alcoholic, and communicating this to him with both verbal and non-verbal cue, the group may have elicited and perpetuated the behavior.

Furthermore, as a result of this pattern of exclusion the president is cut off from vital information concerning the operation of the organization. He knows only what he is told by the group and this information is very sparse indeed, since the group members do not trust the president and fear that he will blurt out some vital information at an inopportune moment. For his part, the president is unwilling to risk the embarrassment of going directly to a subordinate and requesting information since he is supposed to have the information in the first place. A logical outcome of this exclusion process is continued withdrawal of the president from any effective decision making. Thus, through control over the channels of communication and the process of exclusion and exclusiveness, the inner group perpetuates the pathological drinking and retains its hold on the effective power of the organization.

In fact, this close relationship between the president and his advisors may have aided in the precipitation of the drinking problem. For instance, in interviews the president of Organization A reported that he felt very dependent upon his close advisors and dreaded losing them to opportunities elsewhere. On the other hand, he recognized that to keep them he had to provide them with increasing responsibilities and authority. According to the president, this concern of what to do weighed heavily on his mind and was one of the things he drank to forget. His dilemma might be stated as follows: "I need these guys desperately, but they are eating me alive so I retreat into the bottle."

The case of the president of Organization C illustrates a fourth interesting facet of the contribution of organizational factors to the precipitation of alcoholism. The protective clique structure combined with the symbiotic relationship with close associates can aggravate the manifestation of problem drinking. By the same token, the organization can be a potent force for generating the desire to abandon alcohol and the role impairment it engenders.

Fifth, these case studies highlight the findings of previous research. The cover-up aid which these high-status people received from subordinates, the care to maintain normal drinking appearances and the "partial" absenteeism were found by both Trice (3) and Stamps (5). The absence of any real productive activity while at work was another clear finding of this and other studies. Because of the low visibility, the high-status drinker is free to hide his drinking problem for a considerable period of time.

Turning to the work histories of professionals, there were numerous suggestions of job-related factors that could be regarded as forces contributing to alcoholism. In contrast to high-status executives, these factors came more from the intrinsic nature of the job rather than from organizational behavior. The most frequently described experience was occupational obsolescence. Directly related to rapid technological change, this obsolescence confronted the professional with the desperate necessity of trying to "keep up" with younger and more recently trained competitors, while at the same time maintaining his already-achieved position. As this process increased, the professional was left with less and less of a role to perform and more and more of a feeling of uselessness.

Engineers were the best example of this job-related factor, although cases of doctors, professors, dentists and veterinarians showed the same factor. The following subject suggests the specific nature of occupational obsolescence. During college (five-year engineering course at a major university) "engineer D" did superior work in electrical engineering. He drank with his fellow students, but reported no role impairments. In addition he worked part-time for a large electronics firm near the university. Upon graduation he was in great demand and had a pick of numerous offers from leading firms around the country. For approximately seven years his specialty was featured in many company changes and reorganizations. During the time he participated in the planning and execution of revolutionary new processes in radio, TV, and radar production. He advanced rapidly in status and salary.

With the routinization of these changes, however, he described a period of "letdown." Over-all company planning moved to space equipment of a very esoteric sort. Problems of heat control, of metallurgy, and of computer controls rapidly came to the fore. He moved to "brush up" by evening courses, "sitting-in" by his request on planning, and by independent study. None of these sufficed. The competitive positions of the company called for younger, specialized engineers who could rapidly fit the unusual technological demands. Without imputing causal relations, his drinking became heavier and role impairments more noticeable as obsolescence deepened. Paradoxically enough, he moved into an administrative post that did not demand highly specialized technological knowledge approximately eleven years out of college. It was during this period that his alcoholism clearly began to develop.

Accompanying these themes among professionals was a note of subtle status change—a form of demotion. Usually such obsolescence resulted in a decrease in staff and supervisory influence. Rarely was this associated with salary reduction but there were descriptions of separation from the direct line of promotion. An industrial engineer, for example, described entirely new work flows and new production groups to them as his unit shifted to an entirely new product. Promotion priorities went to the new group. He defined the situation as a form of demotion.

An additional factor clustering around obsolescence could be termed "loss of colleagueship." Engineers especially noted that their informal cohort groups were usually weakened by the transfers and cutbacks occasioned by the over-all changes. Clique affiliations were fewer and feelings of being "marginal," as one engineer put it, seemed to increase. As a result, they felt they were "left out" of the communication system and so deprived of the important sources of social reality.

In short, there were few if any links which led from college drinking to alcoholism for the professionals and executives studied. Like the bulk of the college-level subjects, who later develop a drinking problem, there seemed to be scant trace of this problem in college. The more important etiological factors, rather, seem to relate to current "here and now" events, particularly those which cluster around the organization in which the individuals were employed. Four organizational factors, the informal power struggle, the labeling process, personal dependencies and protective clique patterns have been outlined as contributing to the continuation and possible emergence of problem drinking among higher status executives.

In contrast with executives, the occupationally based themes clustered, for professionals, around a marked decline in the demand for specialized knowledge or its replacement by new knowledge and expertise. Thus occupational obsolescence, its implications for demotion and its increased social isolation formed the possible contributing factors. Combined with the three organizational forces described earlier in relation to company presidents, these make up a brace of possible etiological factors. Although we do not, at present, imply any definite causal connection, it does seem reasonable to suggest that future research on alcoholism's etiology explicitly include job and organization forces.

Therapeutic Contribution of Work World

Also indicated is a consideration of the possible motivational and therapeutic potentials in the work world. It seems unusual, for example, that most of the various company policies and programs for the rehabilitation of the alcoholic employee do *not* cover the executive or professional person. Of those who purport to do so, company officials will frankly admit that there are practically no instances in which they have been applied. At the same time, it would seem that such plans might be of greater effectiveness among higher status employees than among those of lower rank. Furthermore, it would seem desirable to devise a company-based approach to rehabilitation for these persons because of their greater all-around cost, both in dollars and cents and in impact on organizational performance.

For example, in an effort to motivate the alcoholic employee to seek therapy, most companies with programs take, as a part of their policies, a "constructive coercion" position. This means that the company intends to treat such persons as suffering from a unique form of illness and to offer them support for therapy without prejudice. At the same time, if the alcoholic does not *reasonably* respond to this offer, he will be discharged, or in some fashion lose a substantial amount of his job investment. Since higher status people typically have greater career investments and fringe benefits in their positions and have higher needs for status maintenance, such an approach might be more crisis-precipitating for them than for lower status persons. In addition, these latter often have union membership that partially insulates them from such a policy.

On the other hand, such a policy suffers from some of the forces described earlier. The alcoholic executives and professionals have much better cover-up opportunities and so are less easily identified. They are more apt than lower status persons to have a coterie of protectors who shield them from such a policy, and they enjoy far greater freedom from supervision. At the same time, the adaptation of a constructive coercion policy to fit the nature of such jobs seems worth exploring. For example, rather than some type of clinic referral that poses threats of disclosure, the use of specialized physicians has proved effective in some instances in carrying out the policy.

In summary, there were few, if any, links between college drinking problems and executive alcoholism. Rather, we suggest that occupational and organizational life may well contain precipitating or contributing factors to the development of alcoholism among college graduates who later become professional and executive employees in complex organizations. This is suggested by the lack of role impairments during college for most of our alcoholic executive subjects. Intense examination of specific cases points to the possible nature of these work world forces: internal power struggle, symbiotic cliques and the executive alcoholic's dependency on them and occupational obsolescence with its various results that impinge on the professional. By the same token, organizational life contains possible forces for motivation and rehabilitation that remain untapped.

REFERENCES

1. STRAUS, ROBERT, and SELDEN BACON. *Drinking in College*. New Haven, Connecticut. Yale University Press, 1953.
2. LEMERT, EDWIN. "Paranoia and the Dynamics of Exclusion," *Sociometry*, 25: 2-20, 1962.
3. TRICE, H. M. "The Job Behavior of Problem Employees," in D. PITTMAN, and C. SNYDER (eds.), *Society, Culture and Drinking Patterns*. New York: John Wiley & Sons, 1962.
4. DALTON, MELVILLE. *Men Who Manage*. New York: John Wiley & Sons, 1959, pp. 57-65.
5. STAMPS, JAMES. "The Alcoholic Employee and Problem Concealment." Unpublished Master's thesis, Washington State University, 1965.

Chapter 10

PRESCRIPTION, PROSCRIPTION AND PERMISSIVENESS: ASPECTS OF NORMS AND DEVIANT DRINKING BEHAVIOR*

EPHRAIM H. MIZRUCHI, *Syracuse University*
ROBERT PERRUCCI, *Purdue University*

Introduction

A MAJOR PROBLEM for contemporary sociologists revolves about the issue of long range vs. short range goals in the solution of perceived social problems. Should the sociologist concern himself primarily with abstract theory which is of a level of generality capable of application to many social settings, once developed and refined? Or, should he apply himself to a particular question yielding more immediate rewards for the process of solving seemingly urgent societal problems? In reality we find only a small number who clearly espouse either one position or the other. More typical of contemporary research is an effort to study the particular in order to cast light on the general.

This chapter attempts to illustrate how the study of normative and deviant drinking behavior yields hypotheses which are explicitly tied to more abstract generalizations which are applicable to a variety of social settings. Thus, research in the sphere of alcohol and society can make simultaneous contributions to the

* From *The Substance of Sociology: Codes, Conduct and Consequences.* Edited by Ephraim H. Mizruchi. Copyright © 1967, Meredith Corporation. Pages 259-270, "Norm Qualities and Deviant Behavior," by Ephraim H. Mizruchi and Robert Perrucci, revised and extended from *American Sociological Review,* 27, 1962, pp. 391-399. Reprinted by permission of Appleton-Century-Crofts and the authors, so far as their rights are concerned. A travel grant from the Syracuse University Research Institute is acknowledged.

solution of immediate social problems and to the development of general theories of societal processes.

Our data are analyzed within a broad framework which embodies questions about the nature of normative integration, deviances, group reactions to deviance and social change.

The organizing concepts emerged both from a study of the data on cultural factors in drinking behavior and further induction into an appropriate theoretical model. The process includes the establishment of ideal-type aspects of norms; providing data illustrating the significance of distinguishing these aspects from other norm qualities; and deriving *explicit* empirically testable hypotheses for the assessment of the original typology. Thus what is being attempted, in addition, is a study of how ideal-type method can be directly integrated with more formal empirical analysis.

Norms and Normative Integration

A fundamental notion embodied in the functional approach to social systems is that certain tasks must be performed in order that a given system may persist. Among the various tasks, or functional prerequisites, is the maintenance of a system of order. Many of the traditional dichotomies associated with the names of eminent forerunners of contemporary sociology reflect explicit and implicit concern with order. Durkheim's mechanical and organic solidarity (12), Tönnies' Gemeinschaft-Gesellschaft (33), Redfield's Folk-Urban (25) and Becker's Sacred-Secular (3) to name only a few, indicate a concern with the fundamental question of how society is organized and changed.

Though there are great divergences of viewpoint among contemporary sociologists regarding which factors are most significant in contrasting relatively simple and complex social organizations, few would disagree that the process of group adherence to shared norms represents an important dimension of order. Thus Durkheim (12) and Freedman *et al.* (13) have focused their attention on the contrast between normative and functional integration. These two dimensions as conceived by these writers are to be found in all group structures and represent ideal-typical states of systems. Thus contemporary urban communities, for example, would be expected to be integrated not only in terms of functional integration, i.e., integration based on the interrelated activities of heterogeneous groups, but normatively as well. Consequently, the norms represent crucial factors in the process of maintaining order.

Relatively little attention has been paid to the qualitative nature of the norms themselves as contrasted with the great concern associated with the direct effect of norms in controlling the activities of individuals in groups.[1] This is particularly the case with regard to the role played by the qualitative characteristics of norms in the process of normative integration and the utility of this dimension in empirical analysis.

In terms of the sociocultural system, the problem of order may be analyzed with respect to the particular characteristics of the norms themselves, in addition to the control processes associated with the norms. In other words, the stability or integration of a system is not insured simply because the normative system is effectively transmitted (socialization) or collectively controlled (sanctions). The qualities of the norms themselves provide an inherent potential for system maintenance and system mal-integration.

Proscriptive and Prescriptive Dimensions of Norms

Richard T. Morris (19), in a paper published a decade ago, suggested a classification of norms which focused on four significant aspects: their distribution; the mode of enforcement associated with a given norm; the transmission of norms; and the process of conformity to given norms. Robin M. Williams, Jr. has also incorporated this scheme in his systematic study of American society (36, pp. 26-27). Though there is no shortage of classificatory schemes in this important area of sociological theory, it would seem to us that still another dimension is worthy of consideration as a possible addition to Morris' classification.

Indeed, Morris himself has suggested that "probably the most striking omission . . . [in his typology of norms] . . . is the content of the norms" (19, p. 612).

> "Content" is used here in two senses: classification of norms according to the area of behavior regulated . . ., or classification of norms according to the nature of action called for by the norms . . . (19).

[1] The most conspicuous exceptions are to be found in the work of William Graham Sumner (32), Talcott Parsons (22), Pitirim Sorokin (30), and Robin M. Williams, Jr. (36).

It is the latter to which we are addressing ourselves here.

Our specific objective will be to present an additional typology, to illustrate its potential value by making reference to several sets of data related to the typology, and to suggest how greater attention to this dimension may prove fruitful in assessing the functional significance of certain aspects of norms in social systems.

In discussing norms in general, Williams points out that ". . . norms always carry some prescriptive or proscriptive *quality* . . ." (36, p. 26).[2] Talcott Parsons, in discussing the integration of social systems, has also directed attention to the significance of the proscriptive-prescriptive dimension. He states:

> It is this integration by common values, manifested in the action of solidary groups or collectivities, which characterizes the partial or total integrations of social systems.
>
> Social integration, however much it depends on internalized norms, cannot be achieved by these alone. It requires also some supplementary coordination provided by explicit *prescriptive* or *prohibitory* role-expectations (e.g., laws) (23, pp. 202-203).[3]

This particular dimension appears worthy of further exploration on the level of system-maintenance analysis. A preliminary ideal-typical description should prove sufficient for the first step in our analysis.

Norms in which the proscriptive element is most predominant are those which direct participants in the social structure to avoid, abstain, desist, and reject all forms of behavior associated with a particular potential type of activity. Examples of this dimension are the "thou shalt not" directives of the Ten Commandments and abstention from the pleasures of the flesh as directed by ascetic Protestantism.

The *prescriptive* dimension, on the other hand, directs par-

---

[2] It should be noted that we are not concerned here with *types* of norms as such, but only with specific *aspects* of norms. It should also be kept in mind that the proscriptive-prescriptive notions have existed in the anthropological literature for some time.

[3] It should be noted also that the present writers do not view the significance of the prescriptive and proscriptive dimensions as operative on the external level alone, i.e., external to the internalized norms, as Parsons implies here, but on both the internalized and externalized levels of social control. Note also Robert K. Merton's awareness of the significance of these dimensions (17, p. 133).

ticipants to act in a particular way, spelling out the forms of behavior to which group members must conform. Typical of prescriptive directives are the norms requiring periodical church attendance and confession among Roman Catholics and the elaborate directives associated with the consumption of alcoholic beverages among the Orthodox Jews.

Thus the mandate of the predominantly proscriptive norm is "do not" while the mandate of the predominantly prescriptive norm is "do this" or "do that." The former provides only a goal viewed negatively; the latter provides a goal viewed positively, as well as a set of means for its attainment.

Whether this scheme is worthy of serious attention as a possible addition to the body of theory on norms would seem to depend upon its usefulness as an analytical tool, particularly as a means of organizing empirical findings. We have, with this in mind, selected some studies which help illustrate the possible utility of these notions in the process of relating theory to concrete data.

At least one area of patterned activity which particularly lends itself to analysis in this context has undergone extensive investigation.[4] The several sociological studies of the relationship between sociocultural factors and the consumption of alcoholic beverages should provide us with a "goodness of fit" criterion for our conceptual analysis.[5] The specific studies to which we refer are those of Straus and Bacon (31), Snyder (28), Skolnick (27), Mulford and Miller (21), Allardt, et al. (1), and more recently, Bruun and Hauge (6). All represent a high order of methodological procedure in terms of sampling, question design and data analysis. All of these studies focus on variations in drinking behavior among various social strata and ethnic groups, and provide a broad range of data on norms, beliefs, and sentiments concerning the uses of alcohol. Thus they are particularly valuable for codification. Our first problem, then, is to demonstrate whether the differences between prescriptive and proscriptive dimensions of norms are of significance in the analysis of concrete data.

The above studies report significant differences among the

[4] Note the similarity between our independently conceived approach and the earlier approach of Edwin M. Lemert (15, p. 33).

[5] For a discussion of the "goodness of fit" concept in the verification of typologies, see, for example, James M. Beshers (5).

various groups with regard to pathological reactions resulting from differential patterns of alcohol consumption. By "pathological" we mean the extent to which these behaviors represent deviations which are threats to the personal well-being of group members, e.g., problems of drinking or psychosis. We are suggesting that the extent to which these levels of pathology are present in a given system is directly related to problems of system maintenance although, as we suggest below, these threats may also play a role in attaining greater short-run integration.

Cultural Norms and Drinking Pathology

Three sets of data have been selected to demonstrate the existence of a relationship between types of normative system and drinking pathology. Snyder's study shows that intoxication is related to religio-ethnic group affiliation for college students.[6] As contrasted with the rates for the Jewish students, whose behavior is presumably directed by prescriptive norms, for example, the intoxication rate is much higher for the ascetic Protestant and Mormon groups, for whom the drinking of alcoholic beverages is proscribed. Snyder holds that,

> These data should not be construed as representing the comparative overall effectiveness of the norms of these groups in minimizing intoxication. The percentages . . . are based on the numbers of students in each group who have had some experience in using alcoholic beverages. They, therefore, do not reflect the large numbers of abstainers, especially in the Protestant group, who have never been intoxicated (29, p. 189).

We would hold that Snyder's interpretation is most meaningful within the context of the relationship between group affiliation and over-all drinking behavior. However, it is precisely the question of the "overall effectiveness of the norms" for those who drink which concerns us here; this is the sphere in which the fundamental difference between our concern and that of the various analysts of drinking behavior manifests itself. While their focus is on the relationship between norms and specified features of the social structure, ours is on the qualitative nature of the norms themselves.

[6] Snyder's data were derived from original data gathered by Straus and Bacon for the college drinking study. See Snyder (29, p. 190).

Skolnick's data[7] reveal even more sharply some of the consequences of normative deviation. When one compares the degree of social complications associated with religio-ethnic group affiliation, one finds that social complications tend to increase for selected groups of students. While social complications for the Jewish students are minimal, there is a marked increase for the ascetic Protestant groups. Thus, the data again reflect a relationship between ascetic Protestant affiliation and drinking pathology with respect to the extremities of deviant reactions for these groups.

Still other results that are significant in the context of the present study are the findings of Mulford and Miller in one of the most elaborate and extensive studies of the drinking behavior of an adult population. They approach questions similar to those posed by the other researchers from a social psychological viewpoint. Differentiating between drinking behavior that is directed by normative systems and that which involves idiosyncratic decisions regarding alcohol consumption, they developed a scale of "personal-effects definitions," which makes a distinction between relatively normative and non-normative drinking behavior (20, 21).

Mulford and Miller's interpretation of their findings is consistent with those of Straus and Bacon and Snyder with regard to the non-existence of group norms which characterizes the drinking behavior of respondents with abstinence backgrounds. From their results, it seems clear that the focus on "personal-effects" on the part of the drinker as contrasted with a more normative orientation is associated with problem drinking. An extensive statement by Mulford and Miller with regard to their findings reflects some points of convergence between their viewpoint and our own.

[7] Skolnick's data were derived from original data gathered by Straus and Bacon for the college drinking study. The reader should note a possible objection associated with the groups on which *problem drinking* rates are based. For example, it has been pointed out that comparisons of alcoholism rates can be variously interpreted, depending upon whether the *base* of the comparison is the *total* membership of the two groups, or solely on the *drinkers* in the two groups. It should be clear, however, that (1) we are not speaking of *alcoholism* rates, but *problem drinking* rates; and (2) that we are primarily concerned with comparing alcohol pathology rates in different groups *for those who do drink.* For a discussion of these points, see Skolnick (27, p. 460).

The heavier consumption by the personal-effects drinker may also be a reflection of the *relative absence of social norms* in the situations where he does much of his drinking. Persons who drink primarily for social effects may be presumed to do most of their drinking in more intimate group situations, involving family and friends, where restrictive norms are relatively effective; although, of course, the party norms may permit considerable latitude. The personal-effects drinker who attends parties probably is the one most likely to exceed the party norms, but as he does so repeatedly, he may find that he is not welcome and is then "forced" to do more of his drinking alone and in public places where there is relative freedom from intimate group-norm restrictions.

Finally, the heavy drinking of the individual who is drinking mainly for the personal effects of alcohol may also reflect the likelihood that he does not carry in his mind a conception of *how many drinks* it takes to attain the desired effect, especially since such *prescriptions* are presumably not general in our culture . . . (21, pp. 276-277).[8]

We can conclude from the above studies that normative systems play a role in the consumption of alcoholic beverages, and that pathological reactions to drinking tend to be greater for certain ascetic Protestant and Mormon groups, as compared with other religious groups. We would hold, in general, that pathological drinking behavior is associated with a relative absence of directives for the act of drinking alcoholic beverages itself. The important question then is: What is there about the nature of the normative systems of the ascetic Protestant and Mormon groups that predisposes their deviants to greater pathological reactions and, consequently, their structure to greater strain?

Significance of Prescriptive and Proscriptive Dimension

We have indicated above that there is an absence of directives regarding drinking behavior among the ascetic Protestant and Mormon groups. In contrast to the prescriptive norms associated with drinking by Jews, for example, the ascetic Protestant and Mormon norms may be characterized as primarily *proscriptive*.

---

[8] See also, Allardt, *et al.* (1), which provides additional data to support the hypothesis about the conditions associated with relative lack of drinking norms and our discussion below.

Total abstinence is the norm for these groups. Hence, deviation from the abstinence pattern, even in what is ordinarily recognized as socially approved drinking in the larger society, e.g., before dinner, at parties, and like occasions, is associated with an almost complete absence of directives. As Straus and Bacon have pointed out in discussing the drinking behavior of Mormons, "If drinking behavior is adopted, variation must be the rule since there is no norm. Extremes are likely since the behavior itself represents rejection of social rules" (31, p. 144).[9]

Jewish drinking, as Snyder has shown, is patterned by an elaborate system of explicit directives as to what, when, where, with whom, how much, and why one is expected to consume alcoholic beverages. The norm is predominantly *prescriptive* in nature, and deviation from the drinking norms is associated with gradual and predictable patterns of deviant behavior. Thus Snyder's statistics show that tendencies to alcohol pathology increase in "step-like" fashion from Orthodox Jewish drinking, which is associated with the relative absence of signs of pathology, to the Reform and Secular drinking pattern in which pathology is relatively high. Nevertheless, the highest rate still tends to remain lower than rates for the Protestant group (29, p. 197).

We would hold that it is inherent in the nature of the two sets of norms, the ascetic Protestant and Mormon norms, on the one hand, and the Jewish norms, on the other, that they predispose group members to different kinds of deviant reactions. The consequences of the differential deviant reactions is differential strain for the two subsystems. Alcohol pathology represents not only personal problems, but problems for the group as well. The various efforts to cope with problems of alcohol

---

[9] Skolnick (27, p. 265) makes the point that extreme drinking behavior of those exposed to abstinence teachings is a result of another norm derived from descriptions of the behavior of extreme drinkers, i.e., "the horrible example." Although we see the virtue of his notion of a "negative" role model, we would hold that theoretically, at least, a distinction must be made between role models—both positive and negative—role expectations, and norms. Thus, unless the expected behavior of the role model becomes generalized to the larger group, i.e., becomes an explicit, shared norm, it remains external to a given social system. In the case of drinking norms, Skolnick's observations need not lead to a rejection of our own explanation, since the negative role model, as we see it, may represent an *additional* factor rather than an exclusive causal factor. However, the reader should keep in mind the fact that these notions—both Skolnick's and our own—represent hypotheses rather than conclusive generalizations.

on the part of different groups—governmental agencies, private welfare organizations, and religious groups, to name only a few —suggest that strain exists not only for the subsystems in which they occur, but for larger social systems as well. In general, it can be noted that at least four types of group reactions to system strain can be isolated as indices of the extent of perceived threat to the system or its members. Group reactions may take the form of: (1) *Retrenchment,* in which all deviants are cast out of the group, leaving only a small hard core of adherents; (2) *Regeneration,* in which there is an attempt to revitalize the norm through a cultural renaissance; (3) *Rational-Scientific Innovation,* which includes efforts on the part of persons outside of the group as well as enlightened group participants to adapt new normative patterns to the pre-existing cultural system; and (4) *Permissiveness,* which involves individual determination of limits.[10] Examples of these types of reactions may be found reflected in behavior associated with deviant drinking activities. Retrenchment has manifested itself in the strong reactions to public intoxication on the part of the Chinese in the United States, who, in the past, forced alcoholics and problem drinkers

[10] Merton and Parsons, it should be noted, have focused on deviant reactions to structured strain. Merton's typology is concerned with structured individual reactions to a disjunction between norms and success goals in American Society. Parsons also deals with individual deviant reactions in terms of motivational analysis. The typology presented here differs from both Merton and Parsons in the following respects: (1) our focus is on *collective* reactions rather than *individual* reactions; (2) this typology is concerned with *normative* reactions to strain rather than *deviant* reactions to strain; and (3) whereas Merton's focus is on *chronic* strain, i.e., a persistent element in the system, the above typology, at least in this context, is concerned with *acute* strain. Adding to the above approaches Williams' concept of "patterned norm evasion," we may derive the following classification of approaches to reactions to strain:

Deviant-Individual[a]	Normative-Individual[b]
Deviant-Group[c]	Normative-Group[d]

[a] See, for example, Robert K. Merton (17); Talcott Parsons (23, Ch. 7); Albert K. Cohen (11).

[b] This category is perhaps the most prevalent in the sociological literature. It is characterized by the following sequence: deviant act—group reaction—individual conformity. One of many examples may be found in Fritz J. Roethlisberger and William J. Dickson's description of "binging" as a negative sanction for non-conformity (26).

[c] See, for example, Robin M. Williams, Jr. (36). Chapter 10 is devoted in its entirety to norm evasion.

[d] In addition to our independently conceived notions concerning normative group reactions to strain, Howard Becker's posthumously published paper deals with similar types of problems (4).

to return to the Chinese mainland if they failed to mend their ways, at the same time reinforcing the norms of individual responsibility to the group (14).[11] Regeneration is reflected in the abstinence movement in the United States. The rational-scientific innovation reaction is exemplified in Mulford and Miller's suggestion that prescriptive drinking norms should replace proscriptive drinking norms for the ascetic Protestant groups in the United States (21, p. 498). And the persistence of patternless drinking in a good many American social contexts is a manifestation of permissiveness.[12]

A Typology of Norms

We have suggested above that the proscriptive and prescriptive dimensions of norms do make it possible for us to attain greater understanding of the dynamics of social pathology. We have, up to this point, discussed the two dimensions in very broad terms. To what extent can we specify the nature of these dimensions and place them in a context of social system analysis? With this perspective in view, norms may be classified ideal-typically in terms of the following descriptive characteristics which have emerged from our review of the various studies cited above: (1) the degree of elasticity; (2) the degree of elaboration; (3) the degree of pervasiveness; and (4) the degree of functional interrelatedness.

Table 1 describes those aspects of norms which make them classifiable as either proscriptive or prescriptive.[13] Table 2 shows

[11] In the general context of group reactions to system strain, see Anthony F. C. Wallace (34).

[12] Our usage of "permissiveness," or individual determination of limits, represents what might otherwise be called unresolved *anomie*. However, since the group reactions described above are in effect reactions to an anomic condition, we have attempted to avoid using *anomie* for purposes of clarity. The significance of *permissiveness* as both a norm and as a type of *laissez faire* reaction is dealt with below.

[13] In an initial classification of norms for general purposes, for example, norms may be classified as being predominantly proscriptive or prescriptive according to whether they enjoin or prohibit behavior. For a more complete understanding of the dynamics of normative behavior, especially with reference to problems of social control, a more intensive analysis of the norms themselves is necessary. Our hypothetical scheme, it should be noted, is derived from: (1) inspection of the various monographs cited in Table 2; (2) inspection of unpublished data on the Chinese; and (3) participant observation in various subcultural contexts.

TABLE 1.—*Qualitative Characteristics of Prescriptive and Proscriptive Norms*

Characteristic of Norm	Proscriptive	Prescriptive
Elasticity	Inflexible: Behavior is defined as either compliant or deviant and there are no directives for action	Flexible: Behavior is defined in degree of conformity and directives for how to act are explicit
Elaboration	No ritual, no embellishment associated with act	Great deal of embellishment in ritualized and symbolic acts
Pervasiveness	Focus on a specific act applying to any and all contexts	Focus on a variety of similar acts in specified contexts
Functional interrelatedness	Norm tends to have few or no convergences with other norms in the larger system	Norm tends to converge with other norms in the larger system

how these factors are related, by way of illustration, to drinking behavior. The extent to which these factors, in varying degree, manifest themselves in given normative systems represents, in our judgment, a measure of the relative degree of predisposition to normative mal-integration with respect to a given norm.

The Normative and the Factual

As we have suggested above, the over-all effectiveness of norms in the process of system maintenance can be attributed to at least two characteristics: (1) the extent to which both internal and external sanctions effectively direct the behavior of group members; and (2) the nature of the norms themselves. It is the latter to which we have addressed ourselves in this paper. Although the two are undoubtedly related, we would hold that the qualitative nature of the norm is analytically distinct from the strength of sanctions attached to the norm. Thus, whether controls are internalized or externalized, or whether the sanctioning agents are informally or formally designated does not concern us here. The above data are consistent with our hypothesis that predominantly proscriptive norms are more likely than predominantly prescriptive norms to lead to extreme degrees of pathological reactions when deviation occurs.

TABLE 2.—*Drinking Norms for Selected Groups, by Qualitative Characteristics and Prescriptive-Proscriptive Dimension*

	Elasticity	Elaboration	Pervasiveness	Functional Interrelatedness	
Prescriptive					
	++	++	++	++	Jews[1]
	+	+	+	++	Italians[2]
	−	−	−	+	Mormons[3]
Proscriptive					

[1] For an elaborate description of Orthodox Jewish drinking patterns, see Charles R. Snyder (28).

[2] Wine is viewed by Italians as both a food and as a beverage. It does not, however, embody the sacred element associated with Orthodox Jewish drinking. Italians do not recite blessings over the wine. See, for examples, Phyllis Williams and Robert Straus (35); and Giorgio Lolli, *et al.* (16).

[3] References to Mormon drinking may be found in Robert Straus and Selden Bacon (31).

It is possible to treat the whole matter of the relationship between norms and social pathology in terms of the relationship between the normative and factual orders. While we have indicated that our focus is on the qualitative nature of the norms themselves, our ultimate concern is with social control and group integration. The normative-factual orders lend themselves to analysis within the framework of the prescriptive-proscriptive dimension. Thus, one could interpret our discussion as an attempt to explore the consequences of situations in which the normative order and the factual order are more or less convergent or divergent. Rather than assume that it is simply the divergence between these two orders which is primarily productive of strain, we would hold that it is the quality of the normative order which determines the extent of strain in this context. The following suggestive scheme provides an illustration of a possible systematic approach to these dimensions. Thus, the following table describes a factual order, given a certain prescriptive-proscriptive normative order. The examples represent approximate empirical referents with regard to drinking norms.

NORMS

	Jewish Italian	Mormon Methodist
Normative Order	Highly Prescriptive	Highly Proscriptive
Factual Order	Deviation	Deviation
Level of Pathology	Low Level of Pathology	High Level of Pathology (Anomie)

As this preliminary scheme suggests, the following propositions can be formulated with respect to the aspects of norms referred to above:

1. Given a situation in which there is *proscription* on the *normative* level and *deviation* on the factual level, pathology will be high.

2. Given a situation in which there is *prescription* on the *normative* level and *deviation* on the factual level, pathology will be low.

The above discussion implies that under certain normative conditions behavior which deviated from the norm does not threaten the system of order, while under other conditions it does. It should be added that the present analysis does not include a discussion of the relative effectiveness of each type of norm under conditions of normative integration without strain. Presumably, pathology is minimized as a result of conformity to both the predominantly proscriptive and prescriptive norms referred to above. Stated as a third proposition:

3. Given a situation in which there is *either* prescription or *proscription* on the *normative* level and *conformity* on the *factual* level, pathology will be *low*.

Thus, this approach is systematic and directly lends itself to empirical analysis.

Permissiveness and Anomie

A third general aspect, to which we referred only briefly, is permissiveness. Although the evidence with respect to this pattern or lack of pattern is scanty, permissiveness appears to be characteristic of periods of normative transformation. Thus, in the United States the shift from proscription among Protestant abstentionist groups *without the provision of a corresponding set of clear directives* for drinking behavior appears to represent a period of *anomic* behavior which will, in time, become organized into a new pattern. In this context, directives tend to be vague injunctions to avoid immoderate drinking and to "stay out of trouble." That this condition may persist over very long periods of time without becoming organized, thus enhancing the anomic condition and consequent deviant behavior, is illustrated by studies of Finnish drinking.

In Finland, where religious groups preach proscription and where the sale and distribution of alcohol is carefully controlled, the arrests for drunkenness rate in 1959 was 72.0 per 1,000 inhabitants compared with 26.0 for Norway, 17.2 for Sweden and 6.3 for Denmark. Finland and Norway, it should be noted, are countries which had prohibition laws following World War I in contrast to Sweden which rejected prohibition as a solution to drinking problems and Denmark which did not even entertain the question of prohibition (6). Assuming that the behaviors associated with efforts to solve problems reflects underlying differences in normative orientations, it seems clear that arrests for drunkenness as a reflection of deviant behavior are higher where a background of proscription is greater.

Straus and Bacon (31), and Mulford and Miller (21), as we noted above, held that when those who were reared as abstainers drink there are no directives for how, when, how much and with whom to drink. Allardt *et al.* (1) explored the intensity of attitude toward drinking in his Finnish sample and found what he described as an intensive negative attitude toward drinking (proscriptive) as contrasted with "an ambivalent one."

> The finding agrees very well with the intuitive picture one gets of the attitudes toward drinking in Finnish society. There are certain people with a strong negative attitude towards drinking, while most other people may show a very positive verbal attitude towards drinking and towards the functions of drinking, but this attitude is not consistent, and it is often expressed in a jocular way (1, p. 26).

Permissive attitudes toward drinking in Finland are also associated with acceptance of the value of occasional unrestrained drinking, suggesting still another link between permissiveness and deviance (1, p. 28). Thus the study of drinking in Finnish culture lends support to our original assumption regarding permissiveness and deviance.

We suggested above that permissiveness represents a condition of unresolved anomie. Recent research in the area of deviant behavior has focused on Merton's hypothesis that strains in social systems lead to deviant behavior and consequent anomie (17, 18, 29). More specifically, in American society the discrepancy between the American desire for success and differential opportunity for the attainment of success goals leads to deviant reactions and, ultimately, to anomie.

Although a thorough discussion of Merton's approach to anomie is beyond our primary concern here, it is well to comment briefly at this point since permissiveness and anomie represent aspects of the same phenomenon.

Our usage of anomie suggests that the source of the weakening of social controls on drinking is a reflection of general societal transformation related to industrialization and urbanization which were the foci of attention of the sociologists to whom we referred at the outset—Durkheim, Tönnies, Redfield and Becker.

Given the kind of rapid transformation which characterizes the responses of subsystems to increase in population, change in type of production and modification of family functions, to suggest only a few consequences of industrialization and urbanization, there is a simultaneous change in group attitudes toward the normative order. Thus, although there still tends to be an awareness of the rules limiting and directing man's desires, there is somewhat less certainty regarding whether or not adherence to these norms should be enforced. As social structures undergo change, so do normative systems. During periods of uncertainty a wider range of deviance is tolerated in the form of permissiveness, which, as we suggested above, allows the person rather than the group to determine the range of appropriate conduct. While all societies and groups must provide for flexibility in order to persist, periods during which permissiveness predominates do not always result in a reinforcement of the original normative system, as we noted above. Thus the uncertainty, i.e., anomie, associated with some of these periods is often the prelude to the emergence of new *normative patterns*.

With respect to drinking behavior in particular, however, the flexibility associated with change, if we are correct in our analysis of deviance, has more profound effects in systems undergoing change from proscription to other normative forms.

Similar to Merton's approach which deals directly with the group's response to deviance is our concern with what we have called permissiveness.

Recently several analysts of deviant drinking behavior, following Merton, have suggested that problem drinking represents a *retreatist* reaction to the strain associated with the discrepancy between success goals and opportunity to attain them. Thus the retreatist, having failed to reach his goal, withdraws from the race and turns to excessive drinking and, finally, to problem drinking (29, pp. 202-205). This in turn leads to more deviant drinking on the part of others who observe the toleration of deviance. Given the paucity of empirical data on this aspect of anomie, it is not possible to draw any conclusions at this time. If, however, patterns of deviant drinking can be linked to more general societal processes and their impact on normative systems, then our objectives in this paper will have been served.

We have suggested that proscriptive and prescriptive dimensions are to be found in the analysis of other normative systems and data other than those dealing with alcohol pathology alone. We would suggest that sexual behavior may be a fruitful area of investigation.[14] Some specific examples of other problems that would seem to lend themselves to this type of analysis would be studies of norms proscribing aggression among Jews; norms proscribing female premarital intercourse among Italians; and norms proscribing the acquisition of material luxuries among the Older Order Amish.

Finally, although we have abstracted norm qualities as our focus of attention and hold that they are an essential aspect of the processes enhancing and inhibiting deviance and pathology, we do not feel that this approach is alone sufficient to understand these phenomena. Thus the subsequent experiences of persons reared in proscriptive cultures and subcultures play an important role in decisions to conform or deviate. Ernest Campbell (7, pp. 406-407)[15] in a recent study, for example, presents data which indicate that college students who have internalized proscriptive drinking norms are more likely to form peer group associations that encourage personal abstinence; and non-drinkers are less likely to pledge fraternities and sororities than drinkers. The study of the effects of drinking norms on behavior, then, also provides entree into the sphere of group formation studies. In short, the study of drinking behavior is not only significant because it contributes directly to the solution of social problems, but also for its contribution to the understanding of basic societal processes.

REFERENCES

1. ALLARDT, E., T. MARKANEN, and M. TAKALA. *Drinking and Drinkers*. Helsinki: The Finnish Foundation for Alcohol Studies, 1963.
2. BALES, ROBERT F. "Cultural Differences in Rates of Alcoholism," *Quarterly Journal of Studies on Alcohol*, 6: 480-499, 1946.
3. BECKER, HOWARD. "Ionia and Athens: Studies in Secularization." Unpublished Ph.D. dissertation, University of Chicago, 1930.
4. BECKER, HOWARD. "Normative Reactions to Normlessness," *American Sociological Review*, 25: 803-810, 1960.

[14] Christensen has noted the possible connection between proscription and extreme reactions, and has suggested that sex behavior and drinking behavior may be analogous in this respect. See Harold T. Christensen (8, 9).

[15] See chapter 5 in this volume.

5. BESHERS, JAMES M. "Pragmatic Criteria in Typology Construction." Paper read at the annual meeting of the American Sociological Association, New York City, August, 1960.

6. BRUUN, K., and R. HAUGE. *Drinking of Northern Youth: A Cross-Cultural Survey.* Helsinki: The Finnish Foundation for Alcohol Studies, 1963.

7. CAMPBELL, ERNEST. "The Internalization of Moral Norms," *Sociometry,* 27: 391-412, 1964.

8. CHRISTENSEN, HAROLD T. "Cultural Relativism and Premarital Sex Norms," *American Sociological Review,* 25: 31-39, 1960.

9. CHRISTENSEN, HAROLD T. "Child Spacing Analysis Via Record Linkage," *Marriage and Family Living,* 25: 272-280, 1963.

10. CLINARD, MARSHALL (ed.). *Deviant Behavior and Anomie.* New York: The Free Press, 1964.

11. COHEN, ALBERT K. "The Study of Social Disorganization and Deviant Behavior," in ROBERT K. MERTON, *et al.* (eds.), *Sociology Today.* New York: Basic Books, 1959.

12. DURKHEIM, EMILE. *The Division of Labor in Society* (1893), translated by George Simpson. New York: Macmillan, 1933.

13. FREEDMAN, RONALD, *et al. Principles of Sociology.* New York: Henry Holt, 1952.

14. LEE, ROSE HUM, and EPHRAIM H. MIZRUCHI. "A Study of Drinking Behavior and Attitudes toward Alcohol of the Chinese in the United States." Unpublished manuscript.

15. LEMERT, EDWIN M. *Social Pathology.* New York: McGraw-Hill, 1951.

16. LOLLI, GIORGIO, *et al. Alcohol in Italian Culture.* Glencoe, Illinois: Free Press, 1958.

17. MERTON, ROBERT K. "Social Structure and Anomie," in *Social Theory and Social Structure.* Glencoe, Illinois: Free Press, 1957.

18. MIZRUCHI, EPHRAIM H. *Success and Opportunity.* New York: The Free Press, 1964.

19. MORRIS, RICHARD T. "A Typology of Norms," *American Sociological Review,* 21: 610-613, 1956.

20. MULFORD, HAROLD A., and DONALD A. MILLER. "Drinking Behavior Related to Definitions of Alcohol: A Report of Research in Progress," *American Sociological Review,* 24: 385-289, 1959.

21. MULFORD, HAROLD A., and DONALD A. MILLER. "Drinking in Iowa." Five articles appearing in separate numbers of Volume 21 (1960), *Quarterly Journal of Studies on Alcohol.*

22. PARSONS, TALCOTT. *The Structure of Social Action.* New York: McGraw-Hill, 1937.

23. PARSONS, TALCOTT. *The Social System.* Glencoe, Illinois: The Free Press, 1951.

24. PARSONS, TALCOTT. "The Social System," in TALCOTT PARSONS and EDWARD A. SHILS (eds.), *Toward a General Theory of Action.* Cambridge: Harvard University Press, 1951.
25. REDFIELD, ROBERT. *The Folk Culture of Yucatan.* Chicago: University of Chicago Press, 1941.
26. ROETHLISBERGER, FRITZ J., and WILLIAM J. DICKSON. *Management and the Worker.* Cambridge: Harvard University Press, 1939.
27. SKOLNICK, JEROME H. "Religious Affiliation and Drinking Behavior," *Quarterly Journal of Studies on Alcohol,* 19: 452-470, 1958.
28. SNYDER, CHARLES R. *Alcohol and the Jews.* Glencoe, Illinois: The Free Press, 1958.
29. SNYDER, CHARLES R. "Inebriety, Alcoholism and Anomie," in MARSHALL CLINARD (ed.), *Deviant Behavior and Anomie.* New York: The Free Press, 1964.
30. SOROKIN, PITIRIM. *Society, Culture and Personality.* New York: Harper, 1947.
31. STRAUS, ROBERT, and SELDEN D. BACON. *Drinking in College.* New Haven: Yale University Press, 1954.
32. SUMNER, WILLIAM GRAHAM. *Folkways.* Boston: Ginn, 1906.
33. TÖNNIES, FERDINAND. *Gemeinschaft und Gesellschaft* (1887), translated by CHARLES P. LOOMIS as *Community and Society.* East Lansing, Michigan: Michigan State University Press, 1957.
34. WALLACE, ANTHONY F. C. "Revitalization Movements," in SEYMOUR M. LIPSET and NEIL J. SMELSER (eds.), *Sociology, the Progress of a Decade.* Englewood Cliffs, New Jersey: Prentice-Hall, Inc., 1961.
35. WILLIAMS, PHYLLIS, and ROBERT STRAUS. "Drinking Patterns of Italians in New Haven," *Quarterly Journal of Studies on Alcohol,* 11 (1950), 4 papers.
36. WILLIAMS, ROBIN M., JR. *American Society.* New York: Knopf, 1960 revision.

Chapter 11

DRINKING REGULATIONS OF COLLEGES AND NATIONAL COLLEGE FRATERNITIES*

University of Georgia

ONE ASPECT of formal organizations usually of great interest to sociologists is the set of organizational norms governing behavior of members (1-4). Yet we know almost nothing about the organizational norms regulating the drinking behavior of college students. Perhaps this reflects a lack of interest in academic organizations, or perhaps it reflects the greater fascination of more esoteric and extreme aspects of drinking behavior, such as skid row drinking, rather than the much more frequent and commonplace patterns of alcohol consumption among collegians. Whatever the explanation, the fact is that we are almost totally ignorant of those organizational rules that deal with college students' drinking activities. Our ignorance in this regard is especially interesting insofar as college students have typically been favorite subjects for research on a wide variety of topics. Our ignorance is all the more interesting in light of a recent study by Gusfield (5) that stresses the importance of social context, of which norms are a major segment, for understanding drinking among collegians and in light of the sizeable proportion of college students who participate in this behavior (6).

Data on drinking norms are needed. The purpose of the research reported here is to describe and suggest an interpretation

* I am indebted to the National Interfraternity Conference and the National Association of Student Personnel Administrators for access to data collected by their organizations and for financial support from the Interfraternity Research and Advisory Council. Partial support from a Public Health Service research grant (MH-2185) is also acknowledged.

of two dimensions of formal norms governing collegiate drinking behavior found in two types of formal organizations, colleges (universities) and national fraternity organizations. The two dimensions of the drinking rules in these types of organizations with which we shall be concerned are the extent to which these rules are possessed and their direction (i.e., whether they proscribe or permit consumption of alcoholic beverages).

Methods

The Data

The data to be considered come from two sources. The first consists of two very similar sets of mailed questionnaires distributed by the National Interfraternity Conference during late summer and early fall of 1963. One set went to colleges and universities which at that time had social fraternities affiliated with them. In nearly all cases these questionnaires were filled out by a Dean of Men or a Dean of Students. The other set was sent to national fraternity organizations which were members of the National Interfraternity Conference. These were completed by the national executive secretary or his equivalent in each organization. Both these questionnaires elicited, among other things, information concerning whether each organization possessed formal statutory provisions in regard to the use of alcoholic beverages by students or fraternity members and, if so, the nature of these provisions. Some information on organizational size was also requested, such as the number of chapters in each national fraternity and the number of fraternity chapters located at a given school. The second source of data was *American Colleges and Universities* (7) from which additional information about size as well as other attributes of the school was obtained.

Usable questionnaires were returned by 62 per cent (N=44) of the national fraternity organizations and 58 per cent (N=242) of the schools. A comparison of certain characteristics of the two samples—the number of chapters in each of the national fraternities and how many chapters of different fraternities were located on each campus; the number of male and female students; type of financial support (public, private-church, private-non-church); and amount of tuition—with those of the non-participating national fraternities and schools revealed no significant differences. Thus, both samples seem representative of their respective populations. With reference to the schools, however, it should be noted that, although this sample may be representative of those schools having social fraternities affiliated with them, some types of academic institutions were systematically excluded. For example, institutions in which the student body is primarily female or Negro are not represented at all; and probably those smaller schools with relatively low tuition as well as certain types of church-related schools are underrepresented. Hence, generalization of the findings to be presented here to all colleges or universities in the United States is definitely not warranted.

Measures of the Two Dimensions of Organizational Drinking Norms

Extent of Possession. For the schools the index of the extent to which formal drinking rules are possessed is based on the number of key words relating to drinking contained in each school's description of its statutory provisions. First, the number of times that each school mentioned the following four types of words was counted:

1. Words which describe WHO is being regulated in connection with drinking, such as students, fraternities, social organizations, or school-sponsored groups.
2. Words which describe what sort of BEVERAGE is being regulated, such as beer, wine, ale, hard liquor, mixed drinks, or just "alcoholic beverages."
3. Words which describe what sort of BEHAVIOR is being regulated, such as consumption, display of alcoholic beverages in bottles, storage in fraternity facilities, purchase by school organizations, serving, possession, or disturbance of others while drinking.
4. Words which describe WHERE behavior is being regulated, such as in fraternity houses, in dormitories, on campus, off campus, at school-sponsored occasions, or in private student residences.

These four totals were then summed, the grand total representing an index of the extent to which each school possessed formal norms concerning drinking. Two examples of rules about drinking from colleges in the sample studied illustrate how the index works. In one school the rule reads "No *intoxicating beverages* shall be *served* by *any student organization* at *any function* regardless of where it is held." Italics indicate the key words used to arrive at a score of 4. In another school the formal drinking rule is even more detailed: *"Possession* or *drinking* of *alcoholic* or *malt beverages* in *fraternity houses* or *premises* or at any *official fraternity function* constitutes a violation of college regulations." Again, italics indicate the key words used to arrive at an index score of 7.

The index of formal rules about drinking had to be modified for use in classifying the rules of national fraternities since 23 of the 44 fraternities had no relevant statutory provision. An additional five noted nothing more than "Each chapter will be governed by the rules and regulations of its respective college or university." Even among the remaining 16 fraternities use of the index was limited in that very few had rules which said much more than "Drinking is/is not permitted on fraternity premises," thus decreasing the capacity of this index to distinguish adequately among them. Hence, a more simple procedure was used to index the extent to which national fraternities possessed norms regulating drinking. These organizations were split into two groups, those which did and those which did not possess any statutory provisions concerning drinking. Although this procedure is more crude than the one used to measure this dimension for the schools, it takes advantage of the available data on the possession of formal drinking norms among national fraternity organizations.

Direction. The index of the direction of organizational rules governing drinking was based on the same general procedure for both the national fraternities and the schools. Essentially, this procedure consisted of coding the rules dealing with drinking into two categories: (1) *definitely prohibitory* e.g., those rules prohibiting the drinking behavior in terms of consumption, possession, serving, storage, ungentlemanly conduct, etc., with no exception mentioned; and (2) *not definitely prohibitory* e.g., rules in which (a) exceptions to the prohibition(s) were mentioned, (b) the behavior in question was discouraged but not definitely prohibited, or (c) the behavior was permitted outright.

Most fraternities, as previously noted, had so few formal drinking rules that each could be placed directly into one of these two categories. However, a different strategy had to be adopted for the schools since most of them had multiple rules, with some of the rules of each school being of the "definitely prohibitory" variety and others falling into the "not definitely prohibitory" class. For each school with multiple drinking rules a score of 1 was assigned if a rule was classified as "definitely prohibitory" and a score of 0 being assigned if one of the rules was "not definitely prohibitory." These scores were summed and a mean, ranging from zero to one, computed for each school. This mean is the index of the over-all direction of each school's body of rules dealing with drinking.

Findings

Two sets of data relating to the national fraternities' and schools' statutory provisions on drinking will be described. The first set focuses on the extent to which each of the two types of organizations possessed drinking rules and the direction of the rules they possessed. Attention will be given to over-all variation *between* schools and national fraternities on these two dimensions of drinking norms. Then, the direction and extent of possession of statutory drinking rules as they vary by organizational size *within* each of the two types of organizations will be examined.

Extent of possession. Almost all of the 242 schools in this study (92 per cent) had formal rules regulating drinking. The 44 national fraternities were significantly less likely (48 per cent) to have such rules. Moreover, when rules about drinking were found at all, schools were significantly more likely than national fraternities to have extensive statutory provisions. In terms of the index of extensity, schools had a mean of 12 specifications of key provisions in their drinking rules in contrast to a mean of 2.7 for the national fraternities. Fraternal organizations apparently rely on informal policies rather than formal statutes. All of the 23 national fraternity organizations which reported no statutory provision governing drinking did claim to have an unwritten but understood policy. Perhaps the most striking thing about these policies is their unanimity in deferring to the drinking rules of the host schools. Almost all the national organizations (82 per cent) made it clear that the regulations of the particular schools at which their chapters are located are considered to be a major part of their own rules or policies on drinking.

The comment of one national secretary in describing his national organization's rules is typical: "If the school says 'NO,' we say no! If the school openly or covertly allows drinking, we do not attempt to stop it. . . ." In fact, for a number of national fraternities in our sample (33 per cent) this is their rule or policy in its entirety.

In brief, then, the national fraternity organizations show less of an inclination to have statutory rules concerning drinking than do the schools. Fraternities rely instead on informal "policies" and both their policies and rules are permeated with explicit recognition of the host schools' regulations.

Direction. For the 30 national fraternities who specify their rules or policy in regard to drinking as something other than "the school's rules are our rules," formal rules about drinking tend to be permissive. Among the 16 fraternities having statutory provisions almost two out of three (62.5 per cent) do not definitely prohibit use. Of the 12 with informal policies, only one definitely prohibits use.

The rules of schools are in strange contrast to those of national fraternities. The mean index of definite prohibition scores for all schools was .67, with a score of 1 indicating maximum prohibition. For the sixteen national fraternities with formal rules, the comparable index score was .38. Thus, the general picture projected by an analysis of the data on the variation between fraternities' and schools' drinking rules is one of opposing images: the national fraternities are permissive, the schools prohibitive; the national fraternities have few such rules, the schools many.

Variation within Schools and National Fraternities by Size

Analysis of the variations in drinking rules within the schools and national fraternity organizations in terms of extensity and direction is centered around the variable of size. This is the case primarily because size was the only organizational attribute on which data were available for both schools and fraternities. Also, certain organizational literature (3, 4) as well as an essay by Simmel (8) suggests its connection with organizational norms, especially the extent of such norms.

For the national fraternities, the number of chapters of each organization served as a measure of size.[1] Three separate indices of size were used for the schools: the number of female students, the number of male students, and the number of social fraternities affiliated with each school. Since the number of students in a school correlated highly with the number of male students (+.95) and since the possibility of variations of drinking rules in relation to the male/female ratio of a school warranted exploration, two measures of school size were used. The size of a school in terms of the number of national fraternities operating on its campus was also explored.

Extent of Possession of Drinking Norms by Size. Using a sociological rule of thumb that the larger the organization, the greater its need for and possession of formal rules, one might expect that formal regulations on drinking would be most evident in the largest national fraternity organizations. The data in Table 1 lend only partial support to this notion. While formal rules on drinking were reported by more of the national fraternities in the two larger groups than in the smaller one, such rules are most common among the *medium-sized* national fraternities. Although the difference between the medium and large national fraternity organizations is not statistically significant, neither is the difference between the large and small ones. It seems, then, that small national fraternities are the least likely to have statutory provisions on drinking and medium-sized na-

TABLE 1.—*National Fraternities' Possession of Statutory Provisions on Drinking, by Size*

Size by Number of Chapters	Statutory Provision Present		Statutory Provision Absent		
	%	N	%	N	Total
Small (11-38)	20	3	80	12	15
Medium (39-74)	71	10	29	4	14
Large (75-200)	53	8	47	7	15

χ^2 (total) = 7.964, 2df, P<.02.
χ^2 (small and medium groups only) = 6.044, 1df, P<.02 (corrected for continuity).
All other comparisons non-significant.

[1] Number of chapters and total membership of national fraternities were highly correlated (+.87); since membership ranged from 3,600 to over 114,000, number of chapters was easier to manipulate in the analysis of data.

tional fraternities the most likely, with the larger fraternities falling in between.

Although the use of multiple measures of size complicates the interpretation of the data on size and possession of formal drinking norms among the schools, the various measures cumulatively reinforce the contention that the largest organizations tend to have the greatest number of drinking regulations. The data in Table 2, in which schools are also controlled by major source of financial support,[2] show a gross relationship between size of school and the extent of drinking rules. If the measures of size are dichotomized rather than quartiled, in all nine instances the

TABLE 2.—*Mean Extensity of Formal Drinking Rules, by Source of Support and Size*

Publicly Supported Schools (N=111)

Quartile*	Females†	Males†	Fraternities†
1 (smaller)	8.2	8.8	7.7
2	10.4	11.9	10.6
3	18.2	12.0	15.5
4 (larger)	15.2	20.0	18.4

Privately Supported Schools (N=49)

Quartile*	Females	Males	Fraternities
1 (smaller)	12.7	12.5	14.3
2	11.7	12.3	10.0
3	12.5	12.4	12.3
4 (larger)	13.4	13.7	13.1

Church-Supported Schools (N=56)

Quartile*	Females†	Males	Fraternities
1 (smaller)	10.2	5.9	7.3
2	5.7	9.4	6.8
3	6.1	11.8	15.8
4 (larger)	13.2	8.1	10.0

* The quartiles of the three measures of size are based on the distribution *within* each of the three types of schools. This procedure was necessary in order to obtain quartile groups with N's large enough for meaningful analysis.

† The two most extreme differences between the quartile means are significant at least the .05 level, two-tailed t-test.

[2] Preliminary analysis indicated that publicly supported schools tended to be larger and privately supported schools smaller. The distinctive pattern of relationships found in church-supported schools appeared to warrant retaining this category also.

larger schools exhibit significantly more extensive drinking regulations than the smaller schools. Even when quartiled, in five of nine comparisons the largest schools have the most extensive formal drinking rules. However, in only two of the nine comparisons is there a monotonic increase in the extent of drinking regulations from the first through the fourth quartile. This suggests that, although some relationship between school size and number of drinking rules exists, factors in addition to organizational size must be considered in the explanation of a school's drinking regulations.

Also interesting to note in connection with Table 2 is the extent to which the relationship between size and number of drinking norms varies from one type of school to another. The expected relationship is found among the publicly supported schools, is almost completely absent in the privately supported schools, and appears to be almost without pattern among the church schools. Thus, the relationship between organizational size and the possession of drinking rules would seem in part to be a function of the organizational context in which it occurs.

Direction of Drinking Norms by Size. Most national fraternity organizations studied, if they had statutory provisions or informal policy concerning drinking at all, were permissive. Among those which had statutory provisions, prohibition of use is related to organizational size. The smallest national fraternities appear to be the least prohibitive, the middle-sized ones the most prohibitive, with prohibitiveness higher among the middle-sized than among the large national fraternities. Whether a fraternity had any rules or informal policy regulating drinking also exhibited this same relationship to size, as noted earlier.

The data on size and direction of drinking regulations among the schools repeat the pattern noted earlier. As in the national fraternities, the middle-sized schools are the most prohibitive (Table 3). For example, within each category of school differentiated by source of support, the second quartile in five of nine instances contains those schools which are most prohibitive. However, the similarity between the schools and fraternities ends here. Whereas among the national fraternities the smallest organizations were the most permissive, among the schools the *largest* are the most permissive. If, for example, distributions by size are dichotomized within the type of support categories, in six of nine instances the larger schools have the most permissive

TABLE 3.—*Prohibitiveness of Drinking Regulations, by Type of School Support and Size*

Publicly Supported Schools (N=107)			
Quartile*	Females	Males†	Fraternities†
1 (smaller)	.75	.65	.69
2	.76	.82	.80
3	.66	.67	.65
4 (larger)	.59	.63	.61
Privately Supported Schools (N=46)			
Quartile*	Females†	Males	Fraternities†
1 (smaller)	.29	.75	.76
2	.73	.39	.50
3	.70	.48	.46
4 (larger)	.51	.51	.35
Church-Supported Schools (N=55)			
Quartile*	Females	Males	Fraternities
1 (smaller)	.72	.79	.76
2	.75	.78	.76
3	.71	.73	.83
4 (larger)	.80	.69	.58

* The quartiles of the three measures of size are based on the distribution *within* each of the three types of schools.

† The most extreme difference among the four quartile means is significant at the .05 level, two-tailed t-test.

drinking regulations. Moreover, the largest schools (fourth quartile) are in six of nine instances, significantly more permissive than any of the other three quartiles within the appropriate category. This pattern is especially clear for one measure of size, the number of social fraternities affiliated with a school. In all three types of schools, those having the largest number of social fraternities (fourth quartile) also have the most permissive drinking rules.

The extent to which the association between size and prohibition of drinking varies with the organizational context in which it is embedded is noteworthy. Like the relationship between size and extensity of drinking rules, the association between size and the direction of these rules exhibits a clear pattern among the publicly supported schools and an erratic pattern within the church schools. Although no relationship was found between extensity of rules and size for privately supported schools in the previous analysis, patterns do emerge in the relationship between prohibitiveness and size. When size is measured by the number of female students, the middle-sized schools are the most prohibitive. When the number of males or the number of fraternity chapters on the campus is used, the smallest schools are the most prohibitive.

Summary and Implications

This initial exploration of the normative atmosphere surrounding collegiate drinking has documented the extreme variations in formal drinking regulations among national fraternity organizations and academic institutions in the United States. Comparison of these two types of organizations revealed in general, that schools have formal drinking rules to a much greater extent than the national fraternities, more than half of whom had nothing more than informal policies about drinking. And even when fraternities had formal regulations, in most cases these regulations said little more than "the schools' rules are our rules." The drinking rules of academic institutions were generally prohibitive.

The extensity and prohibitiveness of drinking rules were also found to vary by size among both fraternities and schools and also by source of support among schools. For the national fraternities, formal drinking rules were least extensive and least prohibitive among the small organizations, most prevalent and prohibitive among the medium-sized ones; the large national fraternities were intermediate in terms of extensity and prohibitiveness of rules. Findings relating to the schools were similar to those of the national fraternities in some ways, dissimilar in others. While drinking regulations once again were generally least extensive among the smallest organizations, they were most extensive among the largest rather than the middle-sized schools. Further, whereas drinking rules were, on the whole, most prohibitive among both the middle-sized schools and national fraternities, they were least prohibitive among the largest rather than the smallest schools. This characterization is most applicable to publicly supported schools and less so to the privately supported and church schools. Perhaps the most interesting divergent pattern was found among the privately supported schools. While these schools showed almost no co-variation between school size and the extensity of drinking norms, there was a pronounced inverse relationship between size and prohibitiveness among them.

In sum, an analysis of formal drinking rules in a number of schools and national fraternities reveals substantial differences in the extensity and prohibitiveness of such rules both between these two types of organizations and within them. Size of the organizational units as well as the source of financial support in the case of schools are associated with the observed variations. In general, size is directly related to the extensity and prohibitiveness of drinking rules, although there is the suggestion that the relationship is curvilinear. *Ex post facto*, both interpretations are plausible. A large organization, with size considered as an indicator of possible complexity, probably requires relatively more formal definitions of its norms than a smaller organization. However, very large organizations probably experience some pressures to decentralize administration of its rules and may rely on sub-units for the control of organizational members. This may, for example, explain in part why the largest national fraternities, with chapters operating in quite diverse normative environments, minimize formal drinking rules in the interest of maximizing organizational flexibility (9, 10). On this point, the comment of a national fraternity's executive secretary is suggestive:

> We have eliminated our national statute specifically aimed at drinking per se, and have replaced it with a broader statute of standards of conduct. We have written it so as to tie the group in with campus rules. We have been forced to this by the widely varying campus practices. . . .

In order to understand the complex relationships among school size, source of support, and the extensity/prohibitiveness of drinking rules much more needs to be known than is in fact known about the clients a school administration perceives as relevant. The prohibitiveness of rules probably reflects the cultural prescriptions which administrators, with an eye on their boards of control, perceive as necessary. Both administrators and board members have some idea, correct or incorrect, about the degree of prohibitiveness required by state laws on minimum drinking age and the wishes of the parents whose children constitute the actual or potential student body. In regard to the direct association between the size of a school and the extensity of drinking and the suggestion of a linear relationship between size and prohibitiveness of such rules, it is possible that the extensive rules of larger schools in fact ameliorate their prohibitiveness by specifying the conditions under which drinking may be done as well as the conditions under which drinking is forbidden.

Clearly there is no consistent pattern of norms about drinking to which an American collegian is exposed. Although the data presented here do not permit any generalizations about the enforcement of the formal rules which exist, it is fair to speculate that patterns of enforcement may be even more complex, perhaps even more ambiguous, erratic and situational than the rules themselves (see, for example, 11). The enforcement of drinking rules and the consequences of different patterns of enforcement are probably the issues which most need looking into if the drinking behavior on college campuses is to be understood.

REFERENCES

1. GOULDNER, ALVIN W. *Patterns of Industrial Bureaucracy.* Glencoe, Illinois: Free Press, 1954.
2. GEORGOPOULOS, BASIL S. "Normative Structure Variables and Organizational Behavior," *Human Relations,* 18: 155-169, 1965.
3. RUSHING, WILLIAM A. "Organizational Rules and Surveillance: Propositions in Comparative Organizational Analysis," *Administrative Science Quarterly,* 10: 423-443, 1966.
4. RUSHING, WILLIAM A. "Organizational Size, Rules and Surveillance," *Journal of Experimental Social Psychology,* 2: 11-26, 1966.
5. GUSFIELD, JOSEPH B. "The Structural Context of College Drinking," *Quarterly Journal of Studies on Alcohol,* 22: 428-443, 1961.
6. STRAUS, ROBERT, and SELDEN D. BACON. *Drinking in College.* New Haven: Yale University Press, 1953, chapters 4 and 8.
7. CARTTER, ALLAN M. (ed.). *American Universities and Colleges.* Washington, D.C.: American Council on Higher Education, 1964.
8. SIMMEL, GEORG. "The Number of Members as Determining the Sociological Form of the Group," *American Journal of Sociology,* 8: 1-46, 158-196, 1902.

9. Thompson, J. D., and W. J. McEwen. "Organizational Goals and Environment," *American Sociological Review*, 23: 23-31, 1958.

10. Eisenstadt, S. N. "Bureaucracy, Bureaucratization, and Debureaucratization," *Administrative Science Quarterly*, 4: 302-320, 1959.

11. Clark, Alexander L., and Jack P. Gibbs. "Social Control: A Reformulation," *Social Problems*, 12: 398-415, 1965.

Chapter 12

NORMATIVE MILIEUX AND SOCIAL BEHAVIORS: CHURCH AFFILIATIONS AND COLLEGIATE DRINKING PATTERNS*

C. NORMAN ALEXANDER, JR.
Stanford University

ERNEST Q. CAMPBELL
Vanderbilt University

THE NORMATIVE MILIEU of an area refers to characteristic patterns of attitudes and beliefs that produce a distinctive social climate regarding certain behaviors. We usually become aware of the effects of such basic norms only with the introduction of discrepant perspectives—when change is imminent, when there is salient variation in the nature and content of norms from one setting to another, or when there is noticeable deviation from behavioral prescriptions. In short, some form of challenge to a set of normative expectations is usually associated with their becoming explicit. Interestingly enough, the maintenance of collective normative reality does not always require adherence to the supportive value-system by even a

* This is a revised and extended version of a paper read at the annual meetings of the American Sociological Association, Miami Beach, Florida, August 31, 1966. The research was supported by National Institute of Mental Health Grant #MH-08925, Ernest Q. Campbell and C. Norman Alexander, Jr., co-principal investigators.

We wish to offer special thanks to Robert Stein (Vanderbilt University) whose assistance in data processing and analysis was invaluable; and to Barbara Bright (University of North Carolina) whose service as administrative assistant during the data-gathering phase of the project was largely responsible for our success in contacting senior respondents.

majority in the social system: as studies of pluralistic ignorance have shown,[1] mere recognition that the norms exist and some legitimation of their social validity provides a sufficient condition for their maintenance, regardless of the personal sentiments and behaviors of those affected. To some extent it may be that sheer recognition of belief-systems as social "facts of life" can reinforce and sustain them, even among those who benefit least from their continued existence.

In many respects the "abstinence orientation" that characterizes the southeastern United States illustrates important aspects of this phenomenon. In this region, there exist traditional beliefs about alcohol use that are noticeably discrepant with actual social behaviors in the region itself and with the beliefs and attitudes that typify urban American society. The disparity becomes almost ludicrous at times, as was the case when Mississippi collected state taxes on liquor sold illegally within the state. Less dramatic indications of the strains produced by normative and behavioral incongruities can be seen in the patchwork of wet-damp-dry counties and cities throughout the region and in the often puzzling regulations on the days, hours, and places of legal sale and use of alcoholic beverages. In other words, the ambivalence compelled by socially accepted norms at variance with socially practiced behaviors is well expressed in various institutional arrangements.

It is interesting to find a situation in which norms persist and importantly affect behaviors despite what amounts to deviant behavior by a majority of the population; even more interesting is the fact that this "deviance" is socially recognized and visibly apparent to the minority upholding the norms. Furthermore, these moral prescriptions persist despite an apparently greater incidence of deviation among the upper occupational and educational strata. What is fascinating in the study of drinking behavior focuses on the very dilemma with which societies have found it so difficult to deal: drinking has its personal pleasures and its social functions, but it has as well its *potentially* disruptive consequences for both the individual and the community at large. When the cocktail hour is as

[1] Richard Louis Schanck, "A Study of a Community and Its Groups and Institutions Conceived of as Behaviors of Individuals," *Psychological Monographs,* whole #195, Vol. 43, #2, (1932), 133 pp. See especially chapter 4, pp. 87-109.

well established as the Sunday sermon, and at least as well attended, a region maintaining a religious orientation of moral abstinence poses the question: whose behaviors and/or beliefs are deviant? The fact of majority deviation from accepted beliefs is almost a contradiction in our usual terms of analysis, and deserves an investigation of the possible means by which such institutionalized beliefs are able to survive.

The data to be reported in this chapter are drawn from a larger study of individuals' orientations toward the social use of alcohol in a region where drinking is generally disapproved. In previous works we have maintained that the Southeast is an area in which abstinence proscriptions are dominant and in which attitudes toward alcohol use are importantly connected with church-related norms.[2] Here we want to show that the churches are strong institutional forces shaping and reinforcing this aspect of the normative milieu. Support for this idea will validate an assumption that has guided much of our earlier work in this area.

We assume that traditional beliefs and orientations do not simply persist through inertia, but that they have a basis of social support, usually in a particular institutional setting that legitimates them. The social climate that constitutes the normative milieu is rooted in the attitudes and values created and sustained by such viable and influential institutions as the church. People are expected to be generally, though selectively, aware of churches' positions on alcohol use, and their church participation should be contingent on their behaviors relative to these norms. Such factors of differential affiliation and association should contribute to the structuring of networks of interpersonal relationships and to the emergence of social pressures within the population that reinforce both

[2] Ernest Q. Campbell and David M. Shaw, "Internalization of a Moral Norm and External Supports" *Sociological Quarterly,* 3 (January, 1962), 57-71. C. Norman Alexander, Jr., "Consensus and Mutual Attraction in Natural Cliques: A Study of Adolescent Drinkers," *American Journal of Sociology,* 69 (January, 1964), 395-403. Ernest Q. Campbell, "The Internalization of Moral Norms," *Sociometry,* 27 (December, 1964), 391-412. C. Norman Alexander, Jr., "Alcohol and Adolescent Rebellion," *Social Forces,* (forthcoming), 1967. C. Norman Alexander, Jr. and Ernest Q. Campbell, "Balance Forces and Environmental Effects: Factors Influencing the Cohesiveness of Adolescent Drinking Groups," *Social Forces,* Vol. 46 (March, 1967), pp. 367-74.

behaviors and beliefs. In this way the institution could receive sufficient support from its members to sustain its normative position while insulating itself and its adherent participants from contra-normative influences in the larger social system.

Since we deal with a very selective population of socially mobile and relatively "emancipated" college seniors (many of them from outside the region), the conclusions that we can draw are necessarily limited. However, the very mobility and presumed age-status insulation from regional identification that we suspect characterize college seniors will also make more impressive any "church effects" that we observe among them. If senior college students show the effects of regional church influences, then we suspect that such influences are even more important factors affecting adults whose community status-roles are more closely tied to local religious institutions.

Data Gathering

In connection with a related project, data were secured in the fall of 1961 from all entering freshmen in seventeen senior and four junior colleges throughout the state of North Carolina. These schools included those in the state university and college systems, together with additional private schools selected to represent a range from those without church affiliations to those that are actively church controlled. Questionnaires were administered to freshmen in group assemblies during their orientation sessions before the beginning of classes in the fall of 1961. For the second phase of the study we took all students whom the 17 senior colleges classified as seniors in March of 1965, contacting them by mail. Questionnaires were mailed to students at their campus addresses, except in two schools that could furnish only home addresses.

While we have responses from almost *all* freshmen who were present for registration and orientation as the "entering class of 1965," the representativeness of the senior sample in 1965 depends on the response rate to the questionnaire mailing. In the middle of March approximately 8,500 questionnaires and stamped, return envelopes were mailed to all seniors. Within a week to ten days after this mailing, about 52 per cent had responded. At that time, follow-up letters were mailed to non-respondents, and these reminders helped boost the response rate to approximately two-thirds of those contacted. If a student had still not responded by the first of April, he was remailed a questionnaire and stamped, return envelope, together with a personally signed letter addressed specifically to seniors at his college.

The results of these efforts were impressive: Of 8,382 sample members contacted,[3] 6,750 usable questionnaires were secured, an overall response rate of 78.4 per cent. While this is an excellent return, it actually understates to some extent the exceptional cooperation we received from our respondents. For, as noted, we were forced to use home addresses rather than campus addresses in two schools; and in two others that were on the quarter system, the addresses were those obtained at the beginning of the quarter prior to the one in which our mailing occurred. All four of these schools had response rates below 80 per cent, and their students constituted 42 per cent of the total sample. In the 13 remaining schools, only three others had return rates lower than 80 per cent, while five had better than 85 per cent (including two above 90 per cent). Among panel cases (those also contacted in 1961) response rates were even higher: In ten of the 17 schools, more than 85 per cent responded, and rates ranged from a low of 79.6 per cent to a high of 97.8 per cent.

In brief, these returns indicate that the questionnaire data are quite representative of the senior classes in these colleges. The willingness to participate in the study (filling out and return-

[3] After the initial mailing, we discovered that several categories of persons, classified as seniors at various colleges, were inappropriately included in our sample. Where it was possible to identify them, we systematically eliminated seniors in medical and law schools, extension-course students who were not connected with the campus, and other "special" student classes. The only unsystematic process of eliminating "inappropriate" sample members involved those who responded to our mailing with a written explanation of why they did not feel they could provide valid responses—two nuns and several retired persons taking courses for enjoyment were thus removed.

Naturally, we also omitted any students who had dropped out between registration and the time of mailing. And, finally, we did not include as members of our "contacted sample" about three dozen persons who could simply not be located, despite additional attempts to secure appropriate addresses from college registrars, student information services, prior home addresses, and, as a last resort, local telephone information.

ing a six-page questionnaire) also suggests that our respondents were highly motivated and, thus, likely to have furnished us with data of high quality. We are able, then, to characterize entering freshmen in 1961 and departing seniors in 1965, and our data include 3,936 respondents (47 per cent of the senior population) from whom we have information at both points in time. The following analysis focuses on the responses of seniors, excluding those who graduated from high school before 1959, since we felt that their age would make them somewhat atypical of the "average" senior student.

Data Analysis

These data concern the effects of religious affiliation and participation on college seniors' orientations toward themselves and others regarding the social use of alcohol. First, we shall explore their perceptions of churches' positions on alcohol use, showing that there is general awareness that churches do "take a stand" on drinking in this region. However, we find that there is selectivity in awareness both of whether or not the church has a position and of what that position is. Next, we ask how perceived church position affects attenders' moral attitudes toward alcohol use, and this will demonstrate their salience and importance in the lives of our respondents. Then, the associations between changes in drinking behaviors and changes in affiliation and attendance rates from the freshman to senior year will be investigated. And, finally, we will show that these factors are related to friendship selections and to social pressures in the college setting.

Operationally, we define a senior as a drinker if he responded positively to the following question: "Since the beginning of the year (January 1st), have you used alcoholic beverages socially in any form?" To be classified as a drinker, then, a person must have used alcohol at least once within the two and a half to three months prior to returning the questionnaire. For freshmen the length of time was somewhat longer, since they were asked at the beginning of September if they had used alcohol "during the last few months (roughly, since the middle of May) . . . ." In addition to drinking and reported church denomination, the other major variable of interest is church attendance. A person is classified as a "frequent" attend-

274 C. N. ALEXANDER, JR. AND E. Q. CAMPBELL

er if he reports going to worship services at least once a week (on the average).

The existence of normative standards must be ascertained independently of their relationship to personal attitudes toward or behavioral adherence to the norm. A proscriptive social climate regarding alcohol use can exist whether or not individuals personally accept or adhere to the values promulgated. In societal and institutional settings, no less than in interpersonal relationships, distinctions must be maintained among norms sent, norms received, and the degree of compliance with these normative expectations.[4] Thus, we ask whether or not particular institutions are socially distinguished by their normative definitions of a behavioral area, apart from the effectiveness of these norms in securing personal acceptance or behavioral conformity: Do church members recognize that their church has a position on the social use of alcohol? And do they accurately perceive this position, apart from their own behavioral preferences? In short, do church-related norms regarding alcohol constitute consensually validated "social facts"?

To ascertain whether churches are seen as adopting distinguishable positions on the issue of alcohol use, we asked:

What is the position of your church on the social use of alcohol?
.... I've never been a church member
.... They don't object to moderate use
.... They don't take a stand
.... They are slightly opposed
.... They are strongly opposed
.... They believe it is morally wrong
.... I really don't know their stand

Table 1 presents the percentage who perceive their church as strongly or morally opposed to the social use of alcohol, among those claiming to know their church's position. Respondents were classified by sex, drinking behavior, denomination, and frequency of attendance. Jews, Catholics and Moravians were excluded from this and the following table because of small cell frequencies.

These denominations fall in the expected rank in perceived

[4] Ragnar Rommetveit, *Social Norms and Roles* (Minneapolis: University of Minnesota Press, 1955).

TABLE 1.—*Per Cent Reporting That Their Church's Position on Drinking Is Strongly or Morally Condemnatory, by Sex, Drinking Behavior, Denomination, and Frequency of Attendance*

	Males		Females	
Frequent attenders	Drinkers	Abstainers	Drinkers	Abstainers
Baptist	86.8 (159)	88.4 (276)	87.7 (106)	93.5 (306)
Methodist	68.5 (124)	85.1 (128)	59.3 (81)	82.5 (154)
Presbyterian	23.1 (126)	34.0 (50)	23.6 (55)	46.3 (67)
Lutheran	5.2 (39)	8.3 (24)	5.6 (18)	29.4 (34)
Episcopal	0.0 (66)	...... (9)	0.0 (60)	6.7 (15)
Infrequent attenders				
Baptist	84.6 (300)	81.7 (110)	89.2 (148)	90.6 (106)
Methodist	58.8 (303)	65.2 (72)	67.1 (143)	77.8 (63)
Presbyterian	11.6 (149)	25.1 (12)	18.6 (70)	30.0 (20)
Lutheran	3.2 (31)	...... (4)	4.6 (22)	...... (4)
Episcopal	1.2 (135)	0.0 (10)	0.0 (80)	...... (5)

opposition to social drinking—Baptists clearly perceive their church as strongly opposed, with Methodists a close second; Presbyterians perceive considerably less opposition; Lutherans and, especially, Episcopalians are unlikely to perceive their churches as being opposed. Least variation in perceived opposition by own drinking behavior occurs at the extremes—among Baptists and Episcopalians—with Methodists and Presbyterians being most variable. Considering only frequently attending Methodists, 59.3 per cent of female and 68.5 per cent of male drinkers believe their church to be strongly or morally opposed, while the corresponding figures among abstainers are 82.5 and 85.1 per cent, respectively. Nevertheless, a clear division between "abstinent" and "permissive" denominations seems evident in this table; for in each comparison, fully 40 to 50 percentage points separate Methodists from Presbyterians in attributing strong opposition to drinking to their respective churches.

It is also interesting to note that consistent differences exist by sex, drinking behavior, and attendance: In 13 of the 16 untied comparisons, females attribute greater abstinence to their churches than males; in 16 of 17 comparisons, abstainers see greater condemnation of drinking than drinkers; and in 12 of 15 comparisons frequent attenders are more likely than infrequent attenders to perceive the church as more negative toward alcohol use. The abstainer-drinker differences are quite understandable, but the reasons for the sex and attendance differences may be less transparent. It seems plausible to suppose that females are simply reflecting the "double standard" for alcohol use that is typical in the United States, though perhaps more strongly held in the Southeast. Differences by attendance, however, suggest that something related to church attendance *per se* disposes one to evaluate drinking negatively in this area. As further evidence on this point suggests, attenders' stronger "abstinence" orientations appear to be a reflection of the social relationships they develop by attending, and not simply an indication of greater "traditionalism" among those who go to church.[5]

These data show that among those who claim to know their church's position, there is relative consensus on what that position is. But quite a few frequent attenders claim to be unaware of their church's position. Since they were given an opportunity to assert that their church did not *take* a position on alcohol use, examination of the "unawareness" figures should prove instructive. Table 2 presents the percentage who claim ignorance of their church's position on drinking—among frequent attenders, again classified by sex, drinking behavior, and denomination.

Lack of awareness is clearly selective. Among Baptists and Methodists, whose churches are opposed to drinking, *drinkers* are less likely than abstainers to know the position of the church. And among Lutherans and Episcopalians, whose churches are decidedly permissive, *abstainers* are more likely

[5] See Thomas R. Ford, "Status, Residence, and Fundamentalist Religious Beliefs in the Southern Appalachians," *Social Forces,* 39 (October, 1960), 41-49.

TABLE 2.—*Per Cent of Frequent Attenders Who Don't Know Their Church's Position on Drinking, by Sex, Drinking Behavior, and Denomination*

Denomination	Males		Females	
	Drinkers	Abstainers	Drinkers	Abstainers
Baptist	13.1 (183)	8.0 (300)	12.4 (121)	6.1 (326)
Methodist	18.4 (152)	16.3 (153)	19.0 (100)	13.0 (177)
Presbyterian	30.8 (182)	31.5 (73)	36.1 (86)	33.7 (101)
Lutheran	26.4 (53)	27.3 (33)	18.2 (22)	22.7 (44)
Episcopal	4.4 (69)	18.2 (11)	7.7 (65)	11.8 (17)

than drinkers to claim ignorance. Differences between abstainers and drinkers are greatest when the position of the churches is least ambiguous—among Baptists and Episcopalians. That is, under conditions where perceptual distortion of the church's position would be most difficult, differential avoidance of knowledge is most pronounced; but, note also, the clarity of the position itself apparently makes it more difficult to remain unaware.

Rather clear-cut differences among denominations exist in members' perceptions of church positions on the social use of alcohol. We have shown that drinkers and abstainers, though in general agreement, differ consistently in their perceptions of church opposition to drinking; and they differ, as we would expect, in the direction of perceived support for their own behavioral positions. Furthermore, among those who would be expected to know their churches' positions on alcohol use and to whom that position would be most salient—those who attend frequently—there exists a tendency to avoid awareness when it would result in cognitions that are discrepant with personal behaviors. Both sets of data indicate that perceptions of church positions are selectively self-supportive. Such perceptual subtleties may effectively eliminate conflict for some; people can systematically disattend to or remain ignorant of church norms when these conflict with their behaviors, or they can systematically distort their perceptions of the church's position to avoid the discrepancy.

While these differences show important disparities within the norm-sending and norm-receiving processes, we should expect to find even greater differences when considering norm-acceptance. Rather than distort or deny an unpleasant social reality, a person is more likely to acknowledge its existence but to reject it as a personal perspective for self-evaluation. Here we ask what implications these perceived church positions have for personal beliefs regarding alcohol use as a moral issue. Two questions were asked:

1. Have you ever believed that God will punish you if you drink alcohol?
   ...... Yes, I do now
   .... Yes, I used to but don't anymore
   ...... No, I never did

2. "Drinking is wrong as a matter of principle; people ought not to drink."
   .... Agree strongly
   ...... Agree somewhat
   ...... Disagree somewhat
   ...... Disagree strongly

Naturally, perception of church position would be expected to correlate with personal acceptance of that position, regardless of the respondents' behavior. However, differences in the extent to which the church position is accepted are expected: Drinkers should tend to reject extremely abstinent church positions, producing the greatest differences between abstainers and drinkers when the church is seen as most negative toward alcohol use.

Table 3 presents the percentage who report that they *still* believe that "God will punish" them for socially using alcohol, among those who attend church once a week or more. The data show convincingly the striking variation by perceived church position on alcohol use. Also, disparities between drinkers and abstainers increase regularly with the extent to which the church is perceived as condemnatory. We have repeatedly characterized the southeastern region as an "absti-

TABLE 3.—*Per Cent Who Still Believe That God Will Punish Them for Drinking, by Sex, Drinking Behavior and Perceived Position of Church*

Position	Frequently Attending	
	Drinkers	Abstainers
Male		
Neutral	1.0	9.1
	(313)	(88)
Slightly opposed	2.3	21.2
	(87)	(52)
Strongly opposed	12.0	36.9
	(183)	(255)
Morally opposed	20.8	44.0
	(96)	(134)
Female		
Neutral	0.0	6.4
	(179)	(78)
Slightly opposed	0.0	9.8
	(45)	(61)
Strongly opposed	5.1	31.6
	(99)	(313)
Morally opposed	12.7	50.9
	(71)	(175)

nent" one, but most readers will probably be surprised at just how abstinent it is, as indicated by these data. Recalling that this is only "border" southeast and that our respondents are seniors in college, it is surprising that fully 44 per cent of males and 51 per cent of females *still* believe that God will punish them for drinking, if they abstain and attend churches seen as morally opposed to alcohol use. This is a high percentage, and, as cell frequencies show, it includes a sizeable proportion of the total sample.

The response tendencies evident in these data are confirmed by those in Table 4, reporting the percentages who feel that drinking is morally wrong. Fully three-fourths of abstainers who perceive their churches to be morally opposed to alcohol agree with this position. Although data are not shown in the table, it is worth noting that 43 per cent of males and 48 per cent of females agree with this statement, even if they no longer attend frequently. Now if college seniors report such attitudes, one can imagine the social climate among their less well-

TABLE 4.—*Per Cent Agreeing with the Statement "Drinking Is Wrong as a Matter of Principle; People Ought Not to Drink," by Sex, Drinking Behavior, and Perceived Position of Church*

Position	Frequently Attending Drinkers	Abstainers
Male		
Neutral	7.0	27.6
	(312)	(87)
Slightly opposed	11.5	50.0
	(87)	(54)
Strongly opposed	20.0	67.3
	(190)	(266)
Morally opposed	35.8	71.4
	(98)	(140)
Female		
Neutral	5.7	42.3
	(177)	(78)
Slightly opposed	17.8	50.0
	(45)	(62)
Strongly opposed	24.2	72.7
	(99)	(319)
Morally opposed	27.4	78.5
	(73)	(186)

educated parents and the even less well-educated and more fundamentalist members of the older generation whose children could not afford to attend college.

Considering only the college environment, however, it is clear that there is a rather strong contingent of church-attending students whose attitudes toward alcohol use are unfavorable. Even if they avoid intrapersonal conflict by rejecting such beliefs, drinkers who find themselves in such an interpersonal atmosphere are likely to feel some discomfort. Thus far, processes of selective avoidance of "sent" norms and rejection of "received" norms have proved to be consistent with a general expectation that people avoid personally relevant condemnation. Nevertheless, there are rather large numbers who both receive and *accept* normative pressures in areas where their personal behaviors are consequently self-defined as deviant.

Despite these indications that some individuals tolerate ambivalence or imbalance between their beliefs and their behaviors, we have yet to consider the most obvious means of controlling exposure to church-related normative influences. If the institutional milieu confronts the individual with a normative climate that is disparate with his personal attitudes and/or behaviors, he can simply withdraw. That is, when his church's position is at variance with his personal preferences, he can stop attending, or he can change his affiliation to a church whose views are more compatible with his own. To examine this tendency, churches were classified as either abstinent or permissive, placing Baptists, Methodists and Moravians in the former category and all others, including Jews and Catholics, in the latter.

First, changes in affiliation were investigated with the subsample of panel cases from whom we secured responses at the beginning of their freshman year and during the spring of their senior year. This analysis could not be pursued beyond a simple tabulation because of the very small number who reported changes in church affiliation. Differences that could be observed are nevertheless in the expected direction: Taking only males who changed from one denomination to another during the four college years, we find that 24.1 per cent of senior drinkers who drank as freshmen (N=29) and 32.0 per cent of those who did not (N=25) moved into abstinent denominations. By contrast, 78.6 per cent (N=14) of those who remained abstainers throughout college changed into abstinent rather than permissive denominations.

Simply considering those who leave their denomination (either to affiliate with another church or simply to disaffiliate), we find the same direction of relationships; but only small percentage differences exist. Senior drinkers, both those who drank and those who abstained as freshmen, are more likely to leave abstinent than permissive denominations, while continuing abstainers are more likely to leave permissive than abstinent denominations. Even if it is directionally consistent, however, the percentage differences in changes are so small that we cannot regard the data as support. Lack of change was a disappointment; but, in retrospect, it is not too surprising in view of the simultaneously sparse attendance and virtually unanimous affiliative claims of the U. S. population as a whole.

Thus, we must turn to data on changes in attendance rates for any convincing evidence that church positions on alcohol use influence selective exposure to church norms.

All seniors were asked:

On the average, how often have you attended worship services during *each* year in college?

...... Twice a week or more
.... Once a week
...... Several times a month
.... Once a month
...... Less than once a month

We are concerned with their reported attendance during their freshman and senior years. To simplify treatment of the data, we arbitrarily scored these five response categories from 0 to 4 so that the highest score indicates the most frequent attendance. Table 5 presents these mean attendance level scores for the senior year—by sex, church position, frequency of attendance during the freshman year, and changes in drinking behavior during college. We predicted that those who remained abstainers would be more likely to decrease attendance at permissive churches than at abstinent churches, holding constant their initial levels of attendance. Exactly the reverse should be true for those who became or remained drinkers during college: they should be more likely to decrease their attendance at abstinent rather than permissive churches. And this is exactly what happens. Abstainers' attendance rates are lower at permissive than at abstinent churches in 7 of 9 comparisons; those who become drinkers and those who remain drinkers during college show lower levels of attendance at abstinent than at permissive churches in 9 of 10 and 8 of 10 comparisons, respectively.

Thus, the church's position on drinking relates consistently to changes in attendance by drinkers and abstainers. However, the table also reveals another trend of considerable importance. While abstainers are more frequent attenders than drinkers in 18 of 18 comparisons among those in abstinent churches, they are also more likely than drinkers to attend permissive churches (14 of 18 comparisons). Selective differences by drinking behavior in attendance frequency indicate

TABLE 5.—*Mean Levels of Senior Church Attendance, by Sex, Drinking Behaviors, Church Position, and Freshman Attendance*

Drinking Behaviors During College	Freshman Frequency of Church Attendance	Males		Females	
		Church Permissive	Church Abstinent	Church Permissive	Church Abstinent
Stays Abstainer					
	Twice a week	3.06 (16)	3.35 (102)	3.73 (15)	3.25 (160)
	Once a week	2.54 (57)	2.61 (272)	1.67 (59)	2.30 (348)
	Several a month	1.74 (27)	1.60 (151)	1.62 (24)	1.75 (159)
	Once a month	1.00 (10)	1.04 (69)	.33 (15)	.92 (73)
	Less often	.42 (24)	.70 (50)		
Becomes Drinker					
	Twice a week	2.45 (11)	2.11 (18)	2.79 (14)	2.31 (26)
	Once a week	2.12 (34)	1.90 (98)	1.85 (48)	1.29 (117)
	Several a month	1.33 (27)	1.13 (69)	1.33 (30)	.98 (92)
	Once a month	.50 (12)	.86 (43)	1.10 (10)	.79 (29)
	Less often	.41 (22)	.39 (38)	.53 (19)	.37 (32)
Stays Drinker					
	Twice a week	2.33 (21)	2.22 (23)	1.67 (49)	1.68 (19)
	Once a week	2.14 (139)	1.94 (124)	2.00 (55)	1.48 (52)
	Several a month	1.43 (103)	1.26 (147)	1.04 (50)	1.24 (63)
	Once a month	.72 (67)	.64 (125)	.80 (35)	.63 (38)
	Less often	.27 (206)	.23 (206)	.49 (67)	.18 (57)

that there is *relatively* increasing correspondence between the behavioral activities of students and the normative regulations of their churches. This is shown both in data on the very few respondents who report changes in affiliation and in the general changes that occur in attendance. However, the increase in correspondence is due to sharp decreases in attendance by drinkers; for, regardless of the church's position on alcohol use, we find that abstainers have higher levels of attendance than those who drink.

It appears that there is a general association between church attendance and abstinence, one which, of course, is stronger for abstinent denominations. This has implications for the friendships that frequent and infrequent attenders are likely to form and for the informal pressures to drink or to abstain that they are likely to experience and exert in relationships with peers. Such differences might also be expected from the differential perceptions of church positions shown initially. Hence, let us examine data relevant to interpersonal relations.

Respondents were asked:

> Thinking now of the sort of people you enjoy being with, how many of them drink at least occasionally?
>
> ...... All of them
> .... Over half
> ...... About half
> .... Less than half
> .... None of them

Table 6 presents the percentage who report that over half their friends drink—by sex, drinking behavior, church position, and frequency of attendance. The consistent differences by church position are in the expected direction: frequent and infrequent attenders are more likely to have a majority of drinking friends if they belong to permissive rather than abstinent churches. However, note that infrequent attenders who belong to abstinent churches are more likely than frequent attenders at permissive churches to have a majority of drinking friends, and this is true whether or not they drink. Going to church, even to a permissive one, is associated with a greater likelihood of close contact with abstainers.

TABLE 6.—*Per Cent with a Majority of Drinking Friends, by Sex, Drinking Behavior, Church Position, and Frequency of Attendance*

Attendance Frequency	Church Position	Male		Female	
		Drinkers	Abstainers	Drinkers	Abstainers
Frequent	Abstinent	64.4 (354)	22.6 (469)	63.2 (228)	12.9 (519)
Frequent	Permissive	80.9 (397)	37.0 (135)	73.3 (217)	22.9 (170)
Infrequent	Abstinent	82.4 (814)	41.3 (240)	80.7 (388)	29.3 (215)
Infrequent	Permissive	89.0 (564)	43.9 (57)	88.4 (302)	43.9 (57)

The same relationships are seen in students' preferences that their friends share their drinking behaviors. We asked:

Would you prefer your own friends to drink socially or not to drink at all?

...... Definitely not drink
.... Preferably not drink, but it's not important
...... Doesn't really matter
.... Preferably drink, but it's not important
...... Definitely drink

Preference for conformity by drinkers would be indicated by a response in the last two categories; for abstainers, by checking the first two.

Table 7 shows the percentages of drinkers and abstainers who prefer behavioral conformity from their friends—by sex, church position, and frequency of attendance. Frequent attenders at abstinent churches are least likely to assert a preference regarding their friends' behaviors if they drink, but most likely to express definite preferences if they abstain. Drinkers are most likely and abstainers least likely to prefer friends' conformity if they are infrequent attenders at permissive churches. Once again, frequent church attendance, particularly at an abstinent church but also at a permissive one, appears to support an abstinent orientation and to discourage the emergence of pressures to drink.

TABLE 7.—*Per Cent Wanting Friends to Conform to Own Drinking Behavior, by Sex, Drinking Behavior, Church Position, and Frequency of Attendance*

Attendance Frequency	Church Position	Male		Female	
		Drinkers	Abstainers	Drinkers	Abstainers
Frequent	Abstinent	14.3 (356)	79.3 (474)	8.3 (228)	87.0 (522)
Frequent	Permissive	25.5 (396)	68.9 (135)	15.1 (219)	74.7 (170)
Infrequent	Abstinent	27.3 (813)	60.0 (240)	21.1 (388)	67.9 (215)
Infrequent	Permissive	39.8 (563)	49.1 (57)	27.7 (303)	47.4 (57)

The role of the church in supporting abstinence orientations and insulating against pressures to drink is well illustrated in the data for abstainers reported in Table 8. All abstainers were asked two questions about pressures exerted on them to drink and about pressures they exerted on drinkers to abstain:

(1) Have you ever tried to discourage people you were with from having a drink or going to a place where liquor was served?

...... Yes

...... No

(2) Do your friends who drink ever encourage you to have a drink with them?

...... Frequently

.... Occasionally

...... Once in a while

.... Never

...... I don't have any friends who drink

The first two columns of the table contain the percentage who report that they have never been encouraged by their friends to drink or have no friends who drink, while the last two show the percentage who say they have tried on occasion to discourage the people they were with from having a drink or going to a place where liquor was served.

Figures in this table are particularly striking, for they re-

TABLE 8.—*Per Cent of Abstainers Who Experience and Exert Pressures Regarding Drinking, by Sex, Church Position, and Frequency of Attendance*

Attendance Frequency	Church Position	Per Cent Never Encouraged by Their Friends to Drink		Per Cent Who Have Discouraged Others From Drinking	
		Male	Female	Male	Female
Frequent	Abstinent	31.2 (446)	56.1 (435)	52.8 (464)	66.3 (516)
Frequent	Permissive	26.1 (134)	47.7 (151)	42.5 (134)	60.7 (163)
Infrequent	Abstinent	18.3 (230)	39.4 (203)	37.3 (236)	49.8 (211)
Infrequent	Permissive	21.4 (56)	34.0 (53)	28.1 (57)	38.2 (55)

veal differences between frequent and infrequent attenders that are quite large compared to the differences by church position with frequency of attendance held constant. Abstainers who attend church frequently, regardless of the church's position on alcohol use, are less likely than infrequent attenders to experience pressures to drink, and at the same time they are considerably more likely to exert pressures on drinkers to abstain. These data stand in contrast to results previously reported by Bacon and Straus,[6] for, while they found little indication of counter-pressures on drinkers, our findings indicate considerable pressures toward abstinence in this region, particularly among frequent attenders at abstinent churches.

It seems that churches generally, but especially those with abstinence norms, are associated with interpersonal environments socially supporting negative orientations toward alcohol and drinkers. Whatever the church's position on the use of alcohol, the person who attends church frequently is more likely than the infrequent attender to be associated with non-drinkers. He is likely to encounter drinkers who refrain from expressing preferences that their own friends drink and abstainers who decidedly prefer abstinence in their friends. If he abstains, he is likely to be relatively insulated from

[6] Robert Straus and Selden Bacon, *Drinking in College* (New Haven: Yale University Press, 1951).

pressures to drink and to be supported in his attempts to influence those who do use alcohol to stop drinking. But, if he drinks, the frequent attender confronts an environment in which fellow drinkers provide little support in the form of overt pressures supporting drinking behaviors and in which the (usual) majority of abstainers appears to advocate openly the abstinence orientation of the region. We may conclude that church attenders as a whole, and particularly those in abstinent churches, differ importantly from those who attend infrequently in their orientations toward alcohol—not only in their behaviors and personal attitudes, but in their public expressions of social pressures.

Conclusion

The population with which we have dealt is composed of senior college students, a group that is undoubtedly more "sophisticated" and less abstinent than the population of this Southern region as a whole.[7] Yet, the majority of non-drinkers in this sample agrees with moral condemnation of drinking as wrong in principle. Among abstaining females who frequently attend churches perceived to be morally opposed to the use of alcohol, approximately half still believe that God will punish them for using alcohol; and fully three-fourths believe that drinking is wrong as a matter of principle, that people ought not to drink. Although abstainers are a minority in our sample, they are a sizeable minority, and their responses show the strong role that the church in this region has as the institutional agent that formulates and reinforces normative proscriptions maintaining an abstinent social milieu.

Despite majority deviance, abstinence norms expressed in church positions and in overall regional climate are maintained with sufficient social pressures to sustain their validity as normative forces and with sufficient social support to sustain abstinent individuals in their conduct. Drinkers and abstainers alike selectively perceive and expose themselves to the normative influences of the church. Due to changes in attendance, those who go to church often are most likely to be those who are negative toward alcohol use, and who find in—

[7] Ford, *op. cit.*

or make of—the church both a source of normative support from institutional doctrine and a focal point for the formation of an interpersonal environment of like-minded others. Such an environment apparently serves to insulate its members from the pressures to drink in the larger social situation and to support them in exerting pressures toward abstinence on those who do drink.

The institutional support for the "condemn and forbid" abstinence orientation is centered largely in the Methodist and Baptist (generally Southern Baptist) churches attended by those in our sample. Even within these groups, however, the "condemn" is more effective than the "forbid" in affecting personal perspectives. These moral proscriptions fail to prohibit drinking but do largely prohibit normative regulation of the drinking behaviors that result when alcohol is used. A similar approach to alcohol is seen in the restrictions on drinking that college administrations adopt (and rather unsystematically enforce). Along with absolutist church positions this factor also contributes to a rather unrealistic "public morality" on the issue.

From both personal and social standpoints, an abstinent normative milieu tends to create problems in dealing with alcohol use, principally among those who do drink while sustaining negative moral attitudes toward alcohol and (more or less implicitly) toward themselves as drinkers. As previous findings indicate,[8] and as analysis in progress with these data tend to confirm, this is an unhealthy situation. For believing that "God will punish" may well be a *self*-fulfilling prophecy for the believing drinker. And such "punishment" is not only wrought on the individual, as statistics on the "social costs" of alcoholism have shown.

---

[8] Alexander, *op. cit.*, (1967). Robert F. Bales, "Cultural Differences in Rates of Alcoholism," in Raymond G. McCarthy (ed.), *Drinking and Intoxication* (Glencoe, Illinois: The Free Press, 1959), pp. 263-277. Jerome H. Skolnick, "Religious Affiliation and Drinking Behavior," in Richard L. Simpson and Ida Harper Simpson (eds.), *Social Organization and Behavior* (New York: John Wiley and Sons, 1964, pp. 432-439. Straus and Bacon, *op. cit.*

Chapter 13

THE STRUCTURAL CONTEXT OF COLLEGE DRINKING*

JOSEPH R. GUSFIELD
University of Illinois

THE DRINKING PATTERNS of college students provide an excellent opportunity to study the role of colleges in influencing styles of leisure and consumership. The use of alcoholic beverages is an important component of the mores and leisure habits of American classes and cultural groups. A number of studies have shown high correlations between social class, ethnic groups and religious cultures, on the one hand, and behavioral patterns of amount and frequency of drinking, attitudes toward moderate and excessive drinking, and rates of alcoholism, on the other hand (1-6).

It is often thought that colleges serve important acculturating functions by socializing entrants into styles of life practiced in the social class to which they will belong or to which they aspire. Mobile students might be expected to learn new styles from elite models, while elite students might be expected to reinforce and ramify consumer and leisure habits congruent with social class patterns. If this view of the socializing and acculturating functions of college education is correct, we should expect common patterns of drinking to emerge in specific colleges.

Past studies of drinking among college students cast much doubt on this theory of college culture, just as the Jacob report (7) casts doubt on the role of colleges in establishing basic political and social values in its graduates. The most definitive study of college drinking, that by Straus and Bacon (8), was

* Reprinted from *Quarterly Journal of Studies on Alcohol*, Vol. 22, No. 3 (September 1961), 428-443.

unable to discover a common "college drinking pattern." Based on their study of 27 colleges, these investigators concluded that background variables of religion, economic status, family drinking habits and ethnic affiliation were more closely related to the student's drinking habits than were facts of college residence. Either "college culture" was a myth or the hard shell of home and community breeding was impervious to change.

The present study is an effort to understand the transmission of campus cultural norms by reference to the social organization of the college campus. Granted that drinking behavior does not appear to be the homogeneous affair that popular thought would have it, what are the elements which bring about this result? The research reported here follows the method and techniques of the Straus and Bacon study as much as possible. It seeks to elucidate the apparent discrepancy between the empirical facts uncovered by that study and the theoretical view of colleges as acculturating and socializing agents.

The study was designed specifically to determine the relative importance of community cultures and campus cultures in student drinking behavior. "Community culture" refers to the drinking norms supported by the non-college groups to which the student belongs—his family, ethnic group, religious denomination and other groups external to the campus social system. "Campus culture" refers to the norms supported by the membership groups in the campus society to which the student belongs, such as his school class, social clique or housing unit.

The basic hypothesis to be tested here is that the social organization of the campus deeply affects the ways in which a given "mix" of students of different social classes and cultural groups interact. It is not that students are impervious to college cultures or that such cultures do not exist. It is, rather, that selective factors in the campus social system govern entrance into campus groups and exposure to subcultures in such a way as to affect the fit of campus culture and community culture.

Sample and Method

In the spring of 1955, 185 men in a randomly selected sample at "Canterbury College"[1] (total male student population approx-

[1] Access to data was contingent on maintaining the anonymity of the college.

imately 700) were questioned about their use of beer, wine and whisky. Canterbury is an old, privately endowed liberal arts college, affiliated with a Protestant denomination of high social status. Located in the east and with a high tuition, it attracts a large percentage of students from upper economic and social levels. Its social composition has been changing since World War II. The student body has doubled in size and the percentage of Jews has greatly increased.

On the basis of pre-study diaries, the analysis of drinking frequency was restricted to beer consumption, as indicated in the respondent's report of how often he "usually" drank beer. The student's self-estimation of frequency was also validated by the diaries. Fifty cases of the total sample of respondents were drawn into a subsample, using every nth number. More than a month before the final questionnaires were distributed, these students were asked to cooperate by keeping a daily record of all instances of drinking. The amount, frequency and type of drink were recorded. The respondents were then ranked by amount and frequency of drink. When, unknown to the respondents, the rankings by diary were compared with the rankings later obtained through the questionnaires, no differences were found in the reports on beer drinking. The differences with respect to liquor were not great enough to make ranking feasible. It should be emphasized that the point of interest was not an accurate description of the frequency or amount of drinking but only the accuracy of the rankings. The entire sample was classified into two approximately equal categories of "high users" (reported drinking beer twice a week or more) and "low users" (reported drinking beer less than twice a week).

Results

Canterbury had a reputation among its students and faculty as a "heavy-drinking school" and the questionnaire responses substantiated this image.[2] Only 6 of the 185 students reported that they had never used beer and only 12 said that they seldom or never used it. Among the total respondent group only 10 had never tasted liquor. Less than 20 per cent of the

[2] The percentage of total abstainers among the students in the sample is well below the percentages of the general public (3, 4, 5) and of the college student populations studied elsewhere (8, pp. 110-117).

sample claimed that they seldom or never drink liquor. Only 5 could be classified as total abstainers from all alcoholic drinks.

Analyzed by religious affiliation, the results were similar to those obtained in the Straus-Bacon study of 27 colleges. The Protestant students, largely from high-status denominations, were more often high users than were the Jewish students. The Catholic population was quite small but similar to the Protestants in percentage of high users. Of the 95 Protestant students in the sample,[3] 63 per cent used beer twice a week or more; of the 49 Jews, 29 per cent; and of the 29 Catholics, 66 per cent. (Chi square, with 2 degrees of freedom, is 17.4, $p<.001$ in a two-tailed test.)

In the Straus-Bacon study, socioeconomic status as well as religion was a salient variable. Canterbury, however, has largely an upper and upper-middle class student body and the percentage of lower-middle and lower class students was extremely small. Father's occupation was used as one index of socioeconomic rank. Classifying the students into three such ranks, no statistically significant relationship emerged between drinking frequency and parental status. (Chi square, with 2 degrees of freedom, is 0.38, $p<.70$ in a two-tailed test.) No observable differences were found when parents' education was used as an index of status.

Nor was academic class a significant variable. Age and academic advancement apparently did not result in a changed self-conception supporting more permissive drinking patterns. (As will be seen later, most of these students had had their first drinking experiences in their high school years.) Although the freshmen did show less frequent use of beer than their more advanced classmates, the difference was not statistically significant. (Chi square, with 1 degree of freedom, is 22, $p<.15$ in a two-tailed test.)

The fact of fraternity affiliation or non-affiliation was considered as possibly explaining the differences in drinking behavior by religious categories. Student conversations and observation of Canterbury suggested that a definite set of norms supporting drinking was part of the culture of fraternity life at

[3] The number of students reported as "in the sample" will vary slightly in the several categories of inquiry owing to the differences in the numbers who responded to specific questions.

this college. Furthermore, membership in a fraternity made possible, if not obligatory, a pattern of social activities less open to non-members, most of whom live in student dormitories. In conversations with the investigator, students freely mentioned "fraternity life" as a pattern very different from "non-fraternity life." They also expected that fraternity members would be heavier drinkers than "independents."

The findings supported these impressions. High users of beer were more frequent among fraternity members than among non-members. Of the 126 fraternity members in the sample, 60 per cent were high users; of the 57 non-members, 32 per cent were high users. (Chi square, with 1 degree of freedom, is 11.8, p $<.001$ in a two-tailed test.)

The differences between Protestant fraternity and non-fraternity members were not a result of differences in the denominational characteristics of the two groups. In both, high-status Protestant denominations were dominant. The high-status denomination least objecting to drinking was the religious choice of approximately 40 per cent of the fraternity members and 50 per cent of the non-fraternity members.

The drinking behavior of the student may be partially attributed to his response to the norms and values of the fraternity or non-fraternity cultures. Upon entering college the student may be exposed to a number of potential structures, each of which may exert an influence upon his behavior: the college religious groups, via chapel, the college drama interests, the athletic teams and the fraternities are instances of the possible structures which are part of the Canterbury social organization. Each of these may be the carrier of a distinctive campus subculture. Some of them never become available to some students, who may not be motivated to enter into them. Those structures which do become accessible to a student and to which he becomes affiliated may be seen as his absorptive structures. They absorb his loyalty, his commitment and his activities. To them he refers his behavior for approval or disapproval.

At Canterbury, the fraternity functions as an absorptive structure. It regulates the drinking behavior of members in a fashion not predictable by his membership in a religious subculture. Students of the same religious affiliation but different residence status showed different drinking frequencies. Of the Protestant students in the sample, 73 per cent of the 73 fraternity members and 34 per cent of the 23 non-members were high users. (Chi square, with 1 degree of freedom, is 10.7, p<.001 in a one-tailed test.) Of the Jewish students, 36 per cent of the 22 fraternity members and 23 per cent of the 26 non-members were high users. (Chi square, with 1 degree of freedom, is 1.0, p<.15 in a one-tailed test.) Among the Catholic students in the sample, 66 per cent of the 21 members and 50 per cent of the 8 non-members were high users.

It should be noted that Jewish students (the low-drinking group) who belong to fraternities had higher drinking frequencies than Protestant students (the high-drinking group) who are non-members. The differences are small (36 per cent of the Jewish members and 34 per cent of the Protestant non-members) but in the expected direction. In each religious group, fraternity membership was positively associated with high beer use.

A style of life involves more than frequency or quantity of consumption. Among other things, it also involves the way in which consumer goods are used. Cultural norms about drinking usually involve norms about the limits of drinking as a leisure pattern. Another facet of drinking behavior, the way in which alcoholic beverages are used on campus, was examined by inquiry about the frequency with which the students were usually "high, tight or drunk." Two categories of "abusers" were defined: "high abusers" (high, tight or drunk twice a month or oftener) and "low abusers" (high, tight or drunk less than twice a month). As was the case in beer-drinking frequency, this ranking was validated by the diaries of a subsample of the questionnaire respondents.

Previous studies of college students (8) had found significant differences between religious groups in response to questions about frequency of drinking to excess. The present findings are similar in content and direction. Of the 96 Protestant students in the sample, 42 per cent were "high abusers"; of the 51 Jewish students, 35 per cent; and of the 30 Catholics, 63 per cent. The importance of the fraternity subculture is indicated in the wide difference between Protestant fraternity members and non-members. Of the 73 Protestant students who were fraternity members, 52 per cent were classified as "high abusers," of the 23 who were not members, 13 per cent (chi square, with 1 degree of freedom, is 11.0, p<.001 in a two-tailed test). The same difference appeared among the Jewish students. Of the 25 fraternity members, 48 per cent were "high abusers"; of the 26 non-members, 23 per cent (chi square, with 1 degree of freedom, is 3.5, p<.06 in a two-tailed test). Among the Catholic students there was no difference in proportion of "high abusers" between fraternity members and non-members, although the numbers are quite small in the non-member group. To an even greater degree than in frequency of drinking, fraternity members as a group are more alike in habits of excessive drinking than are students of the same religious affiliation. Thus 48 per cent of the Jewish fraternity members were "high abusers" but only 13 per cent of the Protestant non-members.

Each of these groups apparently differs in the extent to which drinking is permitted or enjoined as obligatory behavior. The general function of the fraternity as a teaching mechanism for drinking is seen in the fact that of the 40 students who said that they had first used alcohol in excess after they entered college, 75 per cent had their first such experience at a fraternity party. As will be seen below, even non-fraternity members were affected by the drinking habits and mores of the fraternities. Drinking was part of campus culture.

Before the contexts of drinking can be examined as possible sources of differences in drinking behavior, it is necessary to consider a further problem. While the differences in fraternity membership help explain the findings of differences among religious groups, religion is only one form of non-campus subculture membership. Recruitment patterns might result in the selection of heavier drinkers into fraternities and the exclusion of lighter drinkers. Students from families which were less permissive toward drinking might share less of other cultural values essential for fraternity selection. In this case, the fraternity-non-fraternity differences would be manifestations of subcultural differences other than religion. In other words, the findings already presented are consistent with the hypothesis that the college institutional structure was a significant factor in influencing student drinking patterns. They are inconsistent with the hypothesis that religious differences were crucial or sufficient to explain them. But they are also consistent with the hypothesis that cultural memberships related to fraternity recruitment explain the findings. In this case the fraternity-non-fraternity differences would be spurious.

The respondents were questioned about the frequency of use of beer, wine and liquor by their parents. No appreciable difference was discovered between religious groups in the percentage of parents who were abstainers. Neither was any relationship discovered between parental abstinence and degree of student use. The findings are more complex, however, when degree of parental use is examined in relation to degree of student use.

Previous studies (2, 8) of drinking among college students have indicated that children whose parents were "high users" of alcohol were also likely to be high users. This finding was confirmed at Canterbury. High users of beer were more likely than low users to have parents who were adjudged as high users of beer on a very-often-never continuum. (Chi square, with 1 degree of freedom, is 9.70, p<.01 in a two-tailed test.)

Analysis of the responses indicates that this difference was related to recruitment into fraternities. Students whose parents were adjudged as high beer users were more likely to belong to fraternities than were the opposite category of students. (Chi square, with 1 degree of freedom, is 6.7, p<.02 in a two-tailed test.) However, the real crux of this finding lies in its ability to differentiate between high and low users of beer among the students. Assuming that the external subculture manifested by parental drinking habits explains student drinking, then fraternity members with high-user parents would themselves be high users more frequently than members with low-user parents. This is not the case. Among the 103 students in the sample whose parents were high users of beer, 66 per cent of the 77 fraternity members were themselves high users while only 39 per cent of the 26 non-members were also high users (chi square, with 1 degree of freedom, is 7.1, p<.01 in a one-tailed test). Among the 68 students in the sample whose parents were low users of beer, 55 per cent of the 38 fraternity members were themselves high users while 27 per cent of the 30 non-members were so classified (chi square, with 1 degree of freedom, is 5.6, p<.01 in a one-tailed test). Statistically significant differences between fraternity and non-fraternity members do not disappear when parental use patterns are held constant.

It appears, thus, that membership or non-membership in that campus subculture which is represented by fraternities was a factor in the frequency and excessiveness of drinking. The structures represented by the college social organization must be taken into account in assessing the forces at work in determining student drinking behavior.

The similarity between the present findings of religious group differences and the general results of previous studies can be accounted for by the distribution of the religious groups in the various structures. A much higher proportion of the Protestant students were members of fraternities than were Jewish students. This is not unique for an old college with long-established national fraternities whose policies and traditions sanctioned exclusive membership. The development of a large Jewish campus component was relatively new in the history of the college. Only the more recently established fraternities contained proportions of Jewish students equal to the campus proportions. A general census of fraternity membership and religious affiliation, taken at the same time, showed that 74 per cent of the non-Jewish students were fraternity members, compared to 41 per cent of the Jewish students. The conclusion remains that the social organization of the campus was a factor in the generation of drinking behavior and a factor in the selection of students into absorptive structures whose culture maximized or minimized those generative forces. The sober facts of social differentiation channelize the opportunities for drunkenness.

Primary Groups and Drinking Behavior

The primary interest of this study has been to test the proposition that institutional forces must be considered in the analysis of college drinking behavior. Some attention to the ways in which these forces operate on the student may, however, help to clarify why communal, external forces seem so closely related to the institutional ones.

Responses to the questionnaire indicated that drinking at Canterbury was decidedly not an isolated individualistic mode of behavior. Very few students reported drinking beer or liquor when alone. Typically they drank in the company of peers—friends, fraternity brothers, a girl friend or "date."

Here, too, sharp differences appear between the fraternity member and the non-member. A routine of activities based on parties and dates is far more frequent in the campus life of the fraternity member. While the latter, like the non-member, most often drinks in the company of male friends, he is the more likely of the two to drink at parties and on dates. (Chi square, with 1 degree of freedom, is 5.4, $p<.02$ in a two-tailed test.)

The more closely the student is committed and attached to the structure, the more responsive he will be in its customs and traditions. Since fraternity culture places a positive premium on drinking (or at least imposes less restrictions on drinking), the more strongly attached fraternity member should show a higher use of beer than the less well-attached one. The number of close friends within the fraternity was used as an index of attachment. Students were asked to list the fraternity or dormitory affiliations of their 3 closest campus friends. The results supported the hypothesis. Among fraternity members, high users more frequently had close friends in the same fraternity than did low users. Of the 77 students in a high-friendship category (at least 2 of 3 named friends were in same fraternity), 85 per cent were high users of beer. Of the 43 students in the low-friendship category (not more than 1 of 3 named friends were in same fraternity), 73 per cent were high users (chi square, with 1 degree of freedom, is 2.6, $p<.05$ in a one-tailed test).

This is one link in a chain of reasoning that points to the importance of the degree of absorption of the person into the campus culture. A question on movie-going and dating frequency revealed a greater degree of cross-sexual activities among fraternity members than among non-members. It is possible that clique relations among the fraternity members may have been weaker, more subject to the loyalties of the larger group, and open to counterloyalties to girl friends, than were clique relations among the non-members. In other words, the complexities of interfraternity or dormitory affiliations may also be an important part of the ways in which each structure plays a part in the process of developing and transmitting drinking norms.

Further analysis of the problem was obtained through the use of sociograms of three campus fraternities.[4] Fraternity A was founded shortly after World War II. It is an interracial and interfaith fraternity. Fraternity B is the newest on the campus, with low prestige and income. Fraternity C is the highest prestige fraternity with a heavy-drinking reputation.

Within each of the fraternities definite cliques were delineated on the basis of sociograms. Each of the fraternities displayed a distinctive drinking pattern. In fraternity A, 63 per cent of the sociogram subjects were in the low-user category of beer drinkers; in fraternity B, 50 per cent and in fraternity C, only 17 per cent. If there is a normative structure at work in the determination of the drinking patterns, the clique members would be expected to show a greater than chance similarity in drinking frequency. Students were asked to name their three best friends within their fraternity. Reciprocal choice pairs were identified and their respective drinking frequencies cross-tabulated. The results are shown in Table 1. Fraternities B and C present results in keeping with the hypothesis. High

TABLE 1.—*Beer Drinking Frequency (High or Low) of Reciprocated Choices, by the Drinking Frequency of the Choosers in Three College Fraternities*

Drinking Frequency of Chooser	Drinking Frequency of Reciprocated Choice			
	High	Low	Total	
Fraternity A				
High	7	22	29	Chi^2 = 10.9
Low	23	13	36	p<.001
Totals	30	35	65	2-tailed test
Fraternity B				
High	11	5	16	Chi^2 = 2.60
Low	7	10	17	p<.05
Totals	18	15	33	1-tailed test
Fraternity C				
High	5	2	7	Chi^2 = 5.4
Low	2	10	12	p<.01
Totals	7	12	19	1-tailed test

[4] The sociogram presented in the original article is omitted here.

users are paired with high users and low users with low users in greater than chance frequency.

In fraternity C, where all but 3 of the 18 members were in the high-user category, the reciprocal choices were examined by each of two high-use frequencies, so that here high use means "more than twice a week" and low use "twice a week or less." The possibility that some of the differences might be a result of only a 1-step difference separating high from low users was also considered, for in the case the user category might hide the greater degree of clique similarity in fraternities A and B. No such differences were found in fraternity B. In fraternity A, however, 22 of the 65 choices were of this nature, involving reciprocal pairs of C and D respondents. C and D respondents were terms designating exact frequencies within high- and low-use categories. C respondents used beer "twice a week," and D respondents "once a week." They represent the "cutting points" between high and low use, this "cut" being the closest point of division of the entire sample into halves. This goes a long way toward explaining the fraternity A results in Table 1. As that table indicates, in fraternity A high users chose low users as reciprocal partners to a greater degree than would be expected by chance. However, when allowance is made for the number of 1-step differences, the relationship is no longer statistically significant (chi square, with 1 degree of freedom, is 0.36, $p < .60$ in a two-tailed test).

The hypothesis appears substantiated in fraternities B and C but not in A. It is difficult to explain these results, but they do suggest that the fraternity membership factor is hardly the end of the analysis of the structural influences for or against drinking on this college campus. Fraternity A is more than twice as large as either fraternity B or C. The clique intensities may be less salient as directive forces. It is also possible that in these groups other factors external to the campus may be at work as determinants of the clique choice.

The latter possibility is an important one from the standpoint of gauging the impact of external cultural affiliations on campus behavior. As was seen earlier, while the Jewish members of fraternities differed from Jewish non-fraternity students, the differences were not as great as those among the Protestants. The differences were slight also among the small number of Catholics. Perhaps part of the explanation lies in the tendency toward concentration of the Jews and Catholics into a small number of housing units and consequent development of cliques along religious lines. Sixty per cent of all the Jewish students who belonged to fraternities were clustered in 2 of the 10 campus fraternities, in which they constituted 59 per cent and 60 per cent of the total membership. Even within the common residence group, conditions exist which facilitate groupings based on external cultural affinities.

It was not possible to obtain information on the religious affiliations of all the subjects of the sociogram analysis. From personal knowledge of the students, however, a number of cliques composed of persons of similar religion can be identified. In fraternity A, cliques of Jews and cliques of Italian Catholics are present. In fraternity B, there is a clearly delineated clique called the "churchy kids," affiliated with the dominant Protestant denomination on campus, and active in campus church affairs. Fraternity C, with its highly uniform drinking patterns, is largely composed of the two most prestigeful Protestant denominations. It is worth noting that the "elite" of fraternity A (Numbers 4, 31, 37, 6, 29 and 13 on the sociogram) were a group of students of diverse religious and racial affiliations. They present a highly diffuse set of drinking frequency choices. It should also be noticed that clique formation in fraternity B is less apparent than in the other two groups.

The sociograms reveal clique patterns based on such community roles as ethnicity and religion. Further analysis might have substantiated other roles, such as urban-rural residence or prep-school–public-school background. While the individual house units selected members from heterogeneous community groups, the large size of fraternity A appears to have promoted a "clustering out" of cliques around community statuses. The "mix" of the heterogeneous student population is not as mixed as appears at first sight.

Discussion

The data presented to this point have not constituted an attempt to establish fraternity membership as the central factor in college drinking, even for the single case of Canterbury College. Many other possible roles and statuses have not been examined. The purpose has been rather to establish the necessity of viewing cultural phenomena in their institutional framework. It is essential also to note the limitations inherent in the arbitrary definitions of "high" and "low" use and abuse of alcoholic beverages in this study. Although the student diaries showed a close association between frequency and quantity of beer consumed in a week, other distinctions may be important for many purposes. Thus any two students who reported consuming the same amount during a week have been equated although one may have consumed his entire quota at one "sitting" while the other did so a little at a time over the entire week. Similarly, frequency of "abuse" tells little about its intensity. Nevertheless, the main interest here is in the source of the drinking norms and not in the amounts consumed per se. The attempt to account for differences in a larger study by looking at a specific campus seemed to require clear indices for which effective "cutting points" could be established. Two findings in the present study support this decision: One is the findings of differences by religious affiliation consistent with the Straus and Bacon study; another is the fact that the findings in this study based on abuse are more definitive than those based on the vaguer concept of amount and frequency of consumption.

It is evident that while institutional factors are influential in this area of behavior, cultural forces still persist. It is the structure, the framework, which here commands attention. The housing unit is hardly the only absorptive structure on the campus. Such groups as the "theater crowd," "the intellectuals," "the churchy kids," and the "athletes" signify the existence of well-delineated and functioning structures based on interests and activities. Each of these has its own culture and social organization. Each is capable of developing strong loyalties among members. The traditions and values of each may clash with or be congruent with the community structure of the member.

All these types can exist as clear alternatives or as competitors for the loyalty of the student. In Canterbury, a sharply recognized status system placed one or two fraternities at the top of a status gradation. Hence an elite was perceived and a "fraternity model" played a role in membership behavior at all levels of the fraternity system. Such a pattern may not exist so clearly in other kinds of college structures such as new colleges, denominational colleges, or the large state or private university.

Where a social elite is mirrored on the campus, the college socialization process is often integrated into the community structure. Here, as in other campus structures extending the person's community structure, the group self-consciously maintains the wider cultural habits of that community. The campus structure functions to isolate members from other influences. Campus structures which have a cross-class or cross-group framework operate in opposite fashion. While athletics may be a vehicle of mobility for the lower-class boy, it has also been one area in which divergent classes have been able to converse with and know each other. The upper-class boy, drawn into athletic activities, may find himself in a more plebeian atmosphere for the first time in his life. Learning may go in more than one direction.

The image of college in American life is often drawn from the small residential college or the state university. Increasing college attendance in the United States is adding new types of institutions, such as the non-residential community college and urban university. A sociology of education concerned with the implications of higher education for cultural styles and status structures must take cognizance of the differences in social organization between various types of campuses.

Summary

Previous studies of college drinking cast doubt on functions of colleges as socializers to status behavior. The present study investigated beer-drinking habits in a random sample (N=185) of male students in a small liberal arts college by means of a questionnaire and a diary study in a subsample of 50. Only 3 per cent were abstainers.

Consistent with past findings, relationship was found between drinking patterns and students' religious affiliation: 63 per cent of 95 Protestants, 29 per cent of 49 Jews and 66 per cent of 29 Catholics ($p<.001$) were classified as "high users" of beer (twice a week or more). Analysis showed this relationship to be a consequence of the use of religious criteria in allocating campus roles. Student drinking was influenced by participation and involvement in the differentiated behavior demanded by fraternity membership: 60 per cent of 126 members but only 32 per cent of 57 non-members were high users ($p < .001$).

Another variable in the transmission process was the "clustering out" of primary groups along communal lines, such as religion: Among Protestants, 73 per cent of 73 fraternity members and 34 per cent of 23 non-members were high users ($p < .001$); among Jews, 36 per cent of 22 members and 23 per cent of 26 non-members ($p < .15$); among Catholics, 66 per cent of 21 members and 50 per cent of 8 non-members.

Of 96 Protestant students 42 per cent were classified as "high abusers" (high, tight or drunk twice a month or oftener), 35 per cent of 51 Jewish students, and 63 per cent of 30 Catholics. Of 73 Protestant fraternity members 52 per cent were high abusers, and of 23 non-members, 13 per cent ($p < .001$); of 25 Jewish fraternity members 48 per cent, of 26 non-members, 23 per cent ($p < .06$); among the Catholic students there was no difference between members and non-members.

High users among students more frequently have parents who were adjudged high users ($p < .01$). Students with high-user parents were also more likely to belong to fraternities ($p < .02$). Of 103 students with high-user parents, 66 per cent of 77 fraternity members and 39 per cent of 26 non-members were high users ($p < .01$). Of 68 students with low-user parents, 55 per cent of 38 fraternity members and 27 per cent of 30 non-members were low users ($p < .01$).

A sociogram study showed that high users significantly more often than low users had the most close friends in the same fraternity.

Findings in earlier studies of drinking patterns among college students are thus believed to result from the congruence between collegiate (fraternity) and communal (religious) structures rather than solely from factors external to campus organization.

REFERENCES

1. DOLLARD, J. "Drinking Mores of the Social Classes," in *Alcohol, Science and Society;* Lecture 8. New Haven. *Quarterly Journal of Studies on Alcohol,* 1945.

2. HAER, J. L. "Drinking Patterns and the Influence of Friends and Family," *Quarterly Journal of Studies on Alcohol,* 16: 178-185, 1955.

3. MAXWELL, M. A. "Drinking Behavior in the State of Washington, "*Quarterly Journal of Studies on Alcohol,* 13: 219-239, 1952.

4. RILEY, J. W., Jr., and C. F. MARDEN. "The Social Pattern of Alcoholic Drinking," *Quarterly Journal of Studies on Alcohol,* 8: 265-273, 1947.

5. RILEY, J. W., Jr., C. F. MARDEN, and M. LIFSHITZ. "The Motivational Pattern of Drinking. Based on the Verbal Responses of a Cross-Section Sample of Users of Alcoholic Beverages," *Quarterly Journal of Studies on Alcohol,* 9: 353-362, 1948.

6. SNYDER, C. R. *Alcohol and the Jews. A Cultural Study of Drinking and Sobriety.* New Haven: Publications Division, Yale Center of Alcohol Studies; and Glencoe, Ill.: Free Press, 1958.

7. JACOB, P. E. *Changing Values in College.* New York: Harper & Bros., 1957.

8. STRAUS, R., and S. D. BACON. *Drinking in College.* New Haven: Yale University Press, 1953.

Chapter 14

GROUP INFLUENCES ON STUDENT
DRINKING BEHAVIOR

EVERETT M. ROGERS
Michigan State University

THE DRINKING BEHAVIOR of college students offers an interesting contradistinction. Legally, most states prohibit the sale or service of alcoholic beverages to persons under 21 years of age. In accordance, oftentimes, college and university regulations threaten the student who drinks with suspension or expulsion. Since many students are not yet 21, we might then say they are "expected" not to drink. In "reality," however, it is apparent that many of today's college students do drink alcoholic beverages. In a sample of students enrolled at one midwestern college more than half reported that they drank alcoholic beverages with at least some degree of regularity. Straus and Bacon (1, p. 46) also reported that 74 per cent of the almost 16,000 college students in their survey had used alcoholic beverages to some extent.

The purpose of the present chapter is not to discuss the gap between (legally) "expected" behavior and "real" behavior, but rather to analyze some of the group pressures that influence the drinking behavior of college students.

Group Influence on Individual Behavior

The drinking of alcoholic beverages by college students is social behavior. We seldom find the typical student drinking in isolation. He drinks at parties and in other group situations. In fact, his decision whether to drink or abstain is for a large part influenced by those reference groups of importance to him.[1]

In our society we are early taught the importance of group sanctions for our behavior. Although we often make strong arguments for the "individual," those individuals that remain truly "individualistic" are often ostracized. How many times have we heard very young children say, "But mother, it's all right. Everybody else is doing it." Our youngsters are really arguing that because the group which is important to me is doing it, therefore I should do it. By their teen years, the group conformity syndrome is even stronger. The recent song "I'm in with the In Crowd" amply expresses many teen sentiments:

> I'm in with the In Crowd
> I go where the In Crowd goes.
> I'm in with the In Crowd
> I do what the In Crowd does.

With these strong group-minded orientations, the individual goes to college and is so placed in a situation where "*the*" group is drinking. Strong pressures are thus brought to bear. This statement from a college student may serve to illustrate the point.

> Before I went, I knew the party was going to be unchaperoned and I thought some drinking would probably go on. At the party it seemed everyone was drinking but me—it was mostly beer. I just had a coke at first but a couple of my friends practically forced a beer on me. I don't like the taste of beer but I had a couple more before the party was over.

[1] The statement that drinking is a group experience is confirmed by the findings of Slater (2, p. 86) who reported that 67 per cent of the Utah high school students he studied said they drank because of social motivations, i.e., to "follow the crowd." Haer (3, p. 184) found that "friendship cliques and the primary family constitute reference groups of great significance in regard to drinking norms and behavior." Riley, Marden and Lifshitz (4, p. 355) reported that 38 per cent of the respondents in a nationwide sample said they drank to be "sociable." Straus and Bacon (1, p. 197) concluded from their study of drinking in college: "Our survey brought out clearly the relative significance, in molding behavior, of cultural forces as opposed to individual determination." Becker (5) described in detail the importance of the group in the process by which individuals become marijuana users.

A reference group is a group to which the individual relates his behavior. Kelley (6, pp. 410-414) distinguishes two functions of reference groups: comparative and normative. The comparative function of a reference group lies in serving the individual as a point of reference in making evaluations of the self or of others. The normative function is defined by Kelley as that of providing a source of norms or standards toward which the individual is influenced to conform. Kelley points out that both functions are frequently but not necessarily served by the same reference group.

Whether the function be normative or comparative, the group exerts its influence on the behavior of the individual. If we agree with Cartwright (7) that "The behavior, attitudes, beliefs and values of the individual are all firmly grounded in the groups to which he belongs," then it would seem relevant to study individuals' drinking behavior under the influences of group pressures. The early Asch (8) study, which provoked much controversy and further research into the effects of group pressures on the individual, concluded that the group (particularly if the majority of the group is of consensus) can modify the judgment of the individual. The Milgram (9) study, which in some ways can be said to further extend Asch's work, demonstrates the relevance of group pressures for the individual, in that the subjects were required to inflict pain, a task which might be considered to produce a high-resistance factor (just as drinking may provoke resistance to an individual who has been brought up to accept legal authority and who was not exposed to drinking in his parental home). Milgram's work further supports the assertion that individuals act in accordance with the suggestions and decisions of the group, even though the group norms may encounter high resistance. We might also conclude from the investigation of Pollis (10), that a decision to change existing patterns of behavior probably is more stable when established via pressure.

The small-group experiments of Lewin (11), Festinger and Thibault (12), and Back (13) all resulted in findings which generally support the proposition that *attitude change of individuals can effectively be brought about via group influence.*

Where the drinking behavior of college students is concerned, we would expect (on the basis of the findings from the small-group research that have just been reviewed) that group influence is likely to be stronger (1) where the group is especially attractive to the individual; (2) where the individual feels strong association with the group; (3) where the group holds high prestige in the eyes of the individual.

If the group sets the model on which the individual bases his behavior, then it is serving a *comparative* function. It influences or exerts pressures to conform by providing a point of reference or orientation for the individual in his decision-making. For example, a student at a cocktail party may gauge his alcoholic intake on the basis of the number of drinks his friends are consuming.

If the group serves to influence the individual in selecting among the alternatives available to him in the decision-making process, i.e., to drink or not to drink, then we might say the group is serving a *normative* function by communicating what it considers to be his most attractive alternative. To the extent that the individual succumbs to the group pressures and acts in accordance with the expectations of the reference group, approval and positive sanctions are accorded. However, should he deviate from the expectations of the group, negative sanctions such as ridicule or "kidding" may follow.

Whether the group serves in a comparative or normative function, the pressures to conform to "important" reference groups is very apparent among college students of today. Their behavior is in many cases the result of pressures to conform to group values, attitudes, and beliefs.

It must be pointed out that it is often difficult to distinguish between the normative and comparative functions of a reference group. Most of the reference group influences upon student drinking behavior to be described herein are of a normative character.

Drinking as Innovative Behavior

For the college student who is engaging in drinking alcohol for the first time, his behavior is analogous to an individual who is adopting an *innovation,* defined as an idea perceived as new by the individual. Thus, findings from investigations of how farmers adopt hybrid seed corn, physicians purchase new medical drugs, and aborigines begin to use steel (rather than stone) axes may have application to analysis of drinking behavior. One generalization that has emerged from the some 715 studies on the diffusion of innovations is that *while mass media communication channels may be important in creating knowledge or awareness of a new idea, interpersonal communication is necessary to change attitudes and to persuade individuals to try innovations* (14, pp. 98-102).

Thus, from the research tradition on diffusion of new ideas, as well as from small-group research studies, we are led to expect that interpersonal influence from fellow group members will be of great importance in student drinking behavior. This point emphasizes the advantage of analyzing drinking from a social-psychological framework.

Method and Sample

The data for this study were secured by means of a mailed questionnaire from a sample of 725 students enrolled at a state-supported Midwestern college during the 1955-56 academic year.[2] This institution will be referred to here as "Midwest College." Responses were received from 88.3 per cent of the 820 students selected on a random ordered basis from the 8,200 enrolled at the time of the study. Mail, telephone, and finally personal follow-up methods were used with non-respondents in the attempt to secure their cooperation in the study. When the 725 respondents were compared with the 95 non-respondents on eight different social characteristics on which data were available, the only significant difference was the place of college residence. Interpretation of the results of this study is limited to the extent that the sample respondents were selected from only one college.

The 725 respondents were asked whether they participated in social drinking "never," "rarely," "occasionally," or "often." Thus, students could be categorized as drinkers or nondrinkers, and the drinkers could be roughly categorized by three frequencies of drinking. Responses to the question about fre-

[2] As compared to other colleges and universities at the time of the data-gathering, Midwest College was probably more parochial in its attitudes toward student drinking. In the ensuing decade, some broadening of college regulations regarding drinking has occurred, and the prevailing norms on drinking among student groups have probably been considerably more favorable.

quency of drinking might be expected to be biased in the direction of socially acceptable answers. However, the confidential nature of the responses was stressed in a covering letter accompanying the mailed questionnaire and anonymity was also assured.

The study was not connected with the college administration in any way and this fact was made known to the respondents. The question about drinking was "buried" in a checklist concerned with other types of social behavior (card playing, sports, and so forth). Only 22 individuals refused to answer the question. Two copies of the questionnaire were completed by each of 15 students at an interval of about a month (because of a mailing error) and a high degree of reliability was noted in comparing the duplicated replies.

Results and Discussion

Personal Characteristics. The main personal characteristics associated with drinking were the following:

1. Males are more likely to drink than females: 61 per cent of the male students and 38 per cent of the female students replied that they drink, making a total of 56 per cent of the entire sample (chi squared = 43.35, p<.01).

2. Married students were more likely to drink than single students: 68 per cent compared to 53 per cent (chi squared = 10.04, p<.01).

3. Armed forces veterans were more likely to be drinkers than those who had not been in the services: 77 compared to 50 per cent (chi squared = 35.01, p<.01).

4. The percentages of drinkers by classes among male students were: freshmen 40, sophomores 58, juniors 62, seniors 75; and among female students: freshmen 20, sophomores 25, juniors 49, and seniors 57. Thus the percentage of each class that were drinkers increased consistently from the freshman to the senior year in both sexes (chi squared = 33.67 for males and 20.40 for females, p<.01 for each sex). At least 36 per cent of the male students and 37 per cent of the female students began to drink while in college. Presumably non-students also begin to drink in the same age period, but the comparative proportions are not known.

The differences in drinking behavior by sex, marital status, veteran status and year in college are in general agreement with those found by Straus and Bacon (1) in their survey of students attending 27 colleges and universities in 1949-50.

The association between tendency to drink and marriage, veteran status, and year in college may be partly a function of the increasing tendency to drink with increasing age from around 15 to 25 as reported by Ley (15). The increase in the percentage who drink with succeeding years in college may also suggest that the students' reference groups in college place a lower value on abstinence than did their pre-college reference groups. As the student is gradually assimilated into college life he is more likely to drink. Changes in social attitudes caused by the different reference groups found in a college as contrasted with a home environment have been reported by Newcomb (16).

Residence Reference Groups. One type of campus group that seems likely to be important as a reference group to many students is the college residence group. To some extent, the residence group replaces the family and the home for most students. The main residence groupings at Midwest College are fraternities, sororities, men's dormitories, women's dormitories, college married housing (for veterans), and private homes in off-campus areas. These residence groupings varied widely in the frequency with which their members drank alcoholic beverages (Table 1).

The public image of the fraternity man as a drinker seemed to be confirmed to some degree. A smaller percentage of fraternity members abstain from drinking than do members of

TABLE 1.—*Frequency of Drinking, by Residence Grouping (in Per Cent)*

	Never	Rarely	Occa-sionally	Often
Fraternities	27	13	48	12
Married veteran housing	29	41	20	10
Off-campus married housing	37	22	32	9
Off-campus single housing	39	20	26	15
Sororities	57	22	14	7
Men's dormitories	60	15	18	7
Women's dormitories	64	19	15	2
All students	44	20	26	10

any other residence grouping. In general, the differences in drinking on the basis of sex, veteran status, marital status, and year in college contributed toward the differences on the basis of residence groupings. For example, the male residence groupings had a higher percentage of drinking members, as did the residence groupings with many veterans and many married students (college married housing and off-campus residence).

On the basis of the differences in actual drinking behavior among the residence groupings, it can be assumed that there are probably differences in their reference norms in regard to drinking. The norm in fraternities seems to place a lower value on abstinence when compared with the norm of another residence grouping, for example men's dormitories. It is assumed that actual behavior of the reference group is one indication of the norm of that reference group. It is, however, difficult to say whether the norm preceded the actual behavior or vice versa.

One method that has been suggested as a means of investigating the nature of reference groups is to study the behavior of individuals who are located within the sphere of influence of two reference norms.[3] A situation of cross-pressures with regard to drinking existed at Midwest College in the cases of both fraternity and sorority pledges.

At Midwest College all women students are required to reside in women's dormitories for their freshman year in college. The several sororities select their pledges during the first week of the fall term but the latter actually reside with non-pledged women freshmen in "freshmen" dormitories. The pledges are expected to attend a weekly meeting at their sorority house and have various other contacts with the sorority activities. As pledges, they are definitely in a power-subordinate relationship to the actives (normative reference group). A pledge's actual residence (dormitory) might also be expected to function as a normative reference group to some extent. Most pledges are members of clique groups containing both pledges and non-pledges which are developed mainly on the basis of location of the individual's room in the dormitory.

[3] This method was utilized to study cross-pressures in voting by Berelson, Lazarsfeld, and McPhee (17).

It has been shown (Table 1) that the two influencing groups differ in their drinking norms (43 per cent of the sorority members and 36 per cent of the women's dormitory residents are drinkers). It might be expected that the actual drinking behavior of the pledges would fall somewhere between these two groups.

Analysis of the responses showed, however, that only 22 per cent of the pledges were drinkers. This finding led to a re-examination of the influencing situation. The pledges' two influencing groups are really sorority actives on the one hand and freshman dormitory residents (not the upper-class residents of other dormitories, with whom they had no contact in their clique groups) on the other.

About 20 per cent of the non-pledged freshman dormitory residents were drinkers. The pledges' drinking behavior might be expected to be somewhere between this figure and the 43 per cent of sorority actives who were drinkers, and is so, since 22 per cent of the pledges were drinking (chi squared = 4.75, p<.10). Perhaps the tendency for the drinking behavior of the pledges to approach more closely that of the other freshman dormitory residents may be explained on the basis of their more intimate contact with that group. It may also be explained on the basis of the age similarity of the sorority pledges to that of the other freshman dormitory residents. Future research should be designed to study reference group influences on drinking with control for the effect of age.

The way in which the sorority members are gradually led to conform to the prevailing drinking norms of their influencing reference group is indicated by the drinking behavior of sorority members through each year in college. The largest increase in percentage of members drinking comes between the sophomore and junior years. Among sorority members, 18 per cent of sophomores, 58 per cent of juniors and 73 per cent of seniors were drinkers (chi squared = 7.90, p<.05).

Another group of students which is located in a position between two reference group influences is the group of fraternity pledges. At Midwest College some of the fraternity pledges reside in their fraternity houses but most of the remainder live in the men's dormitories. They are not housed in dormitories separate from the upperclassmen as are the female students. Hence, it was expected that the fraternity pledges residing in their fraternities (fraternity actives would constitute their reference group) would be more similar to the actives in their drinking behavior than would the fraternity pledges living in men's dormitories (both fraternity actives and dormitory residents might be influencing reference groups). These expectations were supported by the data. Among fraternity actives, 79 per cent were drinkers; among fraternity pledges living in fraternities, 61 per cent; among fraternity pledges living in men's dormitories, 56 per cent; and among the men's dormitory residents, 40 per cent (chi squared = 31.18, p<.01).

The conformity of pledges to the drinking norms of the residence group is largely completed by the sophomore year and the percentage of drinking members then actually decreases in the junior year. Among fraternity members, 59 per cent of all pledges were drinkers, 88 per cent of sophomores, 74 per cent of juniors, and 77 per cent of seniors (chi squared = 8.13, p<.05). This is an interesting contrast to the case of the sorority members where the most sizable increase in drinking behavior occurred between the sophomore and junior years and consistently increased until graduation.

The preceding analysis of college residents as reference group influences on student drinking might raise a logical question. How much of the change in drinking behavior is caused by the influence of the reference groups and how much is due to the "selection factor," the tendency of students to select certain residences because they wanted to learn to drink? There is little question that people tend to seek the association of others with similar opinions, values and behavior. The tendency to interact with others (in a relatively free-choice situation) like oneself is called *homophily*. Probably group influences on drinking behavior and homophilic tendencies both operate (perhaps they produce a "joint effect" greater than either above) to cause the differences in drinking among student groups that we observed in Table 1.

Religious Reference Groups. The nature of influencing group behavior has been investigated in regard to a situation in which the individuals (fraternity and sorority pledges) were in a position of "cross-pressures" between two reference groups with different norms regarding drinking. Another situation of this kind existed on the Midwest campus.

Many of the students with active membership in fraternities and sororities (relatively low value on abstinence) were also active in varying degrees in religious groups, such as YMCA, YWCA, and church fellowship groups, which place a higher value on abstinence. An association was found to exist between participation in religious reference groups and the drinking behavior of sorority actives. Of the sorority actives who were participating in religious groups, 15 per cent drank; while of those who were not active in religious groups 54 per cent drank (chi squared = 6.33, p<.05).

A similar analysis was performed for fraternity actives with the same general findings. Of the fraternity members who were very active in religious groups, 43 per cent drank; of those who were slightly active, 74 per cent; and of those who did not participate in religious groups, 73 per cent (chi squared = 7.23, p<.05).

Cross-Pressures. Individuals who are located in a situation where the influences from two normative reference groups operate as cross-pressures seem to compromise their behavior for both groups. Stouffer (18, p. 707) has suggested the proposition that an individual in cross-pressures will either conform to the expectations of one reference group and take the consequences from the other or seek a compromise position by which he conforms in part to each group's expectations and hopes that sanctions will be minimal.

An alternative is available to some individuals in cross-pressures. They can reject one of the reference groups and thus eliminate the cross-pressures. The problems of adjustment to the expectations of two contrasting reference groups are interesting ones. Two brief case histories are presented to illustrate reactions to this conflict situation.

Don was the son of a Lutheran minister in a small Midwestern town. He felt that drinking was morally wrong. When he was pledged by a fraternity he knew that a number of the active members drank regularly but this did not greatly disturb him. Then, during the second week of fall term, his roommate returned from a trip "downtown" and began to vomit out of the window. His roommate was so nauseated that if Don had not held him by the legs he would have fallen out the window.

The next weekend, Don and his fellow pledges went on a "walkout" to a neighboring "wet state." His experiences that weekend helped Don decide that he must move out of the fraternity house. He soon moved to a private room in a house with three graduate students, against the wishes of his fraternity brothers. At the end of fall term Don turned in his pledge pin. He liked many aspects of fraternity life but revolted against the drinking that went on.

Wilbur was the son of a Midwest College history professor. During his freshman year he was pledged by a local fraternity, but continued to live at home with his parents. In the course of the fraternity social functions, Wilbur took part in some drinking both at mixed parties and at stag affairs. Wilbur's parents were strongly opposed to drinking and threatened to report the drinking incidents to college authorities. (The regulations of Midwest College prohibited student drinking.)

The topic of drinking continued to be a source of conflict between Wilbur and his parents until the beginning of his sophomore year, when his parents offered Wilbur a new car on his 21st birthday if he would cease drinking. Wilbur did continue to do some social drinking, but always discreetly and he actually received the car. Guilt feelings were usually associated with the drinking, however, and Wilbur never felt that he really enjoyed social drinking.

These two case histories illustrate the two solutions to cross-pressures regarding drinking, a withdrawal from one group or a solution of partial compromise with the expectations of both groups.

Summary

Anonymous responses of a random sample of students at a Midwestern college to questions about their drinking behavior were analyzed by various categories. The proportion of drinkers increased with each higher college class in both sexes. Proportionately more fraternity than non-fraternity members were drinkers, more men than women, more single than married students, more veterans than non-veterans, more fraternity than dormitory residents, and more religiously inactive than active students.

The findings were discussed in terms of group influence on individual decisions. The behavior of individuals between the cross-pressures of two or more reference groups with conflicting norms regarding drinking was described and illustrated with two case histories.

If the drinking of alcoholic beverages is essentially a social experience, then the application of group influence theorems is relevant to situations in which individuals are deciding (a) whether or not to abstain or (b) how much to consume. The tentative findings from the present study suggest a need for further research on group influences on drinking, both among college students and in other segments of the population.

REFERENCES

1. STRAUS, R., and S. D. BACON. *Drinking in College*. New Haven: Yale University Press, 1953.
2. SLATER, A. D. "A Study of the Use of Alcoholic Beverages among High School Students in Utah," *Quarterly Journal of Studies on Alcohol*, 13: 78-86, 1952.
3. HAER, J. L. "Drinking Patterns and the Influences of Friends and Family," *Quarterly Journal of Studies on Alcohol*, 16: 178-185, 1955.
4. RILEY, J. W., C. F. MARDEN and M. LIFSHITZ. "The Motivational Pattern of Drinking," *Quarterly Journal of Studies on Alcohol*, 9: 353-362, 1948.
5. BECKER, H. S. "Becoming a Marihuana User," *American Journal of Sociology*, 59: 235-242, 1953.
6. KELLEY, H. H. "Two Functions of Reference Groups," in G. E. SWANSON, T. M. NEWCOMB, and E. L. HARTLEY (eds.), *Readings in Social Psychology*; pp. 410-414. Rev. ed. New York: Holt, 1952.
7. CARTWRIGHT, D. "Achieving Change in People: Some Application Group Dynamic Theory," *Human Relations*, 4: 381-392, 1951.
8. ASCH, S. E. "Effects of Group Pressures upon the Modification and Distortion of Judgments," in E. MACCOBY, T. M. NEWCOMB, and E. L. HARTLEY (eds.), *Readings in Social Psychology*; pp. 174-183. 3rd ed. New York: Holt, Rinehart and Winston, 1958.
9. MILGRAM, S. "Group Pressure and Action Against a Person," *Journal of Abnormal and Social Psychology*, 69: 137-143, 1964.

10. Pollis, N. "Relative Stability of Reference Scales Formed under Individual, Togetherness, and Group Situations," *Dissertation Abstracts,* 1: 669, 1964.

11. Lewin, K. "Forces behind Food Habits and Methods of Change," *Bulletin of the National Research Council,* 8: 36-65, 1943.

12. Festinger, L., and J. Thibault. "Interpersonal Communication in Small Group," *Journal of Abnormal and Social Psychology,* 46: 92-99, 1951.

13. Back, K. "Influence through Social Communication," in E. Mac-Coby, T. M. Newcomb, and E. L. Hartley (eds.), *Readings in Social Psychology;* pp. 183-191. 3rd ed. New York: Holt, Rinehart and Winston, 1958.

14. Rogers, E. *Diffusion of Innovations.* New York: Free Press of Glencoe, 1962.

15. Ley, H. A. "The Incidence of Smoking and Drinking among 10,000 Examinees," *Proc. Life Ext. Exam.,* 2: 57-53, 1940.

16. Newcomb, T. M. "Attitude Development as a Function of Reference Groups: The Bennington Study," in G. E. Swanson, T. M. Newcomb, and E. L. Hartley (eds.), *Readings in Social Psychology;* pp. 420-430. Rev. ed. New York: Holt, 1952.

17. Berelson, B. R., P. F. Lazarsfeld, and W. N. McPhee. *Voting.* Chicago: University of Chicago Press, 1953.

18. Stouffer, S. A. "An Analysis of Conflicting Social Norms," *American Sociological Review,* 14: 707-717, 1949.

Section C. Drinking Means Many Things

Chapter 15

EXPECTATIONS FOR NEED SATISFACTION
AND PATTERNS OF ALCOHOL USE IN
COLLEGE*

RICHARD JESSOR, RODERICK S. CARMAN
University of Colorado
and PETER H. GROSSMAN
*Community Mental Health Service,
Santa Clara County, California*

THE VARIETY of social and psychological functions served by drinking seems to be limited only by the social definitions and the personal learnings within which alcohol use is embedded. The role of alcohol in the process of solving personal problems and in coping with frustration, failure, and the anticipation of failure has long been stressed in the literature. It was the aim of the present research to investigate this particular function of alcohol use in the adaptation of college students to the demands and opportunities of the college environment.

* This paper was prepared during the first author's tenure as a National Institute of Mental Health Special Research Fellow at the Harvard-Florence Research Project, Florence, Italy.

Concepts and measures employed in the present research were developed within the Tri-Ethnic Research Project which was supported by NIMH Grant No. 3M-9156. Analysis of a portion of the present data was facilitated by a Grant-in-Aid to the first author from the University of Colorado Council on Research and Creative Work.

The bulk of the data reported in this paper is drawn from the second author's Master's thesis (1). The remaining data derive from the third author's doctoral dissertation (2).

This paper is Publication No. 101 of the Institute of Behavioral Science, University of Colorado.

Reprinted by permission. © Quart. J. of Stud. Alc., 29 (1968), pp. 101-116.

Enough research and observation in different cultures and social structures has accumulated to make clear that drinking behavior is usually institutionalized and regulated by tradition, by its relation to religious ceremonies, by its contribution to diet, and by its definition as a symbol of group solidarity. An account of much of the variation in drinking can be provided by reference to concepts at this level of analysis. Nevertheless, the properties of alcohol and the nature of individual experience with it are such as to make possible *personal* variation in its use, and an account of this type of variation would seem to require concepts at the level of personality. Such an account draws attention to the processes which mediate between society and behavior, and it can help to explain individual variation where the sociocultural context remains generally the same.

The present research was conducted within the framework of a social learning theory of personality (3, 4). In this approach, behavior is construed as the outcome of the tendency to maximize expectations of attaining valued goals in any given situation or over time. Most crucial to the point of departure of our own research was the following general formulation which is central in Rotter's social learning theory of personality: *where certain behaviors have come, through experience, to have a relatively low expectation of leading to goals which are valued by the person, other, alternative behaviors which have a relatively higher expectation of leading to these goals, or of coping with the failure to attain them, will tend to occur.*

Within the college environment the goals toward which students strive can be referred to a large variety of need or motivational systems. Two categories of goals seem, however, to be of pervasive importance in college life: the goal of academic achievement or recognition, and the goal of social affection or interpersonal liking. Since the formal structure of the college institutionalizes the goal of achievement in the pursuit of learning, college life is organized to a large extent in relation to this objective. At the same time, especially within the informal structures of college life, both on and off campus, it is being liked by others, having friends, and belonging to social groups which are emphasized as important and widely shared goals.

Because of the significance of these goals in the campus setting and at this stage of life, failure to attain academic success, or peer affection, or both, should have major consequences for the student. Beyond lowering his expectations for future attainment in these areas, failure should result, theoretically, in recourse to other behaviors learned in the past to be ways of achieving the same or similar goals. Among these are likely to be such instrumental behaviors as redoubling one's efforts, spending more time at studying, doing extra work, preparing further in advance for exams, seeking out new groups to join with, being more friendly and warm in social contacts, going out of one's way to help others, and the like. It was our basic thesis that one of the learned behaviors available to college students for dealing with low expectations of attaining valued goals is the behavior of drinking or the use of alcohol.

Opportunities for learning that drinking can be a technically effective alternative means when other behaviors have been unsuccessful are recurrent throughout the socialization of alcohol use and through exposure to social models whose use of alcohol can be observed. The young person has the opportunity to learn, for example, that in drinking situations certain goals are more easily available than otherwise. Thus, dating which is accompanied by drinking may more readily yield communications and expressions of affection and intimacy than dates where no drinking occurs.

The interpretation of alcohol use as an effective alternative means of goal striving is not limited to the kind of example just cited, a situation where the *same* goal, not felt to be attainable otherwise, can be attained through drinking. It is also possible to learn that drinking situations provide *other*, *new* or *different* goals than the ones toward which the person has been unsuccessfully striving. Thus the student who has been frustrated in the pursuit of academic success may have learned that drinking situations provide other goals which can also be satisfying—affection, dominance, independence—and the attainment of these latter goals may substitute or compensate for lack of attainment of the objectives of the original striving.

A further aspect of the present interpretation of drinking depends at least in part on the physiological properties of alcohol, the fact that alcohol, especially in large quantities, may affect internal cognitive processes such as memory and recall and thereby enable the person to avoid or inhibit thinking about his failures and inadequacies. This "narcotization" function of alcohol can also be seen to be a learned way of coping with expectations of adversity. Since narcotization depends upon drinking relatively large amounts of alcohol relatively frequently, it tends to be a pattern of use which is associated with drunkenness and complications. Because of the social disapproval attendant upon the latter when recurrent, the use of alcohol as a way of coping with failure through narcotization is likely to occur only where expectations of attaining satisfactions in most other ways have come to be thought of as minimal. This function of alcohol, then, serves to facilitate retreat from instrumentally-oriented, goal-striving behavior, and represents a way of coping with failure, or its anticipation, by withdrawal.

Drinking behavior can be seen, in short, as essentially adaptive. The socialization of alcohol use makes possible the learning to use drinking as a way of attaining goals otherwise felt to be unattainable, as a way of attaining substitute goals for those for which the expectation of attainment is low, and as a way of coping with failure or its anticipation through forgetting or through inhibiting or interfering with the relevant thought processes. Given the sharp competition in the academic and social spheres of campus life, low expectations for attaining academic success and peer affection are inevitable among certain members of the college community. Given also the general availability of alcohol to persons of college age, some degree of relationship should exist between expectations for goal attainment or need satisfaction and the pattern of drinking behavior among college students.

The investigation of this general hypothesis was dealt with in two phases. The first phase involved assessment of the relation between expectations for need satisfaction, on the one hand, and certain aspects of the pattern of drinking behavior, on the other. The assumption was that students with low expectations of need satisfaction should show greater recourse to alcohol; therefore they should have greater intake, be drunk more often, and have more drinking-related social complications. If this relation can be shown to hold, there would be an initial basis for inferring that drinking may serve as an alternative way of gaining goals, solving problems, or coping with failure.

But such an inference, even if strongly supported by the data, would remain relatively indirect. A more direct assessment of the *meaning* which alcohol has, or of the actual psychological *functions it serves* for students, would need to be made. This was the concern of the second phase of the present study. In this second phase the relation between expectations for need satisfaction, on the one hand, and the functions of alcohol which the subject describes as applying to his own use, on the other, was investigated. The assumption was that subjects with low expectations for need satisfaction should more frequently describe or define alcohol as providing them with alternatives for goal attainment or with ways of coping with frustration and failure.

PART I

Subjects

The subjects of the research were students selected from the introductory psychology classes at the University of Colorado. The personality questionnaire for the measurement of expectations was administered during regular class hour to approximately 300 students. About two weeks later a drinking questionnaire was administered, outside of class, in groups of 20, to those students from the original group who had volunteered to participate in "a drinking study." The administrator was a different person on the second occasion than on the first in order to avoid any connection between the two measures. The voluntary nature of the second session reduced the size of the group on which *both* personality and drinking data were available to 110. Further reduction occurred when married students and non-drinkers were excluded from the sample.

The final sample consisted, then, of a total of 88 undergraduate students. Of these, 38 were male and 50 were female. The mean age of the student group, 19.2 years, showed no difference between the sexes. Subjects had attended college on the average of just under two years.

The Measurement of Expectations of Need Satisfaction

Expectations for goal attainment or need satisfaction in the two areas of academic achievement (ACH) and peer affection (AFF) were assessed by means of a 30-item questionnaire. Fifteen items were referents for academic achievement, and fifteen were referents for peer affection or interpersonal liking. Each item involved the presentation of a verbal referent for one of the goal areas and a linear rating scale along which the subject marked the degree to which he expected to attain that referent or that specific goal.

The item format used was as follows:

2. How strongly do I expect:

   To be in the top half of the class at graduation.

   0   100

   | | | | | | | | |
   Sure it will   Even chance   Sure it *will*
   not happen   "fifty-fifty"   happen

The referent in the example is for the need area of academic achievement.[1] The 15 ACH items and the 15 AFF items were interspersed in order of appearance in the questionnaire.

For each item, the level of expectation of occurrence or goal attainment was given by the category checked on the linear scale. The item scores assigned ranged from 1 to 10. When these scores were summed across the 15 items in each need area, a total expectation score for that area was obtained. Thus, the measure of expectations of need satisfaction yielded

[1] The other ACH referents were the following: To be able to get my ideas across in class; To get on the Dean's list during the year; To be able to answer other students' questions about school work; To be thought most likely to amount to something by my instructors; To understand new material quickly in class; To be well-prepared for class discussion; To win a scholarship while in college; To get at least a B average this year; To be considered a bright student by my instructors; To have good enough grades to go on to graduate school if I want to; To be thought of as a good student by my classmates; To be encouraged by my instructors to go on to graduate school; To do well in some of the more difficult courses here; To come out near the top of the class on mid-term exams. The 15 AFF referents were the following: To be well-liked by most of the people around here; To be

two scores, one for the ACH need area and one for the AFF area.

This personality measure had been used successfully in a number of studies (5, 6) and had been shown previously to have adequate reliability and validity. Further evidence on these issues was accumulated in the present research. Test–retest reliability, for a sample of 16 of the students retested approximately two weeks after the first administration, was very satisfactory: Expectations for Achievement, $r=.95$; Expectations for Affection, $r=.92$.

With respect to the validity of these scores as measures of expectation, it is important, first, to be confident that the two scores are actually measuring *different* need areas. The relatively low correlation between the E_{ACH} measure and the E_{AFF} measure (despite the method of measurement being common to both), contributes toward confidence in that regard. The Pearson correlation of .36 shows the two scores to have less than 15% of their variance in common.

A further question of interest with respect to the validity of the expectation scores has to do with their relations to relevant external criteria. An external criterion of probable success in academic achievement, namely, grade-point average, and an external criterion of probable success in the peer affection area, namely membership in one of the Greek-letter organizations on campus, were selected. (The latter is admittedly remote and tenuous as an external criterion of expectations for affection, but no other was available and some degree of relevance can be claimed.) The resulting data are of interest. The E_{ACH} score correlates with grade-point average

---

asked to take part in many social activities; To be thought of as a best friend by several persons around here; To have groups show real pleasure when I join them; To be one of the most popular undergrads on campus; To go out of my way to help others; To have friends want to do things with me during vacations; To get along well with most of the students; To be in on the fun that goes on around here; To have other students enjoy having me around; To openly express my appreciation of others; To do things with the group just because I like being with them; To be known as one of the best-liked persons in my class; To have many friends in different groups; To know that the instructor actually likes me as a person.

.55 while the E_{AFF} score correlates about zero $(-.01)$. Not only is this difference in the correlations a source of validity for the E_{ACH} score, but it also adds further evidence that the two expectation scores are not measuring the same need area. With respect to the Greek membership criterion, the pattern is similar although not as striking, and is reversed as expected. The E_{AFF} score is significantly related to the criterion $(r=.20)$, whereas the correlation of the E_{ACH} score is less $(r=.12)$ and falls short of significance.

The Measurement of Drinking Behavior

Three aspects of the pattern of drinking behavior were assessed: intake, reported frequency of drunkenness, and re-reported frequency of drinking-related complications. A large number of additional questions was employed, covering such aspects as the initial drinking experience, the usual context of drinking, and definitions of heavy drinking, but these data will not be dealt with in this paper.

The Measure of Intake

The procedure for obtaining a measure of quantity-frequency of alcohol use has been described in detail elsewhere (7; 5, Chap. 7). Wine, beer, and liquor were dealt with separately. For each beverage, a *frequency* question ("How often do you *usually* drink beer?") and a *quantity* question ("When you drink *beer*, how much do you usually have at *one* time?") were asked, and a series of response categories were provided for each question. The quantity responses were converted to units of absolute alcohol and multiplied by a weighted frequency score to yield a quantity-frequency (Q-F) index for each beverage. The Q-F indexes for the three beverages were summed to yield a Total Q-F index for all alcoholic beverages combined. The interpretation of the Q-F score is given as the average amount of absolute alcohol consumed per day. The index increases with increases in either quantity or frequency of intake, or with greater use of beverages of higher absolute alcohol content.

The Q-F scores for males and females show, as expected,

that males drink more (twice as much), on the average, than females in the college sample. The mean Q-F scores for males were the following: Total Q-F=.72, Q-F Wine=.04, Q-F Beer=.51, and Q-F Liquor=.19. For the females the scores were: Total Q-F=.36, Q-F Wine=.05, Q-F Beer=.15, and Q-F Liquor=.19. The sex difference in total alcohol intake is thus accounted for entirely by the difference in beer consumption.

The Measure of Drunkenness

This measure consisted of a single question in the drinking questionnaire. The item was the following:

How many times have you gotten drunk or pretty high in the last year? Circle *one* only.

a.   10 or more times
b.   8 or 9 times
c.   6 or 7 times
d.   4 or 5 times
e.   2 or 3 times
f.   1 time
g.   never

The item was scored from 0 to 6 with the higher score assigned to the higher reported frequency of drunkenness. The utility of this type of item as a measure of drunkenness had been demonstrated in previous research (5, Chap. 7). As expected, there was a sex difference in reported frequency of having been drunk or pretty high in the past year: mean score for males was 3.0, reflecting the response category of "4 or 5 times"; mean score for females was 2.2, reflecting the response category of "2 or 3 times."

The Measure of Drinking-Related Complications

Specific problems such as loss of status or position, accidents, or damage to social relationships associated with drinking were assessed, relying on Straus and Bacon's (8) four categories of drinking-related problems. These included formal punishment or discipline, accidents or injuries, damage to friendships, and failure to meet everyday obligations. Sixteen items, four for each category, were constructed. The format of each question was as follows:

How many times have you ever lost a job due to drinking?
a. several times
b. once or twice
c. never

An effort was made to score the responses to these 16 questions taking into account seriousness of the reported problem, frequency of occurrence of each problem, and both seriousness and frequency combined. Since the various scores correlated among themselves in the high .90's, the decision was made to use as the drinking-related complications score the simplest and most direct measure, namely, the number of items out of the sixteen to which a response other than "never" was given.

The mean complications score was 2.09 out of a possible 16 (males 2.6, females 1.7). The three measures of drinking behavior show a consistency when treated by sex groups. Males report greater intake of alcohol (higher Q-F scores) and also report more drunkenness and drinking-related complications than females. In Table 1 it can be seen that, for both sexes, the three measures of the pattern of drinking behavior correlate significantly among themselves, the higher the reported intake, the higher the reported drunkenness and drinking-related complications. The correlations for females are all higher than those for males, a fact of interest in relation

TABLE 1.—*Intercorrelations among Three Measures of Drinking Behavior* (*Males=38; Females=50*)

	Total Q-F	Drunkenness
Drunkenness		
Males	.32*	....
Females	.60*	....
Drinking-related complications		
Males	.52*	.54*
Females	.70*	.66*

* Pearson correlation significant at the .05 level or beyond, one-tailed test.

to subsequent results. The consistency among the three scores, as well as the obtained sex differences in magnitude of each score, can be taken, in the absence of outside criteria, as providing a degree of validity for the drinking measures.

Results

As discussed earlier, it was anticipated that where expectations are low the measures of intake, drunkenness, and complications would tend to be higher. Two modes of analysis were carried out to test this hypothesis. First, correlations were run between the two expectations scores and the three drinking measures. Second, students were divided into subgroups depending on the level of *both* of their expectation scores, and the subgroups were then compared in terms of their mean scores on the drinking measures.

It can be seen in Table 2 that all but one of the correlations are in the expected, that is, the negative, direction. For the females, five out of the six predicted relationships are significant, providing strong support for the hypothesis. For males, however, the data are considerably weaker: although three of the six correlations are over .20 in the predicted direction, they nevertheless fall short of significance (an r of .275 is needed for significance at the .05 level, one-tailed test, for an N of 38).

TABLE 2.—*Correlations between Expectations for Need Satisfaction and Measures of Drinking Behavior*

	Total Q-F	Drunkenness	Drinking-Related Complications
Males (N=38)			
E_{ACH}	.11	−.25	−.23
E_{AFF}	−.10	−.08	−.24
Females (N=50)			
E_{ACH}	−.26*	−.33*	−.28*
E_{AFF}	−.26*	−.07	−.39*

* Pearson correlation significant at the .05 level or beyond, one-tailed test.

For the second type of analysis mentioned above, four sub-groups of subjects were constituted within each sex group. The two expectancy scores of each subject were examined to determine whether they were above or below the group mean for that score. Depending on their two scores, subjects were then assigned to one of four groups: (1) High E_{ACH} and High E_{AFF}; (2) High E_{ACH} and Low E_{AFF}; (3) Low E_{ACH} and High E_{AFF}; and (4) Low E_{ACH} and Low E_{AFF}. This analysis, unlike the correlational analysis, considers *both* need areas at the same time. Theoretically, the group which should show the highest scores on the drinking measures is Group 4, the group which is low on *both* expectation measures.

The data relevant to this mode of analysis are presented in Table 3. Despite the small N's which result when each sex group is partitioned into four subgroups, it can be seen in Table 3 that, for both sexes, Group 4, the group which is low on *both* expectation scores, has the highest score on each of the three drinking measures. The finding is clearest on the measure of Drinking-Related Complications where the mean score of Group 4 is significantly higher than the mean score of each of the other three groups; and this finding holds for both sexes. With respect to the other two measures, Total Q-F and Drunkenness, the results for the females are again more supportive than for the males. The female Group 4 mean score on each of these two drinking measures is significantly higher than that of at least one other expectation subgroup; this is not true for males.

With respect to the considerations advanced at the outset of this chapter, there is now available initial evidence for the inference that drinking behavior may function, at least in part, as an alternative mode of striving for goals otherwise unlikely to be attained or as a mode of coping with the lack of their attainment. To make this inference more compelling, more direct knowledge about the way in which alcohol is perceived, described, or defined by the subjects is necessary. Such information should show that students with low expectations for goal attainment actually attribute more problem-solving functions to their use of alcohol than do other students. The next phase of the research is addressed to this objective.

TABLE 3.—*Mean Scores on Drinking Measures of Subgroups Established on Level of Both Expectation Scores*

		Total Q-F	Drunkenness	Drinking-Related Complications
Males				
1.	High E_{ACH} High E_{AFF} (N=13)	.71	2.54	2.15
2.	High E_{ACH} Low E_{AFF} (N=6)	.69	2.33	1.50
3.	Low E_{ACH} High E_{AFF} (N=6)	.54	3.50	1.83
4.	Low E_{ACH} Low E_{AFF} (N=13)	.82	3.54	4.00* [1 2 3]
Females				
1.	High E_{ACH} High E_{AFF} (N=16)	.23	1.94	1.19
2.	High E_{ACH} Low E_{AFF} (N=9)	.19	1.44	1.11
3.	Low E_{ACH} High E_{AFF} (N=9)	.41	2.67	1.11
4.	Low E_{ACH} Low E_{AFF} (N=16)	.57* [1 2]	2.75* [2]	2.81* [1 2 3]

* t-test of the mean difference between Group 4 and the other group or groups whose number is shown in the superscript is significant on this measure at the .05 level or beyond, one-tailed test.

PART II

The Measurement of Drinking Functions

This phase of the research is concerned with the measurement of the meanings which are attached by the subject to alcohol use or the functions which alcohol is subjectively perceived to serve for him. Earlier work by Mulford and Miller (9, 10, 11) as well as analysis of drinking functions provided by Fallding (12) influenced our approach. A measurement technique used in the Tri-Ethnic Research Project (see 5, Chap. 7) was adapted to the present research. The technique presents the subject with a list of drinking functions to which he is asked to respond by checking all of those which characterize his own reasons for drinking. The list of functions was part of the larger drinking behavior questionnaire.

Four categories of drinking functions were defined, and items were made up to represent each category.[2] The categories and their definitions were the following:

Positive Social Functions (PS). Motivations and attitudes which link drinking to activities of a pleasant, festive, sociable nature. Drinking is engaged in largely for the convivial pleasure which surrounds it.

Conforming Social Functions (CS). Motivations and attitudes which link drinking to a sense of obligation for meeting group pressures or expectations with regard to what is seen as appropriate to or necessary for certain social situations.

Psychophysiological Functions (PH). Motivations and attitudes which link drinking to physical aches, pains, fatigue, or other forms of physical discomfort. Drinking is seen as a learned remedy for or relief from such physical symptoms.

Personality Effects Functions (PE). Motivations and attitudes which link drinking to unresolved problems or inadequacies of a psychological nature. Drinking is used as an escape from or relief for such problems or shortcomings, or as a way of achieving goals not otherwise attainable.

Of the four categories, the category of Personality Effects Functions is the one which most directly bears upon our interpretation of alcohol use as a learned way of striving or of coping with failure. Our basic prediction was that a *negative* relationship should obtain between expectations for need satisfaction and the degree to which Personal Effects Functions were attributed to drinking. The possibility of a negative rela-

[2] Obviously there are other ways of categorizing the possible functions of alcohol, and these will likely vary in different cultures or groups. The first author has recently completed a cross-cultural study of functions of alcohol use comparing youth in Palermo, Sicily, in Rome, and in Boston, the latter being of Italian-born grandparents. In this study a category of "dietary" functions was also included, e.g., "it rounds out a good meal," "it's important for a good diet," etc.

tionship obtaining with Conforming Social Functions and with Psychophysiological Functions was also anticipated. Conforming Social Functions suggest a learned reliance on alcohol in dealing with certain social situations, and Psychophysiological Functions, insofar as they represent psychosomatic difficulties, also suggest a possible problem-solving use of alcohol. Finally, Positive Social Functions were expected to have a *positive* relation with expectations for need satisfaction, the higher the expectations the greater the use of alcohol would tend to be for positive social (rather than problem-solving) reasons.

A pool of function items was collected from previous work and from inquiry with selected groups of students other than those used in the later study. The items were sorted into one of the four categories of functions by six research workers familiar with the theory of drinking functions being employed in the research. Agreement was clear-cut on 32 items, and these constituted the final list.[3]

[3] The items, their order in the list, and the category to which they were assigned were the following:

Positive Social Functions — 10 items

1. makes get-togethers fun
7. it's a pleasant way to celebrate
8. just to have a good time
12. because it's a pleasant recreation
14. just because it's fun
18. adds a certain warmth to social occasions
21. it's a nice way to celebrate special occasions
23. makes dinner dates out seem more special
29. because it's enjoyable to join in with people who are enjoying themselves
32. it's often a pleasant part of a congenial, social activity

Conforming Social Functions — 6 items

2. to be part of the group
5. it's the accepted thing to do
9. because everybody does it
13. to be one of the crowd
27. it's just a part of college life
30. the places where I go to be with others serve drinks

Psychophysiological Functions — 6 items

3. helps you get to sleep at night
10. feeling tired

Internal analyses of the function items provide evidence that four different categories of functions were actually being measured. Correlations between the number of items checked in each category are all low, ranging from —.08 to .29, with an average correlation of .13. Further, a Tryon cluster-analysis (13) yielded four virtually uncorrelated cluster-composites. These cluster-composites directly parallel our four function item categories, with five of the positive social items clustering, all six of the social conforming items clustering, three of the psychophysiological items clustering, and five of the personality effects items clustering. The domain validities for the four clusters range from .76 to .94 providing evidence that the items comprising each cluster represent a unidimensional subdomain of drinking motivation.

Two scores were examined for each function category: (1) a *number* of functions score based on sheer number of items checked within each category; (2) a *proportion* of functions score to reflect the differential *importance* to the subject of the four categories of functions while, at the same time, taking into account the fact that the number of items in the different categories is not the same.[4]

---

16.   eases aches and pains
19.   to get over headaches
24.   when I have a cold
31.   it settles your stomach

Personality Effects Functions — 10 items

 4.   feeling lonely
 6.   makes you worry less about what others are thinking about you
11.   gives you more confidence in yourself
15.   helps you forget you're not the kind of person you'd like to be
17.   makes you feel less shy
20.   makes you more satisfied with yourself
22.   feeling under pressure
25.   feeling mad
26.   makes the future seem brighter
28.   to get my mind off failures in course work

[4] This latter score evaluates the proportion of a student's total number of checked functions which is attributable to each of the four categories. The score is the number of functions checked in a category divided by the number there are in that category, and the result is divided further by the total number of functions checked by the student from the entire list.

The drinking functions items showed no appreciable sex differences in our college sample. The average number of items checked by the total group was close to ten, with the items in the Positive Social category being chosen by far the most frequently. Relative frequency of category use, taking into account differential category size, is shown in the following scores: Positive Social .63; Conforming Social .25; Personality Effects .15; and Psychophysiological .08.

Results

The data are analyzed in the same two ways as in Part I. Correlations between the two expectation scores and the eight functions scores (Table 4) lend support to the hypothesis. While none of the men's number of functions scores correlated significantly with their expectation scores, three significant relationships obtain when the proportion of functions scores are considered: the higher the expectation for achievement, the larger the proportion of functions chosen attributable to Positive Social Functions ($r=.30$); the lower the expectation for affection, the higher the proportion of functions chosen which are attributable to the Psychophysiological Function category ($r=-.43$) or to the Personality Effects category ($r=-.28$).

Results for the females are more consistently supportive. The number of functions score that is significantly related, in the direction predicted, to *both* the ACH and the AFF expectation scores is in the Personality Effects Functions category, the one most clearly related to our principal hypothesis ($r=-.40$ with E_{ACH} and $-.36$ with E_{AFF}). When proportion scores are con-

TABLE 4.—*Correlations between Expectation Scores and Number and Proportion of Drinking Function Scores*

	No. PS	No. CS	No. PH	No. PE	Prop. PS	Prop. CS	Prop. PH	Prop. PE
Males (N=38)								
E_{ACH}	.06	−.03	−.04	−.16	.30*	.10	−.11	−.16
E_{AFF}	.08	.17	−.26	−.16	.16	.25	−.43*	−.28*
Females (N=50)								
E_{ACH}	.01	−.17	.05	−.40*	.25*	−.25*	.17	−.34*
E_{AFF}	.07	.02	−.23	−.36*	.34*	−.08	−.08	−.27*

* Pearson correlation significant at the .05 level or beyond, one-tailed test.

sidered, five out of the eight expected relationships are significant, four of the five coming from the Personality Effects and the Positive Social categories. Taken together, these correlational results for both males and females provide additional support for our interpretation of drinking among college students.

The second mode of analysis, that involving groups high on both expectations, low on both, or high on one and low on the other, show no significant differences for the males. For the females, on both the number of functions score and the proportion of functions score, Group 4, the Low E_{ACH} and Low E_{AFF} group, is significantly higher on Personality Effects Functions than any of the other expectation groups. Differences among these other expectation groups tend to be minimal. This mode of analysis is consistent with the findings from the preceding correlational analyses; low expectations in *both* need areas are associated with higher reports of Personality Effects use of alcohol among females.

The data presented thus far in Part II have been concerned with examining the link between expectations and drinking functions. To complete the bridge, the further link between Personality Effects drinking functions and drinking *behavior* needs to be examined.

For the males, intake as measured by Total Q-F shows no significant relation to the Personality Effects function scores (Table 5). With respect to frequency of drunkenness, however,

TABLE 5.—*Correlations between Personality Effects Function Scores and Drinking Behavior*

	Number of Personality Effect Functions	Proportion of Personality Effects Functions
Males (N=38)		
Total Q-F	.10	.13
Drunkenness	.52*	.40*
Drinking-related complications	.23	.20
Females (N=50)		
Total Q-F	.32*	.27*
Drunkenness	.50*	.39*
Drinking-related complications	.41*	.34*

* Pearson correlation significant at the .05 level or beyond, one-tailed test.

the Personality Effects category is a significant predictor, and this is consistent for both number and proportion of functions scores. On the Drinking-Related Complications measure, the correlations are short of significance. For the females, all three of the measures of drinking behavior are significantly predicted by the Personality Effects Functions category. Its relation to the drinking measures holds in all cases, whether the number or the proportion score is considered, and the level of relationship is substantial, and average r for the six Personality Effects correlations being .37.

Discussion

With respect to the college environment, the research has identified as relevant to drinking two major areas of striving for goal attainment or need satisfaction: the achievement area and the affection area. Low expectations in these areas are related not only to the pattern of drinking behavior but, more directly, to the meaning which alcohol has come to have for the user. These relationships lend support to the inference that alcohol use may be a learned behavior for attaining goals otherwise unattainable or for coping with the failure to attain valued goals.

This inference obviously needs to be held tentatively at this point. First of all, the cross-sectional research design employed is incapable of establishing the causal direction contained in the inference, namely that low expectations for goal attainment lead to or result in alcohol use as an alternative behavior. Further, the research focuses on only one interpretation of alcohol use; the applicability of alternative interpretations was not investigated. One direction in which investigation of alternatives might go would be to consider drinking as a satisfying and meaningful activity in its own right, rather than as a problem-solving alternative behavior. Some support for pursuing this notion may be adduced from the data in Table 3 where there is a slight suggestion of curvilinearity, the students having *high* expectations in both need areas having somewhat greater recourse to drinking than those low in one need. Although the data are not clear in this regard, they do emphasize the need for consideration of multiple interpretations in order to exhaust the variance in drinking behavior.

Attention should be called to the fact that only two need areas were dealt with in the present research. Given the large number of need areas in which students of college age tend to seek gratification, it remains possible that stronger and more consistent support for our main hypothesis could be obtained if a larger set of need areas could be taken into consideration at one time. Recourse to alternatives such as drinking may become more probable only when low expectations obtain in all need areas. Support for this possibility derives from the fact that it was Group 4, Low E_{ACH} *and* Low E_{AFF}, which tended to differ from the other three groups. A more comprehensive sampling of need areas would provide an opportunity to locate groups with *generalized* low expectations, and to make a less ambiguous test of the low expectation-high drinking behavior hypothesis.

Next in importance to the obtained support for the research hypothesis was the finding of sex differences in the relationships examined, the fact that the findings for the females were consistently more substantial than for the males. One possible explanation is that the two needs measured were of differential centrality to the sexes. It is possible also that the sexes responded to the inventories with differential truthfulness. A further interpretation, one which draws attention again to the limited nature of our hypothesis, seems worth exploring. Sex differences in alcohol use are ubiquitous; among American youth, these have recently been reported, for example, by Maddox and McCall (14). What seems clear is that social norms exist which regulate alcohol use *differentially* for the sexes, males not only being allowed greater freedom of use but, in certain situations such as college, being *expected* to use alcohol. It may well be that much more of the variance in male drinking than in female drinking is to be accounted for *normatively;* said otherwise, more of the variance in female drinking than in male drinking may be accounted for in terms of personality factors since normative regulation tends simply to emphasize abstinence or restraint. Such an interpretation is not only consistent with our findings but also suggests the utility of more comprehensive explanatory systems, those which simultaneously consider both social and personality determinants.

In the present research, the bridge between expectations for need satisfaction and the pattern of drinking behavior was shown to involve the subjectively defined functions of alcohol. The data support the position of Mulford and Miller (9, 10, 11): definitions held about alcohol should be importantly influential in determining the use which is made of it. The utility of a focus upon the meaning of alcohol is that it enables an approach to the individual, a possibility of dealing with his own idiosyncratic definitions instead of relying upon either the general properties of alcohol or the group's institutionalization of its use. Further work on variation in meanings clearly needs to be done, sampling diverse groups, sampling the different stages of the developmental trajectory to assess age-related changes, and sampling the variation in meanings attributed to alcohol when used in different situations.

The usefulness of the Personality Effects category of functions was strongly demonstrated in this study. It seems to be a worthwhile category of meaning to apply to college drinking. The Positive Social Functions category also proved useful. On the other hand, neither the Conforming Social nor the Psychophysiological Functions categories yielded consistent results. It is possible that neither of these latter categories of functions is central to college student use of alcohol or to this particular age level. Psychophysiological functions may, for example, increase in appropriateness in middle or late-middle age. In any event, further research on drinking functions seems likely to prove fruitful.

Our research, to conclude, represents a start in the direction of relating personality factors to variations in the use of alcohol among youth of college age. Previous research on personality and drinking behavior has not proved too successful. In light of that history, some degree of encouragement is to be taken from the support generated by the present findings.

REFERENCES

1. CARMAN, R. S. "Personality and Drinking Behavior among College Students." Unpublished Master's thesis, University of Colorado, 1965.
2. GROSSMAN, P. H. "Drinking Motivation: A Cluster Analytic

Study of Three Samples." Unpublished doctoral dissertation, University of Colorado, 1965.

3. ROTTER, J. B. *Social Learning and Clinical Psychology*. New York: Prentice-Hall, 1954.

4. ROTTER, J. B. "The Role of the Psychological Situation in Determining the Direction of Human Behavior," in M. R. JONES (ed.), *The Nebraska Symposium on Motivation, 1955*, pp. 245-269. Lincoln, Nebraska: University of Nebraska Press, 1955.

5. JESSOR, R., T. D. GRAVES, R. C. HANSON, and SHIRLEY L. JESSOR. *Society, Personality and Deviant Behavior: A Study of a Tri-Ethnic Community*. New York: Holt, Rinehart & Winston, 1968.

6. OPOCHINSKY, S. "Values, Expectations, and the Formation of Impressions." Unpublished doctoral dissertation, University of Colorado, 1965.

7. GROSSMAN, P. H. "The Establishment of Alcohol Consumption Criterion Groups: Rationale and Associated Characteristics." Research Report No. 18, Tri-Ethnic Research Project. Institute of Behavioral Science, University of Colorado, April 1963. Mimeographed, pp. 1-39.

8. STRAUS, R., and S. D. BACON. *Drinking in College*. New Haven: Yale University Press, 1953.

9. MULFORD, H. A., and D. E. MILLER. "Drinking Behavior Related to Definitions of Alcohol: A Report of Research in Progress," *American Sociological Review*, 24: 385-389, 1959.

10. MULFORD, H. A., and D. E. MILLER. "Drinking in Iowa, III. A Scale of Definitions of Alcohol Related to Drinking Behavior," *Quarterly Journal of Studies on Alcohol*, 21: 267-278, 1960.

11. MULFORD, H. A., and D. E. MILLER. "Drinking in Iowa, IV. Preoccupation with Alcohol and Definitions of Alcohol, Heavy Drinking and Trouble Due to Drinking," *Quarterly Journal of Studies on Alcohol*, 21: 279-291, 1960.

12. FALLDING, H. "The Source and Burden of Civilization Illustrated in the Use of Alcohol," *Quarterly Journal of Studies on Alcohol*, 25: 714-724, 1964.

13. TRYON, R., and D. BAILEY. "Theory of the BC-TRY System: Statistical Theory," in *Cluster and Factor Analysis*. Mimeographed, 1964. Chapter 1.

14. MADDOX, G. L., and B. C. McCALL. *Drinking among Teen-Agers: A Sociological Interpretation of Alcohol-Use in High School*. New Brunswick, N. J.: Rutgers Center of Alcohol Studies, 1964.

Chapter 16

COLLEGE PROBLEM DRINKERS: A PERSONALITY PROFILE[1]

ALLAN F. WILLIAMS

The Medical Foundation, Boston, Mass.

I N THIS CHAPTER a series of personality findings on male college problem drinkers will be presented and discussed. Data from three different samples of college students are included. Each of these samples was measured on a college problem-drinking scale, developed by Park (18) by means of factor analysis of items selected from the Straus and Bacon (21) study of drinking among American college students.[2] The problem-drinking scale is considered to be a measure of predisposition or proneness to alcoholism. The majority of the items making up the scale have been mentioned by Jellinek (10) as characteristics of alcoholism. Problem drinkers have not, how-

---

[1] This chapter was written especially for this book. It includes results also presented in other articles by Williams (22-26).

[2] The problem-drinking scale contains 12 items with positive factor loadings; one with a negative factor loading. The 12 positively loaded items are "has felt that subject might become dependent on or addicted to the use of alcoholic beverages"; "has incurred social complications due to drinking"; "has feared the long-range consequences of own drinking"; "drinks large or medium amount of alcoholic beverages at a sitting and more than once a week"; "likes to be one or two drinks ahead without others knowing it"; "has gone on the water wagon as the result of self-decision or advice of the family or friends"; "has had one or more drinks before or instead of breakfast"; "has become drunk when alone"; "has had one or more drinks alone"; "has gone on week-end drinking sprees"; "has been led by drinking to aggressive, wantonly destructive, or malicious behavior"; "has experienced blackouts in connection with drinking." The last six items are scored if they have occurred one or more times. The negatively loaded item is "drinks to comply with custom."

ever, manifested these behaviors as often as alcoholics would have: the behavior items in the scale are scored as indicating problem drinking if they have occurred one or more times. Validation data reported by Park (18) and Williams (26) support interpretation of the scale as a measure of predisposition to alcoholism. Since the scale is of recent origin, it has not yet been established whether or not a significant proportion of problem drinkers do eventually become alcoholics. However, the validation data indicate that it is likely that problem drinkers constitute a population from which future alcoholics will be drawn.

Since there exists the possibility that the problem-drinking scale identifies pre-alcoholics, college problem drinkers will be compared to alcoholics (as well as to college non-problem drinkers) in order to gain leads to the etiology of alcoholism. Etiologically-oriented investigations using alcoholic subjects are hampered by the possibility that the results obtained are consequences of fifteen to twenty years of excessive drinking and the social and psychological stresses which accompany alcoholism, rather than being antecedents of this disorder. By working with college-age problem drinkers, it may be possible to identify pre-alcoholic personality traits. And by comparing problem drinkers and alcoholics, it may be possible to distinguish pre-alcoholic personality traits from those which are consequences of alcoholism.

In Park's study it was found that problem drinkers deviated from the structural requirements of the adaptive male role in the direction of particularism (subjective evaluation, lack of objective judgment and critical ability) and affectivity (immediate gratification, low frustration threshold). Problem drinkers were also found to be ambivalent in role orientation—that is, not only did they deviate from the male role but they appeared to be unsuited to perform any role adequately.

The main instrument used in the personality assessment of problem drinkers has been the Adjective Check List (ACL) (8). The ACL consists of 300 adjectives, and the respondent is asked to check those adjectives which he considers to be descriptive of him. There are a variety of dimensions of personality which can be measured by this instrument.

One of the personality dimensions which has been of interest in this research is that of self-evaluation. Connor (5), in a study of a variety of alcoholic populations using the ACL, found that alcoholics scored low on a measure of self-acceptance. This finding of negative self-evaluation among alcoholics coincides with other research and clinical observations emphasizing the alcoholic's sense of inferiority and inadequacy (1, 4, 12, 20). However, it seems likely that a person's self-evaluation would be adversely affected by alcoholism; loss of self-esteem has, in fact, been mentioned by Jellinek (10) as a consequence of alcoholism. Thus in terms of the etiology of alcoholism it is important to determine whether or not negative self-evaluation precedes alcoholism or is a consequence of this disorder.

Problem drinkers will be compared to non-problem drinkers on the self-acceptance measure. There are also other ACL variables which are related to self-esteem: personal adjustment, self-confidence, and self-criticality.

Connor (5) also found that alcoholics emphasized ACL adjectives signifying permissive friendliness (e.g., forgiving, affectionate), reflecting a desire to be liked and accepted in primary group roles; and de-emphasized adjectives appropriate to secondary group roles (e.g., capable, responsible). These findings for alcoholics will be checked for college problem drinkers.

The bulk of the rest of the ACL variables are need scales developed by Heilbrun (8) from adjectives categorized in terms of 15 variables from Murray's (17) need-press system. Two major personality themes which will be explored by means of these variables are dependency and interpersonal orientation. Three of the Heilbrun variables (succorance, deference, and autonomy) are related to dependency. Several Heilbrun variables (dominance, intraception, nurturance, affiliation, autonomy, succorance, aggression, deference) plus an additional ACL variable (self-control) refer to some aspect of interpersonal relationships.

In one of the samples to be reported, an adjective check list containing anxiety and depression scales was administered. These scales were developed by Zuckerman and associates (28, 29, 30). Both anxiety (14) and depression (31) have been reported to be characteristics of alcoholics. However, the social isolation and the various personal stresses which accompany alcoholism are likely to produce or aggravate these personality characteristics, and it is important to attempt to determine whether or not anxiety and depression precede alcoholism.

Method

There were three samples used in the research. The first sample (Sample A) (23) was composed of 68 subjects from four fraternities at a New England men's liberal arts college. The mean of problem-drinking scores was 3.3, with a standard deviation of 2.7.[3] The data analysis is based on the 45 subjects who comprised the top and bottom thirds of the problem-drinking distribution. The top third (scores of 5–11, N = 23) were arbitrarily designated as problem drinkers; the bottom third (–1 to +1, N = 22) as non-problem drinkers.[4]

A second sample of male subjects (Sample B) was obtained from a different New England college: a large, predominantly male, engineering school. These subjects had taken part in a study by Kälin (11) which involved parties at which either liquor or soft drinks were served. Several weeks following completion of the parties they filled out a series of questionnaires and tests, including the ACL and the problem-drinking measure. On the basis of problem-drinking scores, the 136 subjects were first divided into three groups which corresponded to the upper, middle, and lower thirds of the Sample A distribution of problem-drinking scores (5 and above, 2–4, and –1 to +1, respectively). There were 24 subjects in the group with scores of 5 or more, and subsamples of 24 were drawn from each of the other groups. The analysis is based on the upper and lower groups.

The third sample is composed of male students from five

[3] Scores of +1 were given to positive responses to the 12 positively loaded items on the scale; a score of −1 was given to a positive response to the negatively loaded item. The theoretical range of scores was therefore −1 to +12.

[4] In this sample as well as in the next two, all of the variables were plotted to check for curvilinearity. There was no evidence of curvilinear effects for any of the variables which significantly differentiated problem and non-problem drinkers.

fraternities at two men's liberal arts colleges in New York State. These subjects participated in a study of psychological effects of social drinking (22). The evening before parties were held they completed a booklet of questionnaires which included the ACL, the anxiety and depression scales, and the problem-drinking measure. Problem-drinking scores of the 91 subjects in this study were somewhat higher than in Samples A and B (mean, 5.3; standard deviation, 2.9), and the analysis reported here is based on the top and bottom 40% of the distribution (problem drinkers: 7–12, N = 36; non-problem drinkers: –1 to +4, N = 36).

It should be pointed out that in Sample A and especially in Sample C, fraternities with reputations for heavy drinking were included in order to insure that there would be a sufficient number of high scorers on the scale to allow comparison between problem drinkers and non-problem drinkers. Thus the distribution of problem-drinking scores reported should not be regarded as representative of colleges from which the samples were drawn.

In scoring the ACL variables, ratio scores were used to compute self-acceptance and self-criticality scores. The self-acceptance index indicates the extent to which a person checks the 75 of 300 ACL adjectives rated as "most favorable" by 30 judges (number of favorable adjectives checked/total number of adjectives checked). The self-criticality index is based on the 75 "least favorable" adjectives (number of unfavorable adjectives checked/total number checked).

For the remainder of the variables there are both indicative and contraindicative adjectives involved. Raw scores for these variables are the algebraic sums of indicative and contraindicative adjectives checked as self-descriptive. These raw scores are then converted to T scores, with the total number of adjectives checked taken into account.

Of the three Heilbrun variables related to a concept of dependency, succorance (soliciting support from others) and deference (subordination to others) refer to dependency; autonomy (acting independently of others) refers to independence. Therefore a total self-descriptive dependency score was computed from the sum of deference and succorance minus autonomy.

The anxiety check list contains 11 anxiety-plus words (e.g., afraid, tense) scored +1 if checked, and 10 anxiety-minus adjectives (e.g., calm, cheerful) scored +1 if not checked. The depression check list, scored in the same manner, contains 20 depression-plus adjectives (e.g., calm, cheerful) and 20 depression-minus adjectives (e.g., active, enthusiastic).

Results

Table 1 presents means of the ACL variables, results of *t* tests for the 3 samples, and a combined two-tailed level of significance for the 3 samples computed by the Stouffer method (16).

The combined results indicated that problem drinkers were significantly higher than non-problem drinkers on self-criticality, lability, autonomy, change, and aggression; and significantly lower than non-problem drinkers on self-acceptance, self-control, personal adjustment, deference, order, affiliation, intraception, endurance, and nurturance. Each of these 14 variables—except for "change" in Sample A, endurance in Sample B, and lability in Samples B and C—reflected the combined results in all three samples (at least p = .20).

Problem drinkers did not differ significantly from non-problem drinkers in the combined results on self-confidence, achievement, exhibition, succorance, dominance, abasement, and heterosexuality.

Using the total dependency score computed from the sum of deference and succorance minus autonomy, problem drinkers were lower than non-problem drinkers on dependency in the combined results ($p < .05$), in Sample B ($p < .20$), and in Sample C ($p < .01$). These results were primarily due to problem drinkers' high autonomy and low deference scores. In Sample A there were no differences since problem drinkers described themselves as both independent (high autonomy, low deference) and dependent (high succorance).

In Sample C, scores on the problem-drinking scale were correlated with anxiety and depression scores in each of the five fraternities, and the five correlations were averaged. Results indicated that problem drinking was positively associated with anxiety ($r = +.37$, $p < .005$, one-tailed) and depression ($r = +.26$, $p < .05$, one-tailed).

TABLE 1.—Means of ACL Variables for Problem Drinkers (PD) and Non-problem Drinkers (NPD) and Results of t Tests

	Sample A (N=23)(N=22)			Sample B (N=24)(N=24)			Sample C (N=36)(N=36)			Combined
	PD	NPD	P	PD	NPD	P	PD	NPD	P	P
Self-acceptance	41.9	54.9	<.0005[b]	43.0	50.0	<.05[b]	45.7	49.5	<.10[b]	<.0005[c]
Self-criticality	13.4	6.4	<.005[b]	14.0	8.5	<.05[b]	13.8	9.8	<.05[b]	<.0005[c]
Self-confidence	43.8	49.6	<.10	49.9	51.3	ns	49.6	46.3	<.20	ns
Self-control	43.4	53.1	<.005	39.7	46.9	<.05	41.5	46.6	<.01	<.0005[c]
Lability	55.3	50.1	<.20	57.1	53.5	<.20	52.1	49.4	ns	.05[c]
Personal Adjustment	43.0	51.8	<.005[b]	40.7	46.5	<.05[b]	43.9	46.0	<.20[b]	<.005[c]
Achievement	45.1	53.2	<.01	49.6	51.6	ns	47.1	46.7	ns	<.10
Deference	47.7	51.5	≡.20	39.0	43.5	<.20	42.3	49.1	<.005	<.005[c]
Order	42.9	54.0	<.01	44.7	50.4	<.10	45.1	51.5	<.005	<.0005[c]
Exhibition	49.8	50.8	ns	57.6	53.6	ns	53.6	48.7	<.05[a]	<.20
Autonomy	51.8	46.7	<.10	60.4	53.7	<.10	57.2	51.9	<.05	<.005[c]
Affiliation	45.8	51.2	<.10	41.7	48.0	<.05	44.9	50.7	<.01	<.0005[c]
Intraception	47.6	54.2	<.10	44.4	50.8	<.10	45.7	52.1	<.005	<.0005[c]
Succorance	53.5	45.9	<.05	46.0	45.4	ns	47.9	48.6	ns	ns
Dominance	44.0	52.1	<.01	50.0	50.5	ns	48.7	48.4	ns	<.20
Abasement	52.1	47.4	<.10	44.4	45.4	<.10	47.2	49.9	ns	ns
Nurturance	46.4	54.0	<.05	40.8	45.7	<.10	42.9	49.7	<.01	<.0005[c]
Change	48.4	45.5	ns	52.4	49.7	≡.20	51.7	46.6	<.05[a]	<.05[c]
Endurance	40.6	54.7	<.001	45.3	48.7	ns	45.4	50.3	<.05	<.0005[c]
Heterosexuality	54.3	50.7	ns	50.8	51.4	ns	51.8	50.4	ns	ns
Aggression	51.8	47.5	<.20	58.0	53.5	<.20	56.7	49.4	<.005	<.005[c]

NOTE: Significance levels for Samples A, B, and the combined results are two-tailed, except where noted. Significance levels for Sample C are one-tailed, except where noted.

[a] Two-tailed
[b] One-tailed
[c] All three samples show same direction of difference

Before discussing the results comment should be made on the similarity of the ACL results in the three different samples. There was a great deal of overlap in the three samples. The results in Samples B and C can be considered as two separate replication studies. Most of the variables which were significant or approached statistical significance in any one sample were also significant or nearly significant in the other two samples. Thus one may have a good deal of confidence that for the variables which were significant in the combined results there are real differences between problem and non-problem drinkers. It should be noted also that the three samples were drawn from four different colleges in three states, with the data being collected under markedly different conditions in each case. Since the results in the three samples were similar, the generality of the findings is thereby increased.

Discussion

Self-evaluation

On three of the four ACL variables which can be considered as measuring some aspect of self-evaluation, problem drinkers were found to have negative self-evaluation. Problem drinkers were lower than non-problem drinkers on self-acceptance and personal adjustment, and higher on self-criticality. Problem drinkers used fewer favorable and more unfavorable words in their self-descriptions than did non-problem drinkers. The personal adjustment variable was developed through item analysis of ACL tests of persons rated high and low on personal adjustment and personal soundness. People who score low on this variable have been found to view themselves as at odds with others, and as moody and dissatisfied. Problem drinkers scored lower than non-problem drinkers on self-confidence only in Sample A. In Sample B there were no differences, and in Sample C problem drinkers tended to score higher than non-problem drinkers on this variable. The self-confidence variable was designed to correspond to the poise and self-assurance scales on the California Psychological Inventory (7). The scale has a strong element of dominance, and high scorers tend to be active, assertive, and outgoing people as well. The self-confidence scale is thus somewhat different from the other scales related to self-evaluation: it is an activity variable or a public personality variable rather than a dimension tapping assessment of or satisfaction with the self. This difference is reflected in the generally low correlations of self-confidence with these other variables, as reported by Gough and Heilbrun (8) and as found in the present samples. Self-acceptance, self-criticality, and personal adjustment are highly intercorrelated in the present samples, and high intercorrelations among these variables are also reported by Gough and Heilbrun. In general it may be said that problem drinkers have negative self-evaluation.[5]

The data thus indicated that the low self-evaluation which has consistently been found to be characteristic of alcoholics is also characteristic of college problem drinkers. If the problem-drinking scale is an adequate prognosticator of alcoholism, it may be concluded that this personality characteristic precedes the development of alcoholism and perhaps plays a role in the development of this disorder.

Dependency

A frequent clinical observation made of alcoholics is that they are dependent, and the concept of dependency has played an important part in theories of the development of alcoholism. The data of the present studies indicated that problem drinkers were independent rather than dependent, although a combination of dependence and independence characterized the Sample A problem drinkers. Problem drinkers were also found to have high scores on aggression in all three samples. These results are of interest in the light of a recent longitudinal study by McCord and McCord (15) and a theory of the development of alcoholism by Lisansky (13). The McCords found that while alcoholics were rated as dependent and were probably basically dependent, as pre-alcoholics they were counterdependent, expressing such traits as aggression, autonomy, and lack of deference as reactions against dependency. Pre-alcoholics, in other

---

[5] Other evidence for this conclusion comes from an additional relationship found in Sample A (23). Subjects in this study completed the ACL for ideal self as well as real self, and problem drinking was found to be negatively associated with real-self–ideal-self correspondence ($r = -.35$, $p < .005$).

words, were characterized by a dependence-independence conflict. Lisansky has theorized that there exists among alcoholics a strong need for dependency which results in an intense dependence-independence conflict for pre-alcoholics coping with the adult male role. Lisansky stresses that by the time an alcoholic is a clinic patient—usually long after the establishment of alcoholism—the conflict is less apparent, having been resolved in favor of dependency. The McCords see loss of control over alcohol and the concomitant role failure dissolving the self-image of independence and self-sufficiency, resulting in the emergence of dependency traits which were formerly repressed.

Although the Sample A problem drinkers' combination of dependence and independence can be interpreted as a direct manifestation of a dependence-independence conflict, in general problem drinkers characterized themselves as independent. The question of whether this is truly independence, or counter-dependence—a reaction formation—cannot be answered on the basis of these findings. However, findings related to dependence-independence are likely to be of major importance in an eventual understanding of the etiology of alcoholism, and the question of which alternative is correct should be a subject of future research on college problem drinkers.

Interpersonal Orientation

When adjectives checked at least 20% more often by either problem drinkers or non-problem drinkers in the 3 samples have been considered (23), problem drinkers have been found to differ from Connor's alcoholics who emphasized primary-relationship terms, adjectives centering around permissive friendliness. There was a scattering of primary-relationship terms in the lists of adjectives endorsed more frequently by problem drinkers, but there were more of these adjectives in the lists of words emphasized by non-problem drinkers. Moreover, problem drinkers (but not non-problem drinkers) used a number of words suggesting the opposite of permissive friendliness (e.g., sarcastic, fault-finding). Problem drinkers thus appeared to de-emphasize primary-relationship terms rather than to emphasize them.

This finding was reinforced when ACL variables having to do with interpersonal relationships were considered. On four of these variables—affiliation, intraception, nurturance, and self-control—problem drinkers scored low in each case. Intraception denotes a subjective concern with others and interest in others' behavior and the motivations for it; affiliation, an active seeking and promoting of personal friendships; and nurturance, an attentiveness to the feelings and wishes of others. The self-control variable was designed to parallel the responsibility–socialization scales of the California Psychological Inventory (7). Those scoring low on this variable have been found to be inadequately socialized and tend to be described by others in unflattering terms. The high scores of problem drinkers on independence (low deference, and high autonomy which involves indifference to the feelings and wants of others as well as independence) also fits into this interpersonal syndrome. Problem drinkers appear to be relatively unconcerned with and uninterested in others. This orientation is consistent with their independence, and these data suggest that problem drinkers are not well liked and that they are apt to be isolated from primary-group relationships. Further evidence for this conclusion derives from the high aggression scores of problem drinkers, aggression denoting a tendency to attack or hurt others.

Thus the interpersonal orientation of problem drinkers conflicts with Connor's finding that alcoholics showed a strong tendency to emphasize in their self-descriptions terms centering around permissive friendliness, qualities which would tend to make them liked and accepted in primary group relations. Connor found that the primary relationship theme remained prominent even after long periods of sobriety had been maintained, suggesting that this theme was of basic importance in the personality structure of alcoholics, and may have preceded alcoholism. If the problem-drinking scale is an adequate prognosticator of alcoholism, exactly the opposite conclusion is reached: pre-alcoholics de-emphasize terms which would make them liked and accepted and appear to be relatively unconcerned with and indifferent to others.

If a change in interpersonal orientation of the sort noted does occur subsequent to alcoholism, the question arises as to why it occurs. Inspection of the literature indicates that the primary-relationship theme manifested by Connor's alco-

holics does not coincide with other findings for alcoholics—
all based on empirical data—which would indicate that alcoholics are like problem drinkers in interpersonal orientation:
preoccupation with self (2, 6, 27); insensitive in relationships
with others (4, 19); asocial, distant in emotional contact (14,
32). These findings suggest that permissive friendliness among
alcoholics does not indicate a deep-seated concern *for* others,
but may be viewed as a strategy for gaining support *from*
others, and perhaps, satisfaction of dependency needs. The
appearance of this theme in behavior subsequent to alcoholism
can be accounted for by (a) the likelihood that the development of alcoholism will severely disrupt existing primary group
ties, thereby making the attainment of nurturant and favorable
responses a matter of some concern; and (b) the possibility
suggested by McCords' data and Lisansky's theory that subsequent to alcoholism dependency conflicts are resolved in
favor of dependency. In such a case, one would expect the
alcoholic to attempt to satisfy dependency needs more openly
than the pre-alcoholic. Moreover, the breakdown subsequent
to alcoholism of a self-image of independence and self-sufficiency—if this does in fact occur—is likely to leave the individual needing friends and emotional nurturance. It should be
noted, however, that the primary-relationship theme among
alcoholics remains an important personality finding, even
though it may be a strategy, and is of special significance for
those who have contact with the alcoholic.

Change, Lability, Endurance, Order

Of the four remaining variables which distinguished problem drinkers and non-problem drinkers, problem drinkers
scored high on change and lability, and low on endurance
and order. Lability denotes a delighting in the new and different and a sensitivity to the unusual and challenging, but
its main facet is that of inner restlessness and an inability to
tolerate consistency and routine. High scorers on change
tend to be perceptive, alert, and spontaneous individuals who
comprehend problems rapidly and incisively and who take
pleasure in change and variety and tend to avoid routine. Endurance denotes persistence in tasks undertaken; low scorers
tend to be intolerant of prolonged effort or attention and to

be erratic, impatient, and changeable. Low scorers on order tend to be quick in temperament and reaction, and impulsive. They prefer complexity and variety, dislike delay, caution, and deliberation. The self-control variable, whose theme of inadequate socialization (for low scorers) includes disorderliness, impulsivity and irresponsibility, is also related to this group of variables.

It may be noted that there are common themes running through these variables: a liking for the new and different, and a corresponding dislike for consistency and routine; and a theme characterized by restlessness, impatience, impulsiveness, spontaneity, and action,[6] with a disliking of prolonged effort or attention, delay or deliberation. For two of these variables—endurance and order—the low scores of problem drinkers make them similar to alcoholics. Lack of perseverance has been attributed to alcoholics by numerous authors (3, 6), and characterizations of the alcoholic as impulsive have been frequent in the literature (9, 19). There have been no reports for alcoholics on such variables as change and lability.

The Secondary-Relationship Theme

In considering the adjectives checked at least 20 per cent more often by either problem drinkers or non-problem drinkers, it was found that non-problem drinkers clearly exceeded problem drinkers in their use of secondary-relationship terms, thus making problem drinkers similar to Connor's alcoholics. Secondary-relationship terms were virtually absent in the self-descriptions of problem drinkers in all three samples when the data were analyzed by means of proportional differences in selection, but are frequently found in the lists of adjectives emphasized by non-problem drinkers. Certainly full-blown alcoholism involves a decrease in participation in secondary relationships as the person tends to become isolated from society. Connor found, in fact, a very nearly linear gradient of secondary-relationship adjective depletion from non-alcoholics through sanatorium patients, A.A., penitentiary prisoners, to

---

[6] The "action" theme is also reflected in problem drinkers' low scores on intraception. Problem drinkers tend not to be reflective; they are "doers."

Skid Row types or jail prisoners. Secondary-relationship terms indicate qualities necessary to the operation of the social structure, and, incidentally, to the pursuance of the male occupational role. Since each of the above groups is likely to be progressively more isolated from secondary relationships as a result of alcoholism, it might well be thought that the depletion of secondary-relationship terms from the self-concept is entirely a result of alcoholism. The fact that this condition is foreshadowed in the self-concepts of college problem drinkers suggests that the pre-alcoholic is predisposed toward difficulties in social adjustment or role adjustment, and that secondary-relationship adjective depletion in alcoholics is not just the result of alcoholism isolating the person from participation in secondary-relationship activities.

It may be noted that both Park's finding of deviation and ambivalence in role orientation among problem drinkers, and the finding in the present studies that problem drinkers do not describe themselves in terms of secondary relationship qualities, indicate future difficulties for problem drinkers in attempting to cope with the responsibilities of the adult male role. At the same time, problem drinkers describe themselves in terms of qualities (aggression, independence, lack of social concern and interest) which are commonly associated with masculinity. This combination of findings is again reminiscent of the McCords' longitudinal study in which pre-alcoholics presented a facade of masculine traits which was a reaction formation and which was broken down by their subsequent failure in carrying out the adult male role. At present, however, this combination of findings for problem drinkers can only be noted; its interpretation awaits further research in this area.

Anxiety and Depression

The findings that problem drinkers are characterized by anxiety and depression correspond to similar findings for alcoholics which were mentioned earlier. Since alcoholism appears capable of producing anxiety and depression, these findings may be important ones, indicating that these aspects of personality precede alcoholism and perhaps contribute to its development.

Summary and Conclusions

In research carried out in three samples of college males, problem drinkers were found to have the following main characteristics: (a) low self-evaluation; (b) anxiety and depression; (c) a de-emphasis on secondary-relationship terms; (d) a liking for the new and different and a corresponding dislike for consistency and routine; and a theme of restlessness, impatience, impulsiveness, spontaneity and action; (e) aggression and independence; and (f) a de-emphasis on primary-relationship terms and a lack of concern and interest in others. There was also evidence that problem drinkers are inadequately socialized and that they are not apt to be well liked by their peers.

Problem drinkers were found to be similar to alcoholics on the first three themes (a-c). They were also similar to alcoholics in having low scores on endurance and order, two of the variables making up the (d) theme. It is not certain that alcoholics would also score high on lability and change, the two other variables of this theme. Problem drinkers were dissimilar to Connor's alcoholics (although not to other alcoholic populations reported on in research studies) in de-emphasizing primary-relationship terms and in their lack of social concern and interest.

It may be noted that problem drinkers were similar to alcoholics on the bulk of the variables under study. If the problem-drinking scale is an adequate prognosticator of alcoholism, these findings are of importance to an investigation of the etiology of alcoholism since they indicate that these traits precede the development of alcoholism. It should be pointed out that most of these traits might well be expected to be consequences of 15-20 years of excessive drinking and loss of control over alcohol. Of perhaps greater interest in terms of the etiology of alcoholism are the findings on variables such as dependence-independence and the primary-relationship theme where there are differences between problem drinkers and alcoholics. Assuming that problem drinkers are pre-alcoholics and that they will become like alcoholics in personality later, attempts were made to integrate these findings into a coherent picture of the development of alcoholism. The important point about finding differences between problem drinkers and non-problem drinkers is, of course, that these findings for problem drinkers may provide new clues to the etiology of alcoholism.

In discussing the personality results, reference has been made to the etiology of alcoholism. That is, it has been noted that personality results on problem drinkers may well represent pre-alcoholic personality traits. However, even if this were so, these findings would represent only a starting point in unraveling the etiology of alcoholism. It is not enough to know that individuals with certain traits become alcoholics. One needs to know also why alcohol is used excessively by persons with these characteristics. This later question—why problem drinkers drink heavily and frequently, become problem drinkers and perhaps eventually become alcoholics—has not been discussed in this chapter. However, it should be pointed out that research on this question has been done by means of investigation of the effects of drinking on the variables presented here (22). The results, while not conclusive, do suggest leads as to possible benefits of alcohol received by problem drinkers which are greater than or not received by non-problem drinkers, benefits which would afford them greater motivation for drinking.

Finally, it must be emphasized that the personality description of problem drinkers given is not a finished, or complete picture. There are gaps to be filled in, other variables to be explored. What has been presented in this chapter represents only a beginning in the elucidation of the personality dynamics of problem drinking, and perhaps of alcoholism.

REFERENCES

1. ALLEN, E. B. "Emotional Factors in Alcoholism," *New York State Journal of Medicine*, 44: 374-378, 1944.
2. BILLIG, O., and D. J. SULLIVAN. "Personality Structure and Prognosis of Alcohol Addiction: A Rorschach Study," *Quarterly Journal of Studies on Alcohol*, 3: 554-573, 1943.
3. BUHLER, CHARLOTTE, and D. W. LEFEVER. "A Rorschach Study on the Psychological Characteristics of Alcoholics," *Quarterly Journal of Studies on Alcohol*, 8: 197-260, 1947.

4. BUTTON, A. D. "The Psychodynamics of Alcoholism: A Survey of 87 Cases," *Quarterly Journal of Studies on Alcohol*, 17: 443-460, 1956.

5. CONNOR, R. G. "The Self-Concepts of Alcoholics," in D. J. PITTMAN and C. R. SNYDER (eds.), *Society, Culture, and Drinking Patterns;* pp. 455-467. New York: Wiley, 1962.

6. FORCE, R. C. "Development of a Covert Test for the Detection of Alcoholism by a Keying of the Kuder Preference Record," *Quarterly Journal of Studies on Alcohol*, 19: 72-78, 1958.

7. GOUGH, H. F. *Manual for the California Psychological Inventory.* Palo Alto, California: Consulting Psychologists Press, 1957.

8. GOUGH, H. G., and A. B. HEILBRUN. *The Adjective Check List Manual.* Palo Alto, California: Consulting Psychologists Press, 1965.

9. HALPERN, FLORENCE. "Studies of Compulsive Drinkers: Psychological Test Results," *Quarterly Journal of Studies on Alcohol*, 6: 468-479, 1946.

10. JELLINEK, E. M. "Phases of Alcohol Addiction," *Quarterly Journal of Studies on Alcohol*, 13: 673-684, 1952.

11. KÄLIN, R. "Alcohol, Sentience, and Inhibition." Unpublished doctoral dissertation, Harvard University, 1964.

12. KLEBANOFF, S. "Personality Factors in Symptomatic Chronic Alcoholism as Indicated by the Thematic Apperception Test," *Journal of Consulting Psychologists*, 11: 111-119, 1947.

13. LISANSKY, EDITH S. "Etiology of Alcoholism: The Role of Psychological Predisposition," *Quarterly Journal of Studies on Alcohol*, 21: 314-344, 1960.

14. MANSON, M. P. "A Psychometric Differentiation of Alcoholics from Nonalcoholics," *Quarterly Journal of Studies on Alcohol*, 9: 176-206, 1948.

15. MCCORD, W., and JOAN MCCORD (with JON GUDEMAN). *Origins of Alcoholism.* Stanford, Calif.: Stanford University Press, 1960.

16. MOSTELLER, F., and R. R. BUSH. "Selected Quantitative Techniques," in G. LINDZEY (ed.), *Handbook of Social Psychology*, Vol. 1, pp. 289-334. Reading, Mass.: Addison-Wesley, 1954.

17. MURRAY, H. A. *Explorations in Personality.* New York: Oxford, 1938.

18. PARK, P. "Problem Drinking and Social Orientation." Unpublished doctoral dissertation, Yale University, 1958.

19. QUARANTA, J. V. "Alcoholism: A Study of Emotional Maturity and Homosexuality as Related Factors in Compulsive Drinking." Unpublished Master's thesis, Fordham University, 1947. Abstracted in *Quarterly Journal of Studies on Alcohol,* 10: 354, 1949.

20. SINGER, E. "Personality Structure of Chronic Alcoholics," *American Psychologist,* 5: 323, 1950.

21. STRAUS, R. and S. D. BACON. *Drinking in College.* New Haven: Yale University Press, 1953.

22. WILLIAMS, A. F. "Psychological Effects of Alcohol in Natural Party Settings." Unpublished doctoral dissertation, Harvard University, 1964.

23. WILLIAMS, A. F. "Self-Concepts of College Problem Drinkers. I. A Comparison with Alcoholics," *Quarterly Journal of Studies on Alcohol,* 26: 586-594, 1965.

24. WILLIAMS, A. F. "Self-Concepts of College Problem Drinkers. II. Heilbrun Need Scales," *Quarterly Journal of Studies on Alcohol,* 28: 267-276, 1967.

25. WILLIAMS, A. F. "Social Drinking, Anxiety, and Depression," *Journal of Personal and Social Psychology,* 3: 689-693, 1966.

26. WILLIAMS, A. F. "Validation of a Problem-Drinking Scale," *Journal of Projective Techniques and Personality Assessment,* 31: 33-40, 1967.

27. WITKIN, H. A., S. A. KARP, and O. R. GOODENOUGH. (unpublished material) cited in J. D. ARMSTRONG, "The Search for the Alcoholic Personality," *Annals of American Academy of Political and Social Science,* 315: 40-47, 1958.

28. ZUCKERMAN, M. "The Development of an Affect Adjective Check List for the Measurement of Anxiety," *Journal of Consulting Psychologists,* 24: 457-462, 1960.

29. ZUCKERMAN, M., and B. LUBIN. *Manual for the Multiple Affect Adjective Check List.* San Diego, Calif.: Educational and Industrial Testing Service, 1963.

30. ZUCKERMAN, M., B. LUBIN, L. VOGEL, and E. VALERIUS. "The Measurement of Experimentally Induced Affects," *Journal of Consulting Psychologists,* 28: 418-425, 1964.

31. ZWERLING, I. "Psychiatric Findings in an Interdisciplinary Study of Forty-six Alcoholic Patients," *Quarterly Journal of Studies on Alcohol,* 20: 543-554, 1959.

32. ZWERLING, I., and M. ROSENBAUM. "Alcohol Addiction and Personality (Nonpsychotic Conditions)," in S. ARIETI (ed.), *American Handbook of Psychiatry,* Vol. I, pp. 623-644. New York: Basic Books, 1959.

Chapter 17

COLLEGE DRINKING PROFILES IN THREE COUNTRIES*

PETER PARK

University of Massachusetts

Dimensions of Drinking

DRINKING is a behavioral complex which is composed of elementary traits such as the act of consuming alcoholic beverages, quantity and frequency of drinking, reasons for drinking, behavior during and after drinking, and so forth. There are a large number of such behavioral traits associated with drinking, but clearly they are not all of equal descriptive significance, nor do they all denote separate and independent aspects of drinking. It is scientifically more meaningful and economical to think of drinking structurally in terms of its main dimensions which can be characterized by clusters of drinking related behaviors.

The research to be reported here was initiated with the objective of identifying the more important of these dimensions of drinking among young people, with a special focus on what might be called the problem dimension. The source of data was the research of Straus and Bacon[1] in the early

* This research was supported by a grant from the National Institute of Mental Health (M-2478). I wish to thank the Finnish Foundation for Alcohol Studies, Centro Italiano Studi e Ricerche, and Massachusetts Division of Alcoholism for their help in gathering and analysis of the data. A portion of this report was presented at the annual meeting of the Society for the Study of Social Problems, Chicago, August, 1965.

[1] R. Straus and S. D. Bacon, *Drinking in College* (New Haven: Yale University Press, 1953).

1950's when they collected and analyzed extensive data on drinking among college students in this country. Some salient aspects of these data were selected and an attempt was made to cull out the dominant dimensions of drinking by means of factor analysis.[2] Subsequently, comparable data from college students in Italy and Finland were analyzed.

Five identifiable factors were obtained from an analysis of 24 drinking associated items, or variables, taken from the Straus-Bacon study.[3] These factors were given the names, the "problem drinking," "social drinking," "relief drinking," "fear," and "conformity" dimensions. The first of these, the problem drinking dimension, was seen to be associated with practically all of the behavioral traits which Straus and Bacon considered symptomatic of incipient alcoholism and little else, which is, of course, what inspired the name "problem drinking." More-

[2] Factor analysis is a mathematical method for uncovering the dimensions underlying surface manifestations. Suppose, for example, that the dimensions inherent in a set of interrelated phenomena are known and that they each have several indicators. It is possible to calculate the correlations among the indicators, both across and within the dimensions. If, in addition, it is known to what degree a dimension is represented by the indicators, it is also possible, on the basis of this information, to reproduce the correlations among the indicators. This is a schematic description of the kind of situation the reverse of which confronts factor analysis. That is, given intercorrelations among a set of variables, factor analysis seeks to discover the dimensions as factors for which the variables are indicators and to determine, at the same time, which dimensions are represented by abstract entities the identities of which can be surmised by the variables which are associated with them. The relationship between a dimension and a variable is thus a very important one; the stronger the relationship the better the variable as an indicator. This relationship is expressed in factor analysis by a number known as the factor coefficient, or usually as the factor loading, which in the most commonly used systems varies between -1 and $+1$. A factor structure displays in matrix form the factor coefficients (loadings) for the factors standing for the underlying dimensions.

For a general treatise on factor analysis, see: H. H. Harman, *Modern Factor Analysis* (Chicago: University of Chicago Press, 1960); L. L. Thurstone, *Multiple Factor Analysis* (Chicago: University of Chicago Press, 1947); G. H. Thomson, *The Factorial Analysis of Human Ability* (London: University of London Press, 1956); and B. Fruchter, *Introduction to Factor Analysis* (Princeton: D. Van Nostrand Co., 1954).

[3] P. Park, "Dimensions of Drinking among Male College Students," *Social Problems*, 141, pp. 474-482, 1967.

over, it was interesting to observe that the other four dimensions of drinking—that is, the social drinking, relief, fear, and conformity dimensions—corresponded in essence to what Robert Bales some years ago called, respectively, the *convivial, utilitarian, abstinence,* and *ritual* attitudes toward drinking. Bales thought that these rounded out salient aspects of drinking which explain much of the cultural differences in the rates of alcoholism.[4]

My initial study demonstrated that what was intuitively thought to be the more important aspects of drinking could also be delineated empirically and quantitatively by means of a mathematical method. In the case of the problem drinking dimension, it was particularly significant that what may be called the incipient alcoholism-potential could be measured by a quantitative index of problem drinking emerging as a dimension in factor analysis. And, this index has been partially validated in independent studies of drinking among college students.[5]

The cross-national research to be reported here was carried out in order to test the generalizability of the structure of drinking revealed in the initial factor analysis cross-nationally. Finland and Italy were chosen primarily because of the contrasting features of these cultures. Together with the United States, they promised a desirable degree of variation in the sociocultural background of drinking. The aim was to see if a general frame of reference constructed of the same dimensions of drinking could be quantitatively discerned in the three different countries. The demonstrated utility of such a measure would facilitate cross-cultural descriptions of drinking as well as reveal something about the structure of drinking.

[4] R. F. Bales, "Cultural Differences in the Rates of Alcoholism," *Quarterly Journal of Studies on Alcohol,* 6, pp. 480-499, 1946, and R. F. Bales, "Attitudes toward Drinking in Irish Culture," in D. J. Pittman and C. R. Snyder (eds.), *Society, Culture, and Drinking Patterns.* New York: John Wiley and Sons, 1962, pp. 157-187.

[5] P. Park, "Problem Drinking and Role Orientation: A Study in Incipient Alcoholism," in Pittman and Snyder, *op. cit.,* pp. 431-454. A. F. Williams, "Self Concepts of College Problem Drinkers," *Quarterly Journal of Studies on Alcohol,* 26, pp. 586-594, 1965, and "Validations of a College Problem-Drinking Scale," in press with the *Journal of Projective Techniques and Personality Assessment.*

Data

The factor analysis of drinking behaviors was initially carried out in the United States on the data from 438 male college students. This number was obtained from a 10 per cent random sample of the Straus-Bacon survey after excluding females, abstainers, and those who have never been drunk.[6] These exclusions were made deliberately in order to prevent unnecessary heterogeneity in the drinking experiences and hence in the structure of drinking. In Finland and Italy the study was carried out on random samples of students at the Universities of Helsinki and Rome, respectively.[7] The Finnish analysis was based on 551 Finnish-speaking[8] students who were enrolled in the University of Helsinki in the fall of 1958. This number was obtained from a random sample of the students in all the faculties of the university; the Finnish students were roughly equivalent to the American students of the Straus-Bacon survey in age and other attributes. Female students, abstainers, and persons who had never been drunk were again excluded for the same reason as in the United States. A similar selection procedure resulted in 219 students in Italy from whom the necessary data were obtained.

The data were collected in Finland by mailed questionnaires,[9] and in Italy by questionnaires administered in class-

---

[6] The term "drunk" was defined in the Straus-Bacon study as "an overstepping of social expectations (short of complete 'passing out'), loss of control in ordinary physical activities, and inability to respond to reactions of others." Straus and Bacon, *op. cit.*, p. 131.

[7] These two universities by no means represent cross sections of the students in their respective countries. And yet, they embody more heterogeneous elements than any other universities in the countries concerned by virtue of their being cosmopolitan universities located in the national capitals. This is especially true in Finland where there is no serious contender to the University of Helsinki as the national university.

[8] Finland is a bilingual country where a minority of the population considers its mother tongue to be Swedish rather than Finnish. A sample of Swedish-speaking students also participated in the study and are included in a later analysis.

[9] Data were collected by interview from about a hundred students. Some of these were used in concluding phase of this study.

rooms to which the selected students came in groups by appointment. These questionnaires contained the behavioral variables dealing with drinking which were taken from the initial American study. This report is based on 22 such variables which are described in Table 1.

Cross-National Comparisons

Factor analysis was carried out on the 22 variables separately in each country to ascertain that comparable dimensions of

TABLE 1.—*Variables Included in the Factor Analysis with Dichotomous Cutting Points*

Variable Number	Variable	Cutting Point +	Cutting Point −
1	*Quantity-Frequency* Index	Much-frequent*	Little-infrequent*
2	Drinking to get along better on *dates*	Some or considerable importance	No importance
3	Drinking to relieve *fatigue* or tension	"	"
4	Drinking to be *gay*	"	"
5	Drinking to relieve *illness* or physical discomforts	"	"
6	Drinking to comply with *custom*	"	"
7	Drinking because of enjoyment of *taste*	"	"

* For U. S. and Finland: "Much-frequent" = consuming on the average more than three 8-oz. glasses of *beer,* two 3.5 oz. glasses of *wine,* or two 1.5-oz. drinks of *hard liquor* at a sitting and drinking more often than once a week.

For Italy: "Much-frequent" = (a) more than 1.5-2 glasses of *wine* (10-13 oz.) at every or nearly every meal (excluding breakfast); or, (b) more than 2-3 glasses of *beer* (13-20 oz.) at a sitting and at least 2-3 times a week outside meals; or (c) more than 1-2 glasses of *aperitif* (1.7-3.4 oz.) at a sitting and at least 2-4 times a month; or, (d) more than 2-3 *highballs* or *cocktails* (3.4-5.0 oz. of hard liquor) at a sitting and at least 2-3 times a month outside meals; or (e) more than 1-2 *liqueurs* (.9-1.7 oz.) at a sitting and at least 2-3 times a week outside meals.

"Little-infrequent" = consuming less of the beverages or less frequently than above.

Table 1 (Continued)

Variable Number	Variable	Cutting Point +	−
8	Drinking in order not to be *shy*	Some or considerable importance	No importance
9	Drinking for sense of *well-being*	"	"
10	Drinking as an aid to forgetting disappointments	"	"
11	Drinking to get *high*†	"	"
12	*Social Complications* Scale‡	Some complications	No complications
13	Has had *weekend* drinking sprees	1 or more times	Never
14	Has had *blackouts*	"	"
15	Has had one or more drinks before or instead of breakfast (*morning drinking*)	"	"
16	Has had one or more drinks alone (*lone drinking*)	"	"
17	Has been *drunk* when *alone*	"	"
18	Drinking has led to *aggressive,* wantonly destructive or malicious *behavior*	"	"

† By Straus and Bacon's definition "*high* indicates a noticeable effect without going beyond socially acceptable behavior, e.g., increased gaiety, slight fuzziness of perception, drowsiness and so on." Straus and Bacon, *op. cit.*

‡ For U. S., Finland, and Italy: "Some complications" = one or more of the following experiences: drinking has interfered with preparation for classes or examination, caused loss of or damage to friendships, led to missing of appointments, or caused accidents, injuries, arrests or disciplinary action.

"No complications" = none of the above experiences.

drinking are manifest in the countries concerned.[10] The resulting factor structures are presented in Table 2. The first three factors, as can be seen from the table, are replicated, with minor variations, in the three countries. They denote, in es-

[10] The tetrachoric correlation and the method of principal axes with the largest correlations in the diagonals were employed. The principal factors were rotated both obliquely and orthogonally with comparable results. Only the results of oblique rotations are reported here.

Table 1 (Continued)

Variable Number	Variable	Cutting Point +	−
19	Drinks sometimes *before* going to a *party*, if not sure of getting anything to drink or enough to drink	Yes	No
20	Has *feared* long-range consequences of one's drinking	Yes	No
21	Has sought *advice* of others about one's drinking	Yes	No
22	Has gone on the *water wagon* as a result of—	own decision parent's advice steady date's advice other friend's advice	doctor's advice religious leader's advice participation in sports high school rules college rules never

sence, the problem, social, and relief dimensions of drinking obtained in the initial study of American college drinking.[11]

The first factor is represented in all three countries by "much and frequent drinking," "social complication," "weekend drinking sprees," "blackouts," "morning drinking," and "aggressive behavior resulting from drinking." These are what Straus and Bacon regarded as behavioral traits symptomatic of problem drinking and figured prominently as characteristics of the problem drinking dimension in the original American study. This label can thus be retained here.

It is, however, noteworthy that "lone drinking," a characteristic of this dimension in the United States, does not appear in either the Finnish or the Italian variant; from the latter, "getting drunk alone" is absent as well. As a matter of fact, what might be called a solitary drinking dimension emerges as a separate factor composed of these two items in Finland and Italy (Factor V), with a connotation of non-conformity (not "drinking to comply with custom") in the former. "Drinking before a party if not sure of getting anything or enough to drink" is associated with this "lone drinking" dimension in Finland and Italy but not in the United States. The Finnish

[11] Park, *op. cit.* (1967).

TABLE 2.—*Factor Structures*

U.S.A. (Critical Value = .22)*

Var. No.	Var. Name	I Problem	II Social	III Relief	IV	V	VI
1.	Quantity-frequency†	.40				.26	
2.	Dates		.64		.28		
3.	Fatigue	.25		.53			
4.	Gay		.71				
5.	Illness			.63			
6.	Custom		.36				
7.	Taste					.63	
8.	Shy		.60			−.40	
9.	Well-being		.26	.34			.32
10.	Disappointment		.29	.44			
11.	High		.66				
12.	Social complications	.31			.41		
13.	Weekend	.59					
14.	Blackout	.22				.39	
15.	Morning drinking	.80					
16.	Lone drinking	.39					.26
17.	Drunk alone	.57					
18.	Aggressive behavior	.48					
19.	Before party		.48		.31		
20.	Fear consequences				.70	−.25	
21.	Advice				.29		
22.	Water wagon						.68

* These "critical values" are defined by the mean correlation coefficient and the size of sample. See Harman, *op. cit.*, p. 441.

† The variables are identified here by the underlined parts of the variable descriptions in Table 1.

problem drinking dimension contains "drinking to get high" and "drinking for the sense of well-being," suggesting touches of hedonism. "Drinking because of fatigue or tension" appears in this factor only in the United States and contributes little to the meaning of this dimension judging from the relatively small factor loading. It thus appears that while the kernel of the first dimension common to the three countries denotes an aspect of drinking symptomatic of problem drinking in all three countries, its more peripheral features acquire something of utilitarian and convivial overtones in Finland and Italy in comparison with the United States.

The second factor is composed of "drinking on dates," "drink-

TABLE 2.—*Factor Structures* (Continued)

Finland (Critical Value = .24)*

Var. No.	Var. Name	I Problem	II Social	III Relief	IV	V	VI
1.	Quantity-frequency†	.74					
2.	Dates		.76				
3.	Fatigue			.54			
4.	Gay		.29				.52
5.	Illness			.41			
6.	Custom				−.25		
7.	Taste			.50			
8.	Shy		.81				
9.	Well-being	.37					.41
10.	Disappointment					.24	.26
11.	High	.60					
12.	Social complications	.47					
13.	Weekend	.39		.33			
14.	Blackout	.40					
15.	Morning drinking	.50					−.25
16.	Lone drinking					.70	
17.	Drunk alone	.29				.61	−.26
18.	Aggressive behavior	.55					
19.	Before party	.24	.40				
20.	Fear consequences				.60		
21.	Advice				.40		
22.	Water wagon				.71		

* These "critical values" are defined by the mean correlation coefficient and the size of sample. See Harman, *op. cit.*, p. 441.

† The variables are identified here by the underlined parts of the variable descriptions in Table 1.

ing to be gay," "drinking not to be shy," and "drinking before a party" in all three countries; these items clearly refer to social drinking with instrumental implications. "Drinking to comply with custom" appears only in the United States, which is perhaps a reflection of the fact that drinking on dates is not an institutionalized behavior among college drinkers in the other countries, especially in Italy, to the extent that it is in the United States. "Drinking to get high," "drinking for the sense of well-being," and "drinking when there are disappointments," are also unique to the United States and two of the three connote instrumentality. Not "seeking advice about one's drinking" which appears in this factor for the

TABLE 2.—*Factor Structures* (Continued)

Var. No.	Var. Name	I Prob- lem	II Social	III Relief	IV	V	VI
				Italy (Critical Value = .31)*			
1.	Quantity-frequency†	.56					
2.	Dates		.76				
3.	Fatigue			.51			
4.	Gay		.55				
5.	Illness			.41			
6.	Custom				−.66		
7.	Taste			.65			
8.	Shy		.80				
9.	Well-being			.44			
10.	Disappointment				.76		
11.	High			.31			
12.	Social complications	.39					
13.	Weekend	.45					.39
14.	Blackout	.66					
15.	Morning drinking	.75					
16.	Lone drinking					.50	
17.	Drunk alone					1.00	
18.	Aggressive behavior	.47					.45
19.	Before party	.48	.58				
20.	Fear consequences						
21.	Advice		−.52				
22.	Water wagon						.79

* These "critical values" are defined by the mean correlation coefficient and the size of sample. See Harman, *op. cit.*, p. 441.

† The variables are identified here by the underlined parts of the variable descriptions in Table 1.

Italians alone neither adds nor detracts from its dominant meaning.

The last of the factors which are shared by the three countries is the third one, which contains, in the United States, "drinking to relieve fatigue or tension," "drinking to relieve illness or physical discomforts," "drinking for the sense of well-being," and "drinking for disappointments." It is not difficult to identify this as a kind of instrumental drinking intended to relieve tensions of both physical and psychic nature. But in Finland and Italy, the psychic element would appear to be separated out and a component suggestive of drinking as an end in itself is added. Thus, in Finland, "taste" and "weekend drinking sprees" emerge with "fatigue" and "illness"; but "well-being" and "disappointments" do not appear in the Finnish patterns. Similarly, in Italy, a strong component of "taste" and "drinking to get high" are added to the base of the American drinking factor, but "disappointments" disappears from it. In fact, there is a faint indication that what may be called psychic relief drinking tends to form a separate factor of its own in Italy, which is the unidentified Factor IV in Table 2.

The remaining factors are fragmentary and would appear to fall short of attaining cross-national significance. The fourth Finnish factor denotes a syndrome of fear concerning drinking, including attempts to stop drinking ("water wagon," i.e., periodic attempts to stop drinking entirely). The would-be American counterpart shows a strong component of "fear" about drinking but does not include going on the "water wagon." This dimension of concern about drinking is almost completely absent in Italy except for a trace of it in Factor VI. In this factor "water wagon" has a high loading. Brief remarks have already been made in passing concerning the emergent indications of solitary drinking factors in Finland (Factor V) and Italy (Factor V) and of psychic relief drinking in Italy (Factor IV). Tentative as these identifications are, the rest of the factors are even more marginal and difficult to interpret at this point.

To summarize, then, there are striking similarities in the way the first three factors are characterized, and, hence, in what they signify in the three countries. But the dimensions of drinking which the factors denote take on different nuances in different countries, which is to be expected in view of the cultural variations. In the United States, the anti-social element of drinking, i.e., drinking alone and getting drunk alone, plays a fairly important role in shaping the problem drinking dimension in comparison with the other countries. In Finland and Italy, the same dimension is suggestive of hedonism with a shade of conviviality. The social drinking dimension includes drinking to facilitate social intercourse, especially with the opposite sex, in all three countries. In the United States, however, its instrumental significance is more articulated and overtly identified with social conventions.

What these observations suggest is that the distinction between the problem and social aspects of drinking pivots more acutely on the social relevance of drinking in the United States than is the case in the other countries. The relief drinking dimension has references to both physical and psychic tensions in the United States, while in Finland and Italy, the psychic element tends to disappear. As a matter of fact, there are intimations that psychic tension release might be embodied in a separate dimension in these two countries.[12]

A Common Frame of Reference and Profiles of Drinking

A common frame of reference can be constructed from these dimensions of drinking for the purpose of comparative description. This objective is attained by a method known as transformation analysis[13] which, in a manner of speaking, pools the factor loadings of the three common factor structures to produce intercorrelations[14] among the drinking variables. Factor analysis performed on these intercorrelations yields sets (one for each country) of what might be called common space factors. Any set of the common space factors, when expressed in empirically meaningful form by a technique known as rotation, defines dimensions of drinking common to the three countries. Transformation analysis was applied to the factor structures of Table 2, and three sets of six common space factors were obtained. Table 3 presents the common dimensions of drinking resulting from a rotation of the American set.[15]

Only the first four dimensions are sizeable and appear to be

[12] This possibility is more strongly suggested in an unpublished analysis of the Italian data including several more variables having to do with reasons for drinking.

[13] Yrjö Ahmavaara, *On the Mathematical Theory of Transformation Analysis.* Alkoholipolitisen Tutkimuslaitoksen Julkaisuja. No. 1 (Helsinki, Finland: o.y. Alkoholiike, A. B., 1963). Touko Markkanen, *On Transformation Analysis.* (Helsinki, Finland: Social Research Institute of Alcohol Studies, 1964). Mimeograph.

[14] These are actually covariances.

[15] These are orthogonal dimensions obtained by varimax rotation.

TABLE 3.—*Common Dimensions of Drinking*

	Variable	I Problem	II Social	III Relief	IV Fear	V	VI
1.	Quantity-frequency	.59	.06	.18	.14	−.32	−.13
2.	Dates	.12	.76	.10	.03	−.03	.07
3.	Fatigue	.19	.28	.46	.07	−.04	−.02
4.	Gay	.06	.64	.22	−.06	−.07	.01
5.	Illness	.14	.15	.49	.02	.11	.07
6.	Custom	−.14	.09	.20	−.10	.01	.21
7.	Taste	.25	.03	.46	−.03	−.24	−.01
8.	Shy	.00	.81	.04	−.03	.11	.07
9.	Well-being	.24	.40	.48	.13	.00	.01
10.	Disappointment	.23	.45	.31	.08	−.04	−.19
11.	High	.35	.42	.25	.06	−.07	−.02
12.	Social complications	.53	.16	.12	.14	−.16	−.09
13.	Weekend	.60	.24	.16	.03	−.01	.04
14.	Blackout	.51	.04	.13	.00	−.16	−.04
15.	Morning drinking	.74	−.01	.08	.04	.01	.00
16.	Lone drinking	.58	.05	.22	.08	.10	−.17
17.	Drunk alone	.64	.09	.08	.19	.29	−.09
18.	Aggressive behavior	.63	.21	.07	.25	.05	.06
19.	Before party	.47	.50	.11	.00	−.13	−.06
20.	Fear consequences	.19	.20	−.14	.52	−.17	−.11
21.	Advice	.12	−.12	.11	.54	−.07	−.14
22.	Water wagon	.07	.03	.02	.62	.16	.09

meaningful. The more important variables[16] associated with the common space factors are, in order of factor loading:

I

15.	morning drinking	(.74)
17.	getting drunk alone	(.64)
18.	aggressive behavior	(.63)
13.	weekend drinking sprees	(.60)
1.	quantity-frequency	(.59)
16.	drinking alone	(.58)
12.	social complications	(.53)
14.	blackouts	(.51)
19.	drinking before a party	(.47)

[16] Here factor loading of .40 in absolute value is used as the "critical value" more or less arbitrarily.

II

8.	drinking not to be shy	(.81)
2.	drinking for dates	(.76)
4.	drinking to be gay	(.64)
19.	drinking before a party	(.50)
10.	drinking for disappointments	(.45)
11.	drinking to get high	(.42)

III

5.	drinking for illness	(.49)
9.	drinking for well-being	(.48)
10.	drinking for fatigue or tension	(.46)
11.	drinking for taste	(.46)

IV

22.	water wagon	(.62)
21.	seeking advice	(.54)
20.	fearing consequences	(.52)

These are virtually the same sets of variables which characterized four of the five drinking dimensions identified in the initial American study, i.e., the problem, social, relief, and fear dimensions of drinking. And the few deviations from the original characterizations which are observable actually tend to strengthen the interpreted meaning of the dimensions. For example, "drinking before a party" was a component of the social but not the problem drinking dimension, contrary to the usual interpretation that this kind of behavior is symptomatic of preoccupation with drinking. In the pooled analysis, this behavior is seen to be relevant to both dimensions, indicating that it has both symptomatic and social significance. "Water wagon," though originally thought to be a correlative of fear about possible consequences of drinking, did not appear as an indicator of the fear dimension in other analyses. Here it shows up as the most prominent feature of the same dimension. In the cross-national setting, "drinking for the sense of well-being" replaces "drinking as aid in forgetting disappointments" in the characterization of the relief drinking dimension. This, together with the other items in the dimension, puts the emphasis on reducing tensions without

emphasizing the social implications of the act. "Drinking because of enjoyment of taste," a new addition, though not
particularly helpful for interpreting the dimension, does not
contradict its emergent sense.

It appears, then, that the dimensions of drinking initially
delineated from drinking patterns among American college
students are generalizable to other countries of different,
though not disparate, cultural backgrounds. These dimensions thus would make a useful general frame of reference
for comparative description of drinking patterns in different
countries, as will be shown presently. It must be borne in
mind, however, that this frame of reference is a superstructure,
a kind of abstraction, fitted over the individual frames of
reference and only hints at the cultural differences in the
meaning of the dimensions of drinking. Moreover, the common frame of reference which is proposed here is one which
is biased toward the American structure of drinking. There are
technical reasons—too complicated to explain fully in this
space—which explain this limitation. Suffice it to say here
that common dimensions of drinking could have been obtained
by rotating the Finnish or Italian common space factors as
the basis as well as the American without altering anything
mathematically. But the results would have had a corresponding bias toward the Finnish or Italian drinking patterns. In
any event, the American bias appears justifiable here in view
of the origin of the study.

Where, then, do the American, Finnish, and Italian students
stand with respect to one another in this frame of reference?
The dimensions of drinking as defined here are variables, and
it is meaningful to think of describing an individual's behavior

[17] In answering this question, a sample of male undergraduates at an
Ivy League university who have had the experience of getting drunk
($N = 604$) has been substituted for the original Straus-Bacon sample.
This substitution was made because the new data were more accessible
and more conveniently processed for the purpose at hand and because
they yielded a structure of drinking factors identical with the original.
In addition, the Finnish and Italian samples have been slightly augmented.
To the initial Finnish sample, which included only Finnish-speaking
students who responded to mail questionnaires, have been increased to
231 by adding the students who had not been previously analyzed
due to insufficient information.

in terms of them. An individual's drinking behavior can be described by his responses to items which are the variables constituting the various dimensions of drinking outlined above.[18] Mean scores for groups of individuals for the various drinking dimensions can be derived.

The mean scores for the four dimensions of drinking are given separately for the American, Finnish and Italian students in Table 4. The same information is presented graphically in Figure 1. It can be seen from this table, and more readily from the bar charts in Figure 1, that the mean problem drinking score for the American students towers over those for the Finnish and Italian students. This clearly means that symptoms of problem drinking are more prevalent among the American students. The Italian students are slightly more likely than Finnish students to exhibit problem drinking behavior. A moment's reflection will show that it is not too surprising a result, since getting drunk, an experience which all the participants in the study shared, is far more uncommon in Italy than in Finland. Hence in Italy the deviant behavior which tends to be associated with drunkenness is also more common.

On the second (social drinking) dimension, the Finnish students have the lead, with the American and Italian students, in that order, trailing behind. A common sense understanding of the cultures concerned might have led one to expect the Italians, supposedly sociable people, to run ahead of the others on this dimension, gratuitously and incorrectly equating the word "social" with sociability. The social drinking dimension indicates the extent to which drinking is used to alleviate awkward social situations ("drinking not to be shy," "drinking to get along better on dates") and even to release socially

TABLE 4.—*Mean Scores for the Common Dimensions of Drinking*

Country	Dimensions			
	I Problem	II Social	III Relief	IV Fear
U. S.	.79	.30	.60	.51
Finland	.22	.36	.46	.31
Italy	.34	.16	.39	.17

[18] For the method of estimating factor scores, see Harman, *op. cit.*, pp. 336-361.

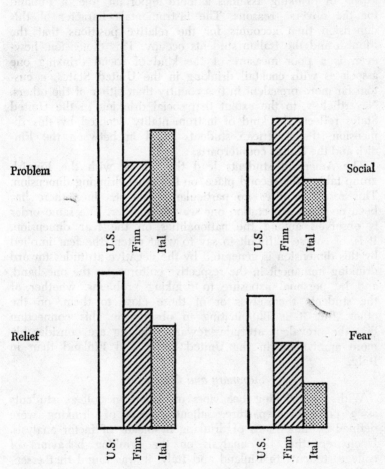

FIGURE 1.—*Mean Scores on the Common Dimensions of Drinking.*

generated tensions ("drinking to forget disappointments").
Italians are presumably less in need of such a change agent
precisely because of their reputed sociability and volatility. This
aspect of drinking assumes a more important role in Finland
for the obverse reasons. The instrumental character of this
dimension then accounts for the relative positions that the
Finnish and the Italian students occupy. This dimension, however, is a poor measure of the kind of social drinking one
associates with cocktail drinking in the United States, a custom far more prevalent in this country than either of the others.
Nevertheless, to the extent that social drinking in the United
States reflects the kind of instrumentality denoted by this dimension, the American students stand in between the Finnish and the Italian counterparts.

The American students lead the others, with the Finnish
group taking the second place, on the relief drinking dimension.
This result requires no particular comment, since there has
been no prior expectation one way or another. The same order
is observed among the nationalities on the fear dimension.
It is, of course, difficult to say to what extent the fear implied
by this dimension is generated by the negative attitudes toward
drinking immanent in the respective cultures, on the one hand,
and by personal exposure to drinking problems, whether of
the students themselves or of those close to them, on the
other. But it is illuminating to observe in this connection
that the prevalent attitudes toward drinking are considerably
more ambivalent in the United States and Finland than in
Italy.

Summary and Conclusion

With the drinking behaviors of American college students
as a point of departure, salient aspects of drinking were
defined as dimensions of drinking by means of factor analysis.
Upon repeating the analysis on the drinking behaviors of
college students in Finland and Italy, it was found that essentially the same dimensions are discernable cross-nationally.
These were identified as the problem, social, and relief drinking dimensions.

In an effort to develop a common descriptive frame of
reference applicable to the countries concerned, the results
of the separate factor analyses were combined and four dimen-

sions were delineated: the problem, social, and relief drinking dimensions plus one more, the fear dimension. These are, it appears, the common denominators of the dimensions in the individual countries, but, of necessity, they ignore the nuances of drinking peculiar to particular countries. Nevertheless, these dimensions provide a convenient set of measuring sticks which can be uniformly applied to the three countries for comparative purposes.

Through the use of these common dimensions of drinking, the average American student can be characterized in comparative terms as being high on the problem, relief, and fear dimensions, and medium on the social. In the same framework, the Finnish profile is low on the problem, high on the social, and medium on both the relief and the fear dimensions; and the Italian is medium on the problem dimension and low on the other dimensions.

The dimensions of drinking identified in this study provide a useful means of describing types of drinkers, including problem drinkers, as the above profiles suggest. And such a typology of drinkers could be a useful tool in the etiology of alcoholism. More generally, these dimensions could be treated as variables and the relationships between these and relevant behavioral and cultural correlates of drinking investigated by multivariate methods. For instance, Bales' hypothesis concerning cultural differences in the rates of alcoholism is predicated on attitudes toward drinking, which have close empirical analogues in the drinking dimensions of this report. Bales' hypothesis, and others like it, could thus be effectively investigated by the cross-nationally developed frame of reference presented here.

PART THREE

IMPLICATIONS

INTRODUCTORY NOTE

THE PARTICIPANTS in the conference on "Alcohol and College Youth," which Bruyn (chapter 18) summarizes, spent a considerable amount of time arguing about whether drinking in college is a problem or produces problems and, if so, what these problems are. Some were convinced that drinking was not a problem on the campus. Where was the evidence, they asked, that there is a high incidence of alcoholism among collegians? Others were convinced that a conference on drug use among collegians was in order but that alcohol was the wrong drug to be concerned about. Wasn't drinking relatively respectable and innocuous when compared with the use of LSD? Most participants seemed to agree eventually that a major dimension of the drinking problem on college campuses was perhaps not so much the behavior of students as the ambiguous, hypocritical rules about drinking perpetuated by the adults responsible for the conduct of collegians. The official campus culture with regard to drinking is as often as not phony and fraudulent. Worse, unhealthy drinking practices which militate against personal development of many collegians are tolerated, if not inadvertently encouraged; moreover, little attention is given to identifying students with a drinking problem or to helping such students work through that problem. While college students are not especially prone to problem drinking, neither are they especially immune. The typical college campus is an environment apparently designed to test the immunity to problems of any young drinker.

It is to the credit of participants at the conference on alcohol and college youth that no one was inclined to propose a simple solution for what was recognized as a complex problem. Riggs (chapter 19) in addition to Bruyn suggests just how complex the issues are. College administrators bear the heavy burden of being *in loco parentis* by tradition, if not in fact, and often find themselves administering unreasonable anti-drinking rules for students which legislators and parents applaud but do not apply to themselves. Riggs calls to our attention that the American college is a peculiar place which is the workshop of academics and of administrators who have their own ideas about what is good for students. While the current generation of students are increasingly aware of and jealous about their rights, they have not been and are not now particularly effective in determining campus policy. Legislators obviously do have some influence on campus policy. So do trustees who have to consider the attitudes of donors, townfolk, and the parents of enrolled or prospective students. There is little indication that most of the adults in a position to influence campus policy on drinking are even considering, much less insisting on, change.

But there are hints of change. Some colleges are revising their drinking rules so as to be no more restrictive than relevant state laws on the legal age for drinking. Others are attempting to distinguish in their disciplinary codes between drinking as an offense *per se* and behavior associated with drinking which would be reprehensible under any circumstances. An undetermined number of institutions permit or encourage formal and informal education about alcohol such as that described by Russell (chapter 20). But these activities remain only ripples in a vast sea of studied indifference. Most college students continue to develop their pattern of drinking in an environment that is officially prohibitive but unofficially permissive. Folklore about drinking and its consequences for the most part remains unchecked and unchallenged by evidence. Problem drinkers tend to remain unidentified unless their behavior is forcefully brought to the attention of administrators. Even this identification is more likely an occasion for disciplinary action than for therapeutic intervention.

What can and ought to be done in institutions of higher learning to minimize the incidence and consequences of problem drinking among collegians are issues which warrant serious consideration, as Bruyn, Riggs, and Russell argue. At this point, consensus on these issues seems unlikely. Colleges and universities are more often creatures of their environments rather than creators of their environments. Policy makers will disagree about the extent to which colleges should concern themselves with the non-academic aspects of student life. They will disagree about the extent to which the college campus is a laboratory in which students experiment with living as well as learning. They will disagree about the extent to which collegians are adults-in-training or adolescents growing up on an installment plan controlled by adults.

Critical inquiry into the drinking behavior of collegians and into the extent to which experience during the college years shapes that behavior for better or worse might well suggest no legitimate basis for concern as some of the chapters in this volume suggest. In a country that has a high incidence of trouble with alcohol, one would expect more than casual interest in such an inquiry. And where would one expect this interest to be if not in the institutions of higher learning themselves?

Chapter 18

YOU'VE GOT TO KNOW THE TERRITORY

Henry B. Bruyn
University of California Medical Center

THE MARKETING of an ethical and well-designed product by a conscientious, honest and enthusiastic, well-trained, intelligent salesman would seem entirely similar to the teaching of a facet of knowledge by a conscientious, honest, enthusiastic, well-trained, intelligent educator or teacher. In each instance, however, the *sine qua non* before stepping before the pupil or the customer is expressed eloquently by Professor Harold Hill in *The Music Man* by the words "You've got to know the territory." Putting these thoughts further into focus, it has been said that it is the recipient of communication that determines whether communication has happened at all (1). The recipient validates communication through his behavior and only through his behavior can we tell whether a communication has been more than interpersonal noise. It is probably true that much of the intended communication of the world misfires, miscarries, or fails entirely because the communicator pays more attention to his bow and arrow than to his target.

A conference on "Alcohol and College Youth" held in June, 1965 and sponsored by the American College Health Association* brought out a variety of opinions and convictions on the topic of "target," "territory," "customer"—or the college student. In the field of alcohol education for the young adult,

* The conference was supported by NIMH Grant MH02009-01. The published proceedings of this conference, entitled *Alcohol and College Youth* (H. B. Bruyn, Ed.), are supplemented by video tapes of the principal participants and appropriate discussion guides. Previous conferences on related topics (7, 8) should be noted. Editor.

the educational community and the family have usually demonstrated remarkable ignorance of the "territory" and thereby have failed to provide a meaningful, honest foundation for the young adult and his attitudes toward a substance—alcohol—which has become firmly placed in our social and cultural world. Before presenting some of the material brought out at this conference it is necessary to briefly review some of the characteristics of the young adult "target" which are of major significance as we consider the interaction between college youth, the college administration, and alcohol.

Erikson (2) has described the developmental process culminating in the young adult of college age as passing through a series of stages from infancy onward. Each of these stages is characterized by problems as well as progress through solutions. Erikson describes the "school age" as a phase of learning how to do things and accomplish projects and a stage in which a sense of inadequacy and inferiority is frequently faced and dealt with. The "adolescent years" introduce the concept of "identity versus identity diffusion." This is a time of physiological revolution with rapid growth and sexual maturity. During these years the emphasis is on questioning all the sameness and all the continuities which have previously been accepted and relied upon. The adolescent refights earlier struggles and battles, especially those of the school age involving inadequacy and inferiority. The diffusion of self-identification results in a negative identity which fights all that parents, adults, and community seem to be expecting. Erikson's next stage brings us to the college years with the young adult whose big struggle is with the problem of "intimacy versus isolation." Security in one's own identity allows for sharing one's identity with others. The young adult may hesitate, according to Erikson, to take on intimate relationships with others because of fear of losing his own identity. He thus develops a deep sense of isolation. Most scholars of young people are aware that the adolescent and young adult are especially sensitive to hypocrisy, bigotry, and the lie. It follows that such attitudes will be especially severe irritants during the young adult years. The idealistic young adult critically evaluates society as he sees it and earnestly, and at times violently, struggles for a better world. It is characteristic that the young adult will try to work out emotional conflicts in dramatic and sometimes anti-social demonstrations. Dr. Dana Farnsworth (3) has emphasized that the application of punitive sanctions at this period in the development of the personality may only perpetuate undesirable behavior and make rebellion more intense. Such punishment seems to justify the young adult's resentment and postpones or prevents the acquisition of self-control.

In a formal presentation to the conference on "Alcohol and College Youth," Dr. Nevitt Sanford (4) presented the classical breakdown of group or individual drinking in three broad categories of integrative, facilitative, and escapist types of drinking behavior. He stressed that integrative drinking, which expresses a solidarity that already exists, favors the identity of the individual. It does not serve to generate solidarity or friendship where none existed before. The integration of drinking and personality must be based first upon a relatively well-developed personality and that this development usually occurs during the college years. While the self-control necessary to accomplish socially acceptable integrated drinking is hardly to be expected in a 14-year-old, on well-established psychological grounds from a wide variety of studies, the 18-year-old is ready to begin the experiences that will make it possible for him to become an integrative drinker with a very healthy prognosis.

The Senate and Assembly Excise Committee of the New York Legislature in 1965 rejected an effort to raise the New York State minimum drinking age to 21 years following careful study and review of expert opinion. This committee expressed concern for clandestine drinking without adult supervision or restrictions on the quantity consumed as well as fear of creating a climate conducive to more serious violations of law and morality. Such a conclusion by a group of responsible citizens would seem of particular significance.

With this brief review of the characteristics and quality of our "target" on the college campus in mind, two examples might illustrate further the concepts and convictions developed at the conference "Alcohol and College Youth."

A salesman is employed by a large and vigorous drug company to promote a new product among the medical profession. The salesman enters a doctor's office, smiles at the receptionist and strides across the room to knock briefly on the doctor's door, open it and walk in. His entrance interrupts a phone conversation between the doctor and a patient which the salesman ignores and launches immediately into his pitch about his product—a hormone preparation for use in elderly women. He is unaware that the physician to whom he is speaking is a gynecologist and very familiar with the product. The salesman's attitude toward his potential customer is imperious and the physician is unable to interrupt him for several minutes. When he asks the physician if he would be willing to place an order for this drug the not unexpected answer is a resounding "no," accompanied by very vigorous and explicit instructions to leave the office. This salesman failed because of his complete ignorance of the "target."

A college decides to put on a series of lectures to the student body on topics of concern to the administration. Among these topics is the use of alcoholic beverages by the students. The student body is rallied by an announcement that the possibility of allowing alcoholic beverages on campus will be discussed. This seductive approach results in a massive turnout. The lecture is given by a member of the faculty in philosophy whose personal religion forbids the use of alcohol in any form. The information presented is poorly disguised temperance material and the use of alcohol by the young adult is presented as a threat to health, both physical and mental, as well as the first step toward alcoholism in later life. Here, too, the teacher or administration demonstrates an equally remarkable ignorance of the "target."

Recognizing the critical importance of student opinion and reaction, conference organizers included four college students among the participants in the "Alcohol and College Youth" conference with the hope that they would remind the other participants of the student viewpoint and also provide new questions, ideas, and opinions. The students were also chosen on the basis of geography and type of college campus without any illusion that they would be "typical American college students." One of the results of the conference was to stimulate more vigorous discussion of alcohol between these students and the other participants.

Some Issues

The following comments were recorded from the many discussions held during this conference and illustrate their substance. The discussion groups were made up of health educators, physicians, and psychiatrists from Student Health Services, counselors and psychiatric social workers, student personnel administrators and students. These participants represented both large and small college and university campuses from various geographical areas of the United States.

. . . .We have only 500 students at our college with a no-drinking rule on campus. They are reported to the Dean if suspected of being drunk. But a survey showed that 50 per cent would take a drink, even though the school is religiously oriented.

. . . .Stanford students have periodically argued this point—that the prohibition of drinking on campus requires going off to drink and driving back; in effect, the rule is encouraging driving after drinking.

. . . .At Ohio University there is no drinking on campus, yet beer is served at all the sorority and fraternity "teas," and they are considered on-campus. I think the trend is for students asking for permission to drink.

. . . .This is one of the areas of selective inattention. In upper middle class suburbia the amount of drinking the house-wife does, and the way she hides the bottles is fantastic, especially in Southern California.

. . . .I wonder if some of the rules and laws about alcohol don't help to create problems of hypocrisy.

. . . .When some Stanford students feel the university is being hypocritical in saying "Thou shalt not obtain, possess, drink, etc." and then steadfastly refuses to really police it—completely looks the other way—some students apparently say, "If *you're* hypocritical it gives me license to be hypocritical too."

. . . .At the University of Pittsburgh we permit drinking for graduate students. Undergraduate students never, even though they are 21.

. . . .What about the student who comes to college whose father is a high-powered executive and comes home three sheets to the wind every day? Not because he's an alcoholic, but business is conducted over two- to three-hour lunches with many martinis. What kind of a model does that boy have for drinking? How does this affect his concept of where it should fit into his life? It's different from the fellow coming to college from a repressive background where drinking of anything alcoholic is forbidden.

. . . .We have a lot of college students who seem to think that getting smashed a couple of times a month is coexistent with, or a corollary to, getting a bachelor's degree. They have to do these things, and they are more important to them as a result of their peer group influence in a college frame of reference at the time. They just do it for the experience. I think a lot of them say, "Well, let's go out and get smashed just for the hell of it. It's a pleasant experience and the big boys do it." This kind of behavior could be an expression of a masculine protest.

. . . .I think the psychologists and psychiatrists would recognize this rebellion against authority through which students pass in this last state of adolescence. Presumably the girls have beaten the boys a few years in getting there.

. . . .In terms of law it seems to be easier for young people to flout the alcohol beverage law than it is to flout the narcotics law. Somehow they are adopting the attitudes of their parents, and parents of their peers, who don't seem to take the same attitude toward the illegal drinking and procuring of alcohol as they do toward procuring and use of drugs.

. . . .It's impossible to call yourself a therapist and at the same time a disciplinarian. These roles have to be strictly segregated in the institutional setting.

. . . .The administration tells the college student "Thou shalt not drink," so they don't serve beer on most campuses. But they can walk right across the street to the basement of the fraternity house and get smashed.

. . . .The university does have a responsibility to learn about alcohol use and to present this information to people. There's at least 35 solid years of research available to impart to students.

. . . .You're suggesting we get away from our puritanical heritage and deal with the more factual kind of thing. What do you think student response would be?

Student: Students might resent any type of instructions. Students learn more by making mistakes of their own.

. . . .In the secondary schools in Florida they finally hired a consultant for alcohol education in the public schools, as required by law. She was apparently doing a good job that the school system liked. But extreme influence of the WCTU put on great pressure to fire her because she wasn't teaching the "evils of drink."

. . . .Student lack of interest in hearing about alcohol because they pretty well know what they're going to hear—the same old temperance lecture. Isn't it possible that interest in this sort of thing might be increased with such titles as "How to Drink Safely"?

. . . .But the essence of the problem boils down to regarding college students as adults. College students regard themselves as adults and are ready to adopt the mores of adult society. In a sense we're here saying "Let's start treating college students that way—leveling with them." But the law and administration say, "No, he's not an adult."

. . . .You're upset by the inconsistency. You can't enforce this rule—don't want to enforce it—yet it's very difficult to change rules.

. . . .I'm upset because I saw an opportunity to sit down with students and discuss a rule that has always been handed down to them but they have not shared in the making. Conversely, they've shared in many other areas—we have a lot of student government. But this "no drinking" rule has been a condition of attendance. Students don't pay any attention to it and enroll anyhow.

. . . .Our Health Service recently drafted a letter which pertained to this area stating that the feeling of the university is that drinking which is not breaking any laws is something that is a private matter, and as long as it doesn't disturb other people and get in other people's way or reflect on the university it is a matter for the student to take care of himself.

. . . .In my experience, all campuses I have been on had rules against drinking in fraternity houses, but it was understood that the rule wouldn't be enforced unless someone got into trouble.

. . . .How in the world can a college cook up a rule about drinking that's going to convince an intelligent undergrad with all this phoniness in front of him?

. . . .Any student on the Berkeley campus who drank very much wouldn't be there very long, regardless of any rules, because he couldn't keep up with the pressure and pace of grades. So we have internal controls in our requirements for efficiency.

Student: Whether rules on campus are liberal or completely restrictive, college is sink or swim in the drinking area because kids are going to get hold of it no matter what, and a restriction doesn't make that much difference.

. . . .But what we're talking about on the Berkeley campus is a state law, not a university regulation. A faculty member could have a seminar in his home, serve drinks to an 18-year-old and go to jail. What you're saying to students by so doing is, "I will violate the law if I don't believe in it. Therefore I suggest you do too."

Student: Perhaps when you have an 18-year-old drinking law you have to start alcohol education about 16, because many 16-year-olds drink if they look old enough. As the saying is, if you can get your hand over the bar you'll get your drink. I'd like to throw in another problem. In your role as counselors and educators you must realize that students are going to drink and the problem is going to be there.

Another student: About 90 per cent of the men students at Amherst are fraternity members. The age for drinking is 21 in Massachusetts. The law states that anyone serving a minor is subject to fines. The Social Chairman takes this responsibility and minors drink, so the law is never enforced. The town police are hired by the college to come in during parties to protect the fraternity property, and stand next to minors drinking, but they don't take any action.

. . . .In the university there is tremendous pressure put upon the administration to do that which the parents didn't feel comfortable about doing themselves.

. . . .It's difficult to get people at administrative or higher curriculum levels to admit that all of this questioning is in itself a valid part of education. Students are asking some very fundamental questions which are handled as unrest or disturbances and not a part of education.

Student: The official university position is no drinking at all, of course.

. . . .But sororities modify that to the extent that moderation is tolerated.

. . . .There's been a tremendous change in the last 25 years.

The white Protestant families used to hide their liquor. Children could grow up without ever knowing their parents drank.

. . . .So we sit on our hands and say we wish we could do more, and let generation after generation of students go out without a possible hope for benefit which could be derived from some level of health education.

. . . .There are laws in every state requiring education along these lines at the high school level. This legislation I'm sure was the result of the WCTU many years ago. But you find very little evidence of teachers being given any special preparation for education along this line.

. . . .We could say that alcohol is here to stay and we can't talk it out of existence or legislate or rule it out of existence. We accept its presence, and having accepted the fact that people drink and alcohol is around, it is incumbent upon us at this state in the lives of college students to teach them how to drink for its best enjoyment and with the least possibility of deleterious effects. If we can go back and present this attitude to our administrations, get them to recognize the same ideas, then look around for a person to develop the right kind of course, we're on the right track.

. . . .In our community, people are more interested in reading about the horrible things that alcohol causes. They're delighted to think that this is what is being taught on college campuses—

how to drink badly. This is because they feel it's a moral issue.

. . . .At Westminister the students like to drink beer, but have to go off in the canyons to do it, as drinking by college students is prohibited, so they feel they've done something wrong.

. . . .Each university should review its rules with respect to drinking and then examine the implications of these rules. Do they want any rules? Are rules necessary? Why can't they review them for their relevance, for their implications as to how consistent the general need for rules in this area is. And whatever rules are adopted should be relevant to the university's goals.

Some Recommendations

The following conclusions and recommendations of the "Alcohol and College Youth" conference group discussion leaders are particularly pertinent to "knowing the territory" of alcohol education.

We produced after these several sessions some recommendations and proposals and some consensus—a good deal of consensus, in fact.

The first, but not necessarily the most outstanding recommendation was that educators, education administrators, faculty in general do have responsibility in their position in our society to help form public opinion, to help form public attitudes, to help form regulations on their campuses and to help form state laws governing the use of alcohol in our society in general, particularly the regulations and rules relative to the use of alcohol on the campuses of this country. We didn't decide how we could best go about forming opinion, but it was agreed that they do have a responsibility and are ready, with the proper mechanisms, to accept that responsibility to implement these objectives.

Another recommendation was that educators do have a responsibility to teach students about alcohol and its use, just as they have the responsibility for teaching any other discipline on the campus. Also the college and university as a whole has a like responsibility. Conference participants

396   HENRY B. BRUYN

felt that the subject of alcohol and its use has a legitimate place on the college campus and should have the consideration and attention that it warrants.

We had a good deal of discussion of ways in which we might implement this warranted consideration and attention. One conclusion was that it is not the responsibility of the administrator or the faculty to teach youth how to drink, but to help the student appreciate the place of alcohol for the individual in the micro-culture of the college and the macro-culture of the larger society in which he lives. In other words, that you can't use any chemical, including alcohol, in any behavior intelligently unless you know in a pretty thorough way its identity and characteristics.

It was agreed that the most effective alcohol education is conducted on the campus by and with student peer groups. With an articulate, skillful, knowledgeable cadre of students on the campus, they themselves are very apt to have more influence on their student peer groups, who in turn would be more apt to be influenced by these knowledgeable and articulate students than lectures from the faculty. Students are a very important link with the faculty in trying to develop the notion among students that civilized drinking is cool, that drunken behavior as a result of alcohol is not something to be sought, and that drunkenness in general is unacceptable behavior.

While concern about alcoholism and other pathological drinking was experienced, there was general acceptance of drinking in the proper context or, to quote Nevitt Sanford, "civilized drinking." There is a difference between drinking and alcoholism, and we should strive for sober drinking, civilized, integrated, drinking.

We proposed that following this conference an effort be made to develop regional working conferences on the subject of alcohol on the campus for student personnel and other appropriate disciplinarians and officers on the campus, including students.

We also proposed that it is a responsibility of college and university administration to create a context in which a dispassionate and objective exploration of facts, values, and attitudes facilitate a thoughtful choice in this matter of alcohol use.

In addition, we proposed that we move forward with consideration of relevant research that will lead toward identification of those students at risk, and that drunkenness and alcoholism are not logical choices.

One discussion group concluded in its summary of the conference that education relative to alcohol use really has to be based on up-to-date scientific facts and data. The concern about alcohol use in the college age group included the implication that most students would become parents at some time. Dr. Lolli, a resource speaker, suggested the etiology of alcoholism might lie in the maternal-child relationship. This group recommended that an intensification of research into the etiology of alcoholism be pursued. We believe, they said, that students are honestly concerned with the problem of drinking, and we must supply scientific facts and useful information concerning the origins and development of pathological drinking.

There was much discussion of the different institutions represented—their policies in regard to use of alcohol, their rules and regulations. It was agreed the rules about alcohol use cannot be generalized. Each institution must set policy, if there is to be one, in accordance with its own background, whether religious or state-supported institution, and its own community setting.

It was agreed the colleges and universities had the right to set their own rules and to help the students maintain them. It was felt that colleges should promote discussion and communication and possibly set their rules on the basis of these discussions and communications. Above all, if rules and policies are set down they should be made very clear and should be enforced. A recommendation was made that all colleges and universities should review their policies at the present time concerning rules about alcohol, look at the implications of these rules, and ask themselves whether they are relevant to their goals. This review should include a look at positive policies, and students should be heavily involved in the discussion.

We also discussed the subcultures on the campus that influence drinking patterns. While we came to no definite conclusions as to whether there was or was not an influence, we wondered if this really isn't an area which deserves a lot of exploration. The changing impact of students on college and university policies should be taken into consideration in our thinking about alcohol usage and education, and the role of subcultures is an important area for research as to their relevance in the development of drinking patterns. We are certainly aware that the subcultures exist. We would like to know how we could utilize them in a positive manner.

We considered the types of health education in our respective institutions—those that had any health education at all—and there are a number of them. We discovered that a great many of the health education courses were in the Physical Education Department, that at least in many instances the instructors were not well prepared, and especially not well prepared on education regarding alcohol use. We felt it fairly urgent at this time that student personnel administrators inform themselves about drinking problems. Generalizations about health education on alcohol proved difficult because of the different levels of development of the institutions involved.

Recognizing that many areas on the campus have to do with health education, we recommended that both formal and informal approaches be exploited, improved, and developed. Alcohol should be high on the list. Administration, faculty, and students should inform themselves by communicating with those who are most knowledgeable. The Student Health Service should play a central role as a source of information.

In regard to institutional rules and attitudes—or publicly expressed attitudes—about drinking, we all agreed quickly that official rules of total proscription were not particularly helpful in what could be more constructive efforts in analyzing and teaching, and were not really realistic in reflecting the situation. Or, as they say at Stanford, there is no drinking on campus except in fact! This immediately brought up another question as to why an institution's authorities generally feel the need to take some stand. There are very real pres-

sures—financial and political—which encourage the administration in taking a somewhat negative stand. This might be
referred to as the "honors sharing in hypocrisy." In other
words, it's possible to say, "Look kids, we have an impossible
situation that we can't presently alter, but let's both admit it,
let's face it, and we'll work out some kind of compromise
together." And at least in one of our institutions represented
at the conference such a compromise had been struck and
seemed to be a fairly successful solution, though perhaps not
an ideal one in the long run. However, it may be an honest
and realistic approach to a situation that cannot be altered
immediately.

We kept coming back to the fact that emphasis on education
for living, as opposed to academic education, poses a real
problem. Nowadays the more an institution claims to be a
"great" university the more emphasis it places on academics
and the more it tends to look at health education for living
as Mickey Mouse, that is, as kid stuff. We discussed various
ways in which this undesirable attitude might be altered or
approached and came up with a series of recommendations.

First, in retrospect we wished there had been college
presidents or academic deans represented at the conference—
people concerned with curriculum. In future conferences we
felt that faculty and administrators responsible for curriculum
should be involved. We could also have learned something
from college security officers and legislators. We look forward
hopefully to changing institutional attitudes toward including
education in living as an explicit part of the curriculum.

We should be inspired opportunists and capitalize on any
opportunity to enter into dialogue with students at any level
on issues that concern them. Alcohol certainly provides such
opportunities in which one might not only discuss drinking
but many other issues that are of vital interest to them. We
tended in the first few sessions of the conference to oversim-
plify, as if students would welcome us with open arms to
discuss alcohol education. Most students may feel that "Well,
I'm living anyway, why do I have to be taught about this?"
The fact is that there are moments and crises for many students which can be used as an occasion for dialogue.

Some of the teaching methods or tools of health educators

should be reviewed, since it seemed unlikely at the moment that the institutions as a whole would regard health education about drinking as a very positive value. The Health Services were seen typically as being enough outside the academic area; and yet they may have enough prestige to begin to serve more as the source of health education than they have in the past. We felt a knowledgeable, active health educator in a college or university setting would stimulate many invitations for all kinds of small conferences or lectures by bringing good speakers on campus in addition to providing the resource material. Although the inclusion of alcohol studies in the content of regular courses in the social sciences was mentioned, the curriculum is already so crowded in most cases that this approach seemed unlikely to succeed.

We were impressed with the wide variation of drinking practices that were reported by the representative institutions at the conference. This wide variability actually ranged from almost no drinking observed by the participant to the other extreme of a great amount of drinking observable on campus. For example, in one institution 13 fraternities budgeted some $3,000 each every academic year for the purchase of beer and liquor. It is common at this college on a Friday and Saturday, or Saturday and Sunday night to tap a keg, and it was estimated that some 10 per cent of the students are drinking to excess. Also at this institution it is common practice for members of the faculty throughout the year to be invited to the various fraternity houses for a beer drinking party or cocktail party. On these occasions it was felt that more is gained from the standpoint of positive faculty-student relationships than is lost in terms of the leveling effect. Under these conditions it was felt that excessive drinking rarely occurred and only under situations where uninvited faculty members dropped in for a free drink was there any loss of respect on the part of faculty members. The representative from this college felt the 10 per cent who did drink excessively also suffered academically.

The amount of drinking that actually goes on by college students in the college setting tends to vary with a number of factors. Among them were living on campus, the values of the students, their cultural background, whether the institution was a private, denominational, or state-supported institution. More research to better define the drinking patterns on the various college campuses is needed, especially research on the factors which promote integrative, in contrast to facilitative and escapist drinking. Does, for example, student-faculty drinking encourage integrative drinking? Many but not all conferees thought it did.

Our list of barriers or problems in achieving integrated, integrative drinking among college students far outnumbered our methods of implementation. The major problems as barriers were strong public opinion and opposition to drinking generally, strong religious beliefs opposing drinking in many college environments, current laws forbidding drinking before the age of 21, the existence of colleges where most students are commuters and there is no college community, and very large colleges where experience in integrative drinking would not be possible and practical.

Drinking is here to stay. It is an integral part of our society. If this is so, there is a need for colleges and universities to come to grips with the cultural ambivalence with regard to the use of alcohol among college students and to address the issues involved. What is to be done will vary with local conditions, and in many instances this whole process of doing something will of necessity be a very long-term process. Of utmost importance, colleges and universities must be candid; they must demonstrate honesty and integrity in dealing with the whole area of alcohol education and student drinking on the campus.

An Illustration

The conference on Alcohol and College Youth illustrated a wide variety of opinions and experiences which suggest the nature of the "target" or "territory" to be addressed by health personnel. As an example of one college's approach to the challenge, the following material is quoted verbatim from an official statement distributed by the college administration to all students. This was supplemented by a major presentation by the Dean of Students and four small group discussion meetings.

The results of an official questionnaire administered on the

Austin College[5] campus early in 1966, and answered by 678 students, indicate that our student body is fairly representative of students across the country and that its members come from homes which are not unlike those in other sections of the country. Only 26 per cent of the students included in this survey indicated that alcoholic beverages are never served in their homes. Only 26 per cent of the students participating stated that they never drink. While 62 per cent stated that they drink socially or occasionally, 12 per cent indicated that they drink regularly. Moreover, in response to a question concerning the degree of agreement between them and their families on their use of alcoholic beverages, 69 per cent of the students stated there was agreement. While 12 per cent stated their families did not know of their drinking habits and 16 per cent indicated there was some degree of difference, only 3 per cent indicated a sharp difference between them and their families on their use of alcoholic beverages. The results of this questionnaire supported the belief that the problems connected with the use of alcohol are not remote from the Austin College campus and that the college regulations concerning the use of alcohol needed to be revised.

In preparing the revised Austin College statement on the use of alcoholic beverages, the following factors have been kept in mind.

1. The college is attempting to deal openly and forthrightly with the problem presented by the use of alcoholic beverages by students.

2. The statement on alcoholic beverages is related to, and based upon, the honor system which, as a continuing program toward the development of honor and mutual trust within the community, is an integral part of the educational program of the college.

3. More and more, the majority of students enrolling at Austin College come from family backgrounds where alcoholic beverages are served at least occasionally.

4. In view of state laws on the possession of alcoholic beverages and due to its location in a "dry" county, Austin College is in a particularly difficult legal position. While it is not the responsibility of the college to serve

as a law enforcement agency, as a law-abiding institution
the college must support the observance of the law.

5. The consumption of alcoholic beverages does not contribute to and has a tendency to deter the educational environment and program of the college. The fact remains
that most colleges in the United States prohibit the use
of alcohol on their campuses, even when the laws of the
state in which they are located would allow them to do
otherwise.

6. The advice and counsel of a lawyer, district attorney, one
of the local judges, and a representative of the local
Liquor Control Board has been sought and taken into
consideration. Administrative officers in other colleges and
universities have also been consulted.

7. While certain authorities claim that alcoholism has nothing
to do with wise and moderate drinking, there is no question that alcoholism is one of the more tragic problems
of our society. The college has a clear responsibility to
try to prevent the development of alcoholism by creating
and supporting an environment where the unreasoned or
excessive use of alcohol is not the accepted norm.

8. While it may be obvious that the statement on the use
of alcoholic beverages is not an ideal solution to the
problem, it certainly attempts to be realistic as well as
pragmatic in facing the problem of student use of alcoholic beverages.

While the Austin College policy on the use of alcoholic
beverages is not based on a denominational or religious stance,
a Christian view of man and of the laws of society demands
a genuine concern for individuals and the excesses to which
man is subject. Within a framework of law, temperance, and
personal discipline, the college recognizes the right and the
responsibility of each individual to arrive at his own decision
concerning the use of alcohol.

At the same time, it is clear that not only individuals but
also institutions are confronted with certain legal and other
limitations. Under present law, Austin College cannot permit the possession or consumption of alcoholic beverages

within the physical confines of the campus. In dealing with students who consume alcohol away from the campus, the emphasis will be placed on the resultant behavior. The legal liability of a group that makes available alcoholic beverages to a person under 21 years of age extends to each member of the group. Regardless of location, an individual 21 years of age or older—whether student, faculty, or staff—who provides or makes available alcoholic beverages to a person under 21 years of age may under state law be charged with contributing to the delinquency of a minor. Austin College expects all members of the college community to understand and comply with existing laws and statutes. Because the consumption of alcoholic beverages by minors is prohibited by law unless minors are in the presence of parents or legal guardians, members of the administrative staff and faculty are advised not to serve alcoholic beverages to students.

The following policy statement for Austin College concerning the use of alcoholic beverages by students has been approved.

The use of intoxicating beverages is not a part of nor does it contribute to the total educational emphasis at Austin College. The use of intoxicants by students is not approved.

The possession or consumption of alcoholic beverages within the boundaries of the campus, or at all-school functions of any type, is prohibited.

The fact that some students may choose to drink alcoholic beverages is a matter of individual responsibility. Although the College acknowledges the student's responsibility to make a personal decision in this matter *when away from the campus*, it expects the student's conduct to be acceptable at all times.

The reader will note several significant things about this statement by college administration to its student body. The first and most important fact is that the statement is open, frank, honest and clear without ambiguity or equivocation. The second important element found in this statement is the frank expression of frustration with which the college administration faces its position in a dry county. The third important fact transmitted to the student body by this college administration is the unavoidable, unalterable reality of the local law. It will be noted that this is presented to the students with ample background reference to advice and counsel from lawyers, the district attorney and the local Liquor Control Board. It cannot, then, be interpreted by the young adult college student as an arbitrary, blind, authoritarian opinion and direction from the college administration. The only spot at which I think the policy of this college could be criticized by most authorities on the subject of alcohol and alcoholism is item 7. The prevention of the development of alcoholism by suppressing and excluding alcohol would certainly not be claimed by many modern authorities in the field, and represents a classical temperance movement philosophy. Perhaps the element of ambiguity in this statement is important. The administration feels that it is creating an environment where "the unreasoned or excessive use of alcohol is not the accepted norm" and yet the policy statement prohibits "the possession or consumption of alcoholic beverages within the boundaries of the campus or at all school functions of any type." This policy certainly goes much further than preventing "unreasoned or excessive use." Nevertheless, this example of attitude on the part of a college administration is refreshingly honest and practical, and I am sure would for the most part be acceptable and understood by the "target" which is the subject of discussion.

Another example of official university statement on the subject of alcoholic beverages is found in a prominent place in the General Catalogue of that university and thereby directed not only to prospective students and their parents but also an official statement to the enrolled student body. This statement reads: "The policy relative to alcoholic beverages involves a minimum of rules and a maximum of individual and group responsibility. The University must at all times uphold the state and city statutes relative to alcoholic beverages. It interprets this to include that the storage, possession, and use of alcoholic beverages is not allowed in University supervised houses, apartments, residence halls, on sorority and fraternity property, on the University campus, or on other University property.

"Any student of legal age who exhibits offensive behavior on University owned or supervised property while under the influence of alcoholic beverages will be subject to severe disciplinary action."

It will be noted that this sort of statement reflects the regulations of the state and city laws and emphasizes that "offensive behavior" under the influence of alcohol will be subject to university action. This type of university policy statement has the advantage of being brief and straightforward with a clear-cut definition of the way in which alcohol and its use is of concern to the institution.

In conclusion, the problems found in the interaction between youth and alcohol, as well as the challenge, would all seem capable of successful solution. Utilizing well-established and widely accepted facts, knowledge, and advice presently available, not only in regard to alcohol itself but most particularly regarding the young adult of college years is part of that solution. These facts require frequent re-emphasis, re-evaluation and critical review, but as they are brought together to establish new programs, new policies, and new laws, changes will take place. Such changes, however, are the duties of a responsible society which looks forward with vision based on knowledge and reason rather than backward and downward with decisions based on emotion, bigotry, insecurity, and ignorance.

REFERENCES

1. SANFORD, F. H. "Inter-personal Communication," *Industrial Medicine and Surgery,* 25: 261, 1956.
2. ERIKSON, E. H. "The Problem of Ego Identity," *Journal of American Psychoanalytic Association,* 4: 75, 1956.
3. FARNSWORTH, D. L. *Psychiatry, Education, and the Young Adult.* Springfield, Illinois: Charles C. Thomas, 1966.
4. SANFORD, N. Proceedings of Conference on Alcohol and College Youth. American College Health Association. University of Miami, Coral Gables, Florida.
5. Basic Decisions Program, Austin College, Sherman, Texas, 1966.
6. General Catalogue, University of Nevada, Reno, Nevada, 1966-67.

7. CAIN, VASHTI (ed.). *Proceedings of a Regional Conference on Alcohol Education in Institutions of Higher Learning,* Biloxi, Mississippi, March 26-28, 1963.

8. McCARTHY, R. G. (ed.). *Proceedings of a Conference on Interpreting Current Knowledge about Alcohol and Alcoholism to a College Community,* Albany, New York, March 28-30, 1963.

Chapter 19

COLLEGE ADMINISTRATION OF ALCOHOLIC BEVERAGE REGULATIONS

Lawrence Riggs
College of Wooster

ATTEMPTS TO CONTROL the use of alcoholic beverages on a college campus present unique and complex problems more acute than those faced in civic life. Because of a growing tradition of drinking strengthened by widespread social and economic pressures, because of the specific purposes and functions of various colleges, and because of a general uncertainty and a vigorous questioning about the authority and responsibility of college officials, the control of the use of alcoholic beverages in relation to college life is certainly not a simple matter of issuing an edict. The college campus of today is reflecting the values and practices of the society from which it draws its constituency. "It should come as no surprise to anyone that large numbers of students bring to their colleges a drinking custom taught by their parents and supported by strong social and economic forces" (1, p. 27). At least sixty-two out of every one hundred American adults use alcoholic beverages on occasion. They annually spend two and one half times more on these drinks than is spent by the total population on religious and welfare activities (2, p. 11).

Current discussions about the proper concerns of college officials range from those who hold that the college is properly concerned about the total behavior of its students to those who hold that the true function of the college is to be concerned only with those matters of the mind that affect the student in his classroom performance. The time-honored principle of the college standing and acting in the place of parents (*in loco parentis*) has been vigorously challenged in the name of what is claimed to be "new understandings" about individual freedom, the invasion of the private lives of students and the proper authority of college officials.

In spite of arguments to the contrary, a rigorous examination of the proper authority and responsibility of college officials leaves no doubt about their jurisdiction in reference to any action affecting the "common good" of the college or the welfare of its students. Likewise there is no doubt about the fact that public opinion, parental attitudes, and the expectancies of those associated with a college point to agreement that the college should, indeed, act in ways that protect the welfare of its students. College officials properly take extensive action for the protection of individuals and groups in cases of emergency that arise on the campus. From a legal point of view the college *is* obliged to act in responsible ways for the protection and welfare of its student body (3, p. 23).

In academic matters extensive efforts are made to assist students in avoiding unnecessary failures by presenting them with legitimate alternatives for the development of their best academic achievement. No one would argue that college officials and faculty members are therefore responsible for forcing learning or personal development on their individual students. There is clear recognition that the central considerations are to present young people with the opportunities for growth and development to which they must individually respond and to encourage positive responses. The final decision for such responses rests squarely with each student. The college is obligated to provide an atmosphere in which responses can be made effectively with increasing maturity of judgment.

College regulation in such matters as might adversely affect students or the college community is clearly proper. Upon choosing to go to college, students voluntarily become members of a corporate group where they come under rules and regulations designed to support the purposes of that group. The college is responsible for making known those limits of behavior beyond which students may expect to receive discipline action.

College controls on the use and possession of alcoholic

beverages must not be contrary to state law. They need not, however, be identical with state law and may extend to situations affecting the campus but not governed by state law.

It must next be pointed out that individual conscience cannot ever be invaded by regulation or law. It is the role of a college to support the development of high moral standards in private behavior and thus encourage individuals and groups to develop a conscience characterized by moral principles as guiding and evaluative determinants of behavior.

I

College officials and the public they serve must more completely understand the peculiar nature of the campus community and how this relates to the control of the use and possession of alcoholic beverages.

The campus community is such that when the use of alcoholic beverages is introduced this practice must be viewed differently from drinking in the larger civic community. The political and social structure of the campus and the developmental needs of the people involved present differences that must be understood. Comparisons with civic communities break down at many points.

At least the following characteristics of the college campus must be thoughtfully considered as being unique aspects of college community life and therefore presenting different problems relating to the use of authority and the assumption of responsibility by administrators in controlling the use of alcoholic beverages. Numerous questions arise.

1. On most campuses there is a special age grouping of people usually ranging from 17 to 25 years of age. Considering state laws, most of which make 21 the legal age for the use of alcoholic beverages, what is the responsibility of the college to see that state laws are observed? How may sensible distinctions be made between those legally able to drink and those not old enough? Should these distinctions apply off as well as on the campus? What authority does the college have over "of age" students in respect to using alcoholic beverages on campus? Off campus?

2. In most instances college students are to a large extent

concentrated in living arrangements of considerable size. Most college students are living in residence units bringing them in daily contact with vastly larger numbers of people than their family groups have provided. This geographic compactness brings about a social compactness with more frequent face to face personal contacts with the same people in this special community than in most civic communities. This indeed becomes a world reduced in geographic limits, but multiplied in terms of individual contact. The potential influences of any individual on others is greater.

To what extent is the introduction of alcoholic beverages in such a closely related group different from the use of alcoholic beverages in society at large? Should the college assume any responsibility for trying to protect students from each other? Are the effects of choosing to drink in this setting the same as choosing to drink in community life? Do these choices have any bearing on the atmosphere and academic quality of the institution? Does the college have the right to act in prohibitive or punitive ways when "wrong" choices are made by individuals? Is choosing to drink a "wrong" or harmful choice in relation to the mission of the institution?

3. The college community is subject to wide geographical influences. Students are more mobile both in and out of this country. Foreign students are present on most campuses, bringing differing cultural backgrounds. Because cultures vary widely regarding the use of alcoholic beverages, this diversity of cultural influence concentrated and reflected on the campus becomes another force for the student meeting a wider scale of values.

To what extent can a college require conformity by individuals to a standard about the use of alcohol that does not reflect the student's customs, traditions, or newly acquired convictions as a result of exposure to other cultures? Should foreign students accustomed to the use of alcoholic beverages be required to observe a limiting and different standard in this respect? Do foreign students require special attention in regard to the institution's regulations on alcoholic beverages?

4. Today's college student presents a different background from his counterpart of only a few years ago. He has had earlier social experiences (dating, social life); earlier, more

advanced and more varied academic experience of a high level (some come with advanced credit and some have had the benefit of more effective teaching methods and equipment than some colleges provide); more sophistication about entertainment, national and international affairs (thanks to television), and earlier drinking (many college students who drink had their first alcoholic beverage at about 14 or 15 years of age). This "adult" experience background, recently thought to be reserved for the college years and beyond, is frequently without the benefit of accompanying maturity of judgment, a sound sense of personal identity, and the ability to respond maturely to freedom in restricted paths. Concepts of the common good are subjugated to concerns for self.

There is at college a new sharp reality to changing relationships with people. Frequently this requires the development of understandings of what to many students appear to be new and foreign authority—responsibility, relationships and a definition (all too often for the first time) of the meanings of social and personal responsibility in the exercise of individual freedom. Individuality has been so strongly stressed and valued that considering the common good becomes less relevant than many administrators understand. Commitments are not so much to institutions (including the college) as to philosophical principles.

What is the rationale for regulations on alcoholic beverages which can be presented so as to be meaningful to students? Does the use of alcoholic beverages reinforce strength or weaknesses in students?

5. Closely related to the comments just made is the matter of self-centered values in an increasingly competitive setting. A kind of "T.V. morality" prevails. The goals of high academic achievement and of personal identity are too often sought without qualms about the methods used to gain these ends. In these instances reaching the goal seems more important than integrity. Stealing examinations, taking books from the library with no intention of returning them, the manufacture of elaborate but false identification, disregard for the comfort and convenience of others when selfish goals are sought, are all too common.

It is now in the college years that many basic values appear to be developing and there is a strong potential for the development of values in the college years. We must not lose sight of this merely because we can no longer assume students bring some of the basic traditional values with them.

Should the use of alcoholic beverages be discussed in terms of moral issues, i.e., issues affecting other people?

How serious is the use of false identification to obtain alcoholic beverages? Should the college be concerned about this (can it properly be?) or should this be a matter of law enforcement?

Is college drinking a status symbol? If so, and if this is considered undesirable in any way, how can this means of achieving status be replaced with something else?

Is there any hope of conformity to mature standards of integrity regarding the acceptance of controls on the use of alcoholic beverages?

Do our rules and regulations in any way add to rather than help solve the problems of values involved?

6. The existence of common goals (to get a degree, to achieve, to be eligible to go to graduate school, or get a good job, etc.) leads to a high degree of competitiveness. Attendance at college is a freely chosen enterprise, but one now accompanied by high financial costs and a high degree of societal and parental expectancy. These are sources of pressure. There is now a demand for intellectual performance on a level never before faced by college students.

To what extent is the use of alcohol a justifiable means of relieving these pressures as a sort of self-medication? What are the advantages of such use? The disadvantages?

Is there any relationship between the use of alcohol and achievement?

7. There are developmental needs characteristic of students in the college community. These needs are met or not in the interaction of individual persons and groups in campus life. Needs for status, recognition, response, identification of self, independence, conformity to and acceptance by peer cultures (at the risk of psychological suicide if one fails), experimentation and adventure, are only a few of the personality needs being introspectively viewed and actively sought for in fulfillment. Everett Tillson has said that students seem

to him sometimes to be "shadows playing at being real; lonely people playing at fellowship."

When beverage alcohol becomes a means of meeting any of these needs, what understandings should accompany its use? Is the college responsible for education along these lines?

Are these limits beyond which experimentation cannot be accepted? How are such limits set? Can the college really control experimentation? If not, what is the stand of the college about experimentation? Is this different for alcohol from attitudes about other drugs, sex, dishonesty?

Are alcoholic beverages an efficient means of meeting these needs?

Does the use of alcohol contribute to a sense of reality? To fellowship?

8. The political "power structure" is unique. Students (the constituency) do not elect the officials of the college who carry final responsibility for administering the affairs of the community. Students cannot vote out the administration, although they have developed means of effective pressure; students are transient members of the college community. Historically, the freedoms that students enjoy have been delegated to them. They may influence decision making concerning college policy, but seldom are they finally responsible for policy development except in areas delegated to them. Students are taxed heavily for participation in the college community but have limited voice in the final determination of policy. In a sense they are buying educational services which they have voluntarily selected to buy inasmuch as they have chosen their college community. Furthermore, there are legal, social, and parental expectancies that the college will act in responsible ways by expressing concern for the welfare of its students (3, p. 23).

How much voice should students have in policy formulation? In disciplinary functions relative to college rules? What obligation has the college to make clear its mission as officially viewed and accepted, and the limits of behavior viewed as inimical to the welfare of the institution? Has the institution any right to set these limits in contradiction to the customs and wishes of its students? Does such a thing as "institutional integrity" really exist, or should the only standards be those formulated by students? What can be done when these are in conflict? In what ways is the college *in loco parentis?* How can concern for students best be expressed and still preserve the rights of students to make choices, to grow in experience?

So much for the setting and some of the worrisome questions that must be faced. The college community is a unique and in some ways a false community if the civic community is the basis of comparison. Administrators must understand this and respond to the campus situation in terms not always apparent in civic life.

What other issues should administrators understand in reference to the many considerations surrounding attempts to control the use of alcoholic beverages in college life?

II

College officials must know why they set limits on the use and possession of alcoholic beverages and they must be able and willing to convey these reasons to students.

For too long institutions have found "tradition" a complete answer and a protective device. Administrators guilty of using tradition as an explanation of their rules may appear to be concealing their reasons for having restrictions about alcoholic beverages, or being ashamed of, or out of agreement with the reasons, or simply not having a sensible rationale.

Basic to any rationale about alcoholic beverages in college life is a concept of the mission of the college. In some cases a view is held that the college mission is sharply limited to goals directly relating to academic performance. In these instances, concerns about alcohol are minimal and relate only to those cases where the student is not able to present himself in the classroom as an effective learner. If the use of alcoholic beverages leads to the student's failure, this is a choice made by him, the consequences of which he must face. In colleges with this view, the rationale can easily be put purely on the basis of effectiveness in attendance and academic response. Because the student's decision about drinking is not the college's concern, there is little if any restriction, and hence no need for more than the minimum explanation that the student is expected to be in class, able to learn.

Another view holds that drunkenness and undesirable behavior resulting from the use of alcohol is beyond acceptance by the college. The rationale for any regulations in such cases can be clearly put in terms of the effect of one's behavior in annoying or inhibiting the learning of others and in terms of accepting responsibility to keep one's drinking within such limits as not to lead to drunkenness or misconduct interfering with others. It is also possible to include an undesirable effect on the general atmosphere of learning as a reason for such a restriction. Some colleges go further in active support of state law, thus outlawing by college rules under-age drinking on the campus or in relation to official college activities.

Private institutions, and some state schools as well, frequently extend their authority to support state law and to ruling out drinking by anyone on campus, in relation to college activities, or student-sponsored activities. This is a more direct opposition to the use of alcoholic beverages by any student. An attempt is made in these cases to keep the restriction in terms of its relation to campus life and to misconduct by any student as long as he is in residence or under the jurisdiction of the college. College officials taking this position feel they are exhibiting a concern for the student as a person as well as the student as a learner. In such instances a more thorough rationale is suggested involving evidence about the pharmaceutical nature and properties of alcohol, its effects on higher processes of judgment, conscience, and personal development. Moral values, social conscience, and personal development are held as valued goals toward which the college feels responsible to work (4).

Administrators working in such a situation cannot properly escape a thorough study of the physiological and psychological effects of alcohol, the moral and social issues involved and the variety of legitimate attitudes about alcohol in our country. College deans and counselors must become more aware of the need for better understanding on their part regarding the nature of alcoholic beverages and their effects on individuals and society.

There is ample material easily available on this subject.[1] Factual information must be the basis for a rationale behind a specific restriction on the use of alcohol. This rationale will not only be in the tradition of good scholarship, but will be the only basis on which students in college will even begin to understand and accept the regulations imposed. They must make sense.

Some colleges associate their regulations on the use of alcoholic beverages with a religious context and tradition. Churches with an abstinence point of view who are supporting or operating colleges can be properly expected to reflect this view in the operation of their schools.

It is clearly established that colleges have a right to set their aims, purposes and goals and the means of achieving these. The mission of the college should set the context for all the programs of the college. Administrators must first of all be able to relate restrictions on the use of alcohol to their particular institutional context and philosophy.

For those who have restrictions on the use of alcohol based in part on the effects of alcohol and the concern of the institution for the influence of alcoholic beverages on individual students, there must be a clear, factual, and specific understanding of what alcohol is and how it does affect individuals and groups.

Recognizing again that ultimately the decision to drink or not is a personal matter of choice, colleges taking a strong stand on this issue are abrogating their educational functions should they fail to provide accurate data for student consideration about the alternatives involved in the choice to use or refrain from using alcoholic beverages. No rule or regulation by itself will insure any particular choice.

There is, furthermore, an obligation to make openly explicit the rationale of the college for its rules on the use and possession of alcoholic beverages to provide unemotional, factual, objective, and completely open discussion including data about the use and influence of alcoholic beverages in our society.

[1] See, for example, 5.

III

The effectiveness of rules and regulations about the use and possession of alcoholic beverages must be viewed in terms of student understandings and misunderstandings.

How do students view college rules on drinking?[2]

The Intercollegiate Association for the Study of the Alcohol Problem sponsored an annual essay contest among college students in the United States and Canada. In 1962 the essay subject was "Are College Drinking Rules Effective?" Three hundred thirty-one college students from the class of 1962 through the class of 1965 representing 20 colleges and universities in the United States responded to this question by submitting essays in the 1962 contest. In this group there were 173 men and 158 women.

Of the 249 essays useful for tabulation 69.5 per cent said, "No, college drinking rules are not effective." Fourteen per cent sidestepped the basic question by submitting short stories, essays on the general problem or irrelevant papers. Eight and a half per cent said, "Yes, drinking rules are effective in college." Eight per cent said, "Yes and no, it depends on what is meant."

Keeping in mind that relatively small numbers are involved, it is interesting to note a tendency for sophomores to side-step the issue more than any other group (27.5 per cent sophomores as compared to 13.33 per cent seniors, 11.59 per cent juniors, and only 9.23 per cent freshmen). This may reflect a certain wisdom after the freshman year! Fewer sophomores than any other group felt drinking rules were effective and only 11 per cent of the seniors, the group most confident about the effectiveness of the rules, consider college drinking rules effective.

The reasoning presented by the students is of interest. Those who said, "Yes, college rules are effective," included some who felt they are effective because they aren't enforced and some who felt the effectiveness to be in terms of pacifying the public. Only a very few of this group really gave unqualified "yes" answers.

---

[2] The material in this section first appeared in Riggs (6, pp. 32-39).

The "yes-*and*-no" answers were largely in terms of meaning "yes" if some control on campus is meant and "no" if the meaning is that college rules cause abstinence. Some indicated the rules were effective for those with abstinence backgrounds who accept this stand, and not effective for others (who choose not to follow the rules).

Many papers approached the problem by raising a question about the purpose of college rules. There was an almost uniform opinion that reasons for rules weren't adequately understood, and a great suspicion existed that many college administrators didn't have a reasoned basis for them either, or were so out of sympathy with the rules they couldn't adequately explain them. Rules on drinking alcoholic beverages were thought by a good portion of students to be for the purpose of protecting the college from embarrassment, to placate wealthy supporters, to conform to church policies (in church-related schools) and in some few cases to help the individual student.

One student observed the dilemma in which administrators find themselves by pointing out that strict enforcement means student resentment and liberal policies bring adverse reactions from the community. She said, "[Our] school copes with these two problems by formalizing a policy, then neglecting to enforce it." This apparently makes everyone happy. Another student wrote, "When college administrators emerge from their fear of public censure, college drinking rules will become truly effective."

With a few notable exceptions there was generally a clear feeling that the whole matter of drinking rule administration is a frustrating reality perpetrated on an unwilling student body by administrators who are under pressure from above (boards, the community, the church and supporters). A strong point was made to the effect that students are going to drink regardless. This embraced a feeling that one need not respect a rule that inconveniences him personally and, indeed, should not be expected to.

Many plead openly for drinking on campus. Said one man, "The alcohol rule is the student's area of rebellion and the pop of the beer can is his call to arms!" Said one woman, "Perhaps if college officials would realize what a clever group they are trying to deal with, they would realize how futile the whole matter is—that of controlling the use and possession of alcoholic beverages by college students." Another wrote, "To American students 'Thou shalt not' means 'I dare you.'" Another said, "Students just naturally rebel against rules."

Other pertinent comments included these:

"Good college student relations depend on some drinking being possible."

"Colleges must tactfully solve the alcohol problem without causing undue criticism from students."

"Drinking is not wrong in the right hands."

Their ability to conduct an adequate personal evaluation was assumed by numerous statements such as these:

"Students want to be treated as adults and have no one telling them what to do."

"Students don't want to be protected from themselves."

Drinking was viewed as having a friendly connotation. It is a symbol of friendship and goodwill and therefore has a place in society and on the campus.

If social pressure to drink "is strong enough to affect a whole nation, people of all social classes and positions in life, then why should the student be the only one strong enough to reject it?"

"When a young man or woman graduates from high school and leaves home to go to a college, he finds himself suddenly free of mental, moral and parental regulations."

"Be sensible, administrators. Be tolerant to the point of being blind to alcohol."

A constructive and realistic approach is viewed as one that would allow drinking off campus under faculty supervision. Drinking with professors and officials would bring drinking into an area of respectability and sensible perspective.

"By leaving the way open for a college student to come into contact with alcoholic beverages, he will be more likely to resist such forces in the future."

Rules should be relaxed because the further a student has to go to drink the more he will drink in order to make the trip worthwhile. Accidents might occur en route and this would be because of the rules making the student travel to get his drinks.

Rules were held responsible for a number of tragedies, including one suicide.

"Lenient rules seem to have the advantage of keeping the individual student in a healthier emotional and mental state."

"One man's rules have no influence over another man's behavior. College drinking rules exist only for the book."

"Rules may create as many cases of personal disorganization and frustration as they are trying to prevent."

College "drinking rules are no more than duck blinds. Students are more intelligent than birds and get around the rules."

"Anxiety or tension is a more decisive factor in college drinking than school rules."

Insofar as these are representative comments, they reveal an acceptance of "a norm of evasion as a societal standard" as one student aptly put it. Revealed also is a distressing need for sounder understanding about the reasons for rules on beverage alcohol in light of what alcohol is and does and what the colleges view as their purposes and aims. Undoubtedly these matters require sounder reasoning and clearer explanations in logical terms by college officials. Recognition must be forthcoming that nowhere else in society do we have communities with such concentration of an age group characterized by all sorts of strains and tensions often producing much anxiety in response to so many status needs. Comparisons of college campuses to civic communities break down at this and other points, as has been pointed out earlier in this chapter.

There were references in the student papers comparing law enforcement in the community and on campus saying "crime flourishes in a community where there is no enforcement of the law." Questions arose about the nature of "adequate punishment" in an educational institution. Only one student pointed out that there is greater centralization of control and geographic concentration on a college campus than in civic community life.

Much was said about enforcement. Comments such as those

reported above spoke for little or no enforcement. Enforcement seems to some to be equated with harsh action—usually dismissal from school. Almost unanimously, those who discussed enforcement wanted *action* and said rules were not effective because they weren't enforced. Some pointed out that proctors, housemothers, faculty, and even deans were sometimes guilty of conscious lack of action in known cases, or of actual participation with students in drinking. Students spoke of offenders "getting off," "being rescued by deans" (an interesting role assignment), and said that "an honest interest in students calls for a strict enforcement of the rules."

It was pointed out that when there was little enforcement of rules students are "overriding the faculty" thus injuring the "prestige and influence" of the school.

"The fault," said one student, "is with the makers of the rules, not the breakers of the rules."

Inconsistent treatment of offenders was criticized. Others pointed out the desirability of each case being handled on its merits even though the outcome may be different for cases that appear on the surface to be the same. A few students advocated weeding out the offenders. Some papers advocated dismissal, then inconsistently stated that fear is not a proper controlling method. "Part-time drinking rules" were lamented. Consistency was called for.

While claiming that many students drink to defy the rules, only a few papers listed this as a student reason for drinking when formally discussing this topic. The "rules are to be broken" approach thus may be a rationalization in support of a desire to drink.

There was much confusion as to what enforcement means, but there was a clear appeal to be consistent in taking some action in the cases of rule violators. Respect is gained as action is taken. Administrators have a responsibility to work with students in clarifying the possibilities and the desirability of various forms of action as being appropriate and real in their effectiveness. Thus "those making the rules [would] believe in them enough to enforce them" as one person put it.

Rules were generally blamed for falsifying I.D. cards and

other evasions. This lack of responsibility for law observance may be quite disturbing, but it is quite real.

There were many suggestions for the improvement of the situation aside from those already covered in relation to rules. Foremost among suggestions for improvement was an almost unanimous agreement that education and open discussion are needed. Students appear to be more interested in this and more ready for it than administrators have generally recognized.

Consider these thoughtful comments: "An uncrystallized set of social values and lack of systematic attention to social drinking in our society may account for the relationship of college administrators and the attitudes and practices of the college student."

Courses were advocated. The integration of useful information into classroom discussions was suggested. The employment of campus leaders in "information giving" positions was recommended (orientation groups, clubs, senates, dorm assistants, etc.).

Informing students more carefully about the existing rules was strongly advocated. One student conducted a survey on his campus asking about knowledge of drinking rules and got these replies, "Pour beer into the side of your glass," "Loosen your tie before drinking," "Turn your glass upside down when you finish."

There was agreement the problem should be brought out into the open, translating, as one student put it, "alcohol education into ethics" by education.

Encouragingly, numerous students saw the basic problem of values and stressed this. Some felt drinking patterns began before college and it was too late to do anything in college, but others were more optimistic.

"Alcohol must be incorporated in our mores not as a symbol of adulthood, but as a symbol of immaturity and weakness." Can college students (so given to conformity) develop a conformity to a no-drinking policy?

Several papers (fewer than one might expect) suggested religious values as a resource for developing a sense of worth and integrity and a feeling of responsibility for others that would rule out alcohol, or be a guide in its use.

"To be effective," said a young man, "rules must appeal to one's sense of honor, dignity, and self respect."

Another added, ". . . the college must replace rules with trust, discipline with direction, and force with faith."

"It will not be a change of rules that will eliminate the drinking problem; instead it will be a strengthening of our moral fiber accompanied by a raising of our standards and ideals."

Another, pointing to the need for students to become interested in their own best development pointed out in a neat phrase that "the wheel of responsibility must come full turn."

One brave student even suggested the campus would be a happier place if students cooperated with administrators in working on this problem!

Another pointed out it is up to the students who abstain to realize that they are the best possible aid to the drinking atmosphere of the campus when they are the silent abstainers. The silence of peers, she pointed out, is damaging. She went on to observe that the concerned student has referral resources in the form of counselors and deans to recommend to fellow students with an alcohol problem.

Only a few students wrote about responsibility to each other as fellow creatures. This is apparently an expression of an attitude characteristic of more maturity than most students possess, but it is an idealistic point that appeals to some.

One paper pointed out that we should use more positive data in our considerations and not lose sight of the 20 per cent of college men and the 39 per cent of college women who she said are and have been abstainers.

Several suggested the possibility of changing community laws or of better community enforcement of under-age drinking statutes to assist in cutting down on the drinking problem. One suggestion was to do away with the by-the-bottle sales and permit less to be sold (by the drink) so one can buy less and hence feel under no compulsion to drink his whole purchase in the form of a bottle of liquor.

Parents were included in many comments. Large numbers of students felt the alcohol beverage problem for youth stems from the home and so placed responsibility and blame with parents. Parental permission nullifies school rules, one said. The high school level needs action in relation to effective education and development of attitudes about alcoholic beverages.

This does indeed pose an interesting problem in values. If behavior is reflective of values, then there must be a value base upon which to develop attitudes about the use of alcoholic beverages. To be sure, facts play an important part in determining values, too, and must be supplied. The question then arises, can there be developed in individuals such a sense of confident judgment that it will become more important than the values of the surrounding social-cultural milieu in determining behavior? This will require stability of personality, a sense of direction in terms of personal and social goals and a kind of self-respect that has an authentic religious quality as man views himself as a creature of God. Are students willing to abdicate the privilege of individual freedom and personal choice in these matters and be buffeted by external forces only? And furthermore, can they extend respect and bestow dignity due their fellow creatures who choose differently than they, so this matter doesn't fracture their fellowship as men?

Freedom can be used in self-preserving and elevating directions, sometimes even against the social stream. There is a possibility of a change in social behavior if we address ourselves to fundamental values in life and appeal to reason with sound understanding of the facts at hand. College students have an unusual opportunity to thus be a creative force in society.

IV

Thoughtful approaches to enforcement of drinking rules must keep humanizing but consistent processes central as in all other areas of effective education.

"College authority cannot be properly extended into personal decisions unrelated to the college. Rules that attempt this are unenforceable, causing campus disciplinary bodies frequently to experience conflict over their feeling of responsibility to act in areas where they do not have proper authority. Colleges must take a strong, clear stand on the limits of behavior acceptable within the college community.

"There seems to be a widespread belief that all one needs to do is to dismiss a few students from school and the problem of drinking alcoholic beverages will be solved. This is completely unrealistic. There must be a procedure by which each particular circumstance is fully reviewed and each case is treated in terms of its own psychological and social aspects, with the best interests of both the particular person and the college community clearly in mind.

"When this is done, the results sometimes seem weak to uninformed observers. The charge is often made that college officials really do not mean to crack down on drinking because they have not taken severe action in every case of known drinking. To be sure, the easiest approach is to exercise the power and authority vested in administration and to take automatic, severe action without regard to the individual situation.

"Those who claim to have no difficulty with their campus drinking problem are usually those who take such arbitrary action. For them, the whole problem is automatically, easily, and—let us emphasize—impersonally handled. This negates our announced purpose to recognize the importance of personality and take individual differences into account. Appropriate action in cases involving violations of drinking regulations may range from counseling to dismissal.

"It is the role of education to insist that recovery is more important than punishment. At the same time, college officials must not be weak or indecisive in declaring a stand and taking action on behavior that is outside the limits of tolerance established and maintained by official campus rules and policies" (1, p. 28).

V

When the student culture is in serious conflict with the college stand on the use of alcoholic beverages, consideration must be given to alternatives to overcome existing ambiguity as far as possible.

Only four alternatives appear to be available. These are not mutually exclusive. Most often a combination of these alternatives is entered into, recognizing various difficulties as presented below (7, pp. 2-3).

It is the responsibility of the institution to see that its rules and regulations, its expectancies regarding the use of alcoholic beverages, are made quite clear to all students beyond a mere statement of these regulations. Interpretation is necessary. This requires repetition and patient discussion. Students who for whatever reason wish to drink, or students who seem to be making an issue of the drinking problem regardless of their own personal feelings in the matter, often seem to be asking the college to tell them how much or where they may drink. Many colleges refuse to enter into either of these questions, although other institutions of higher learning make it quite clear that drinking is not permitted on the campus, in college residences, at college functions, and set no further geographical limits. In such instances, there is usually a statement to the effect that misbehavior and drunkenness are of concern to the college regardless of the place of drinking.

There is an uncomfortable aspect to the conflict which leads students to raise many "red herring questions." Students have pointed out that a rule which is stated in terms that do not give them a clear idea as to where or how much they may drink contributes to uneasy drinking. These students usually then try to infer that their uneasiness and conflict are the responsibility of the college whose rule creates this uneasiness in their minds. If such conflict is present after the rule has been explained, interpreted, and ample discussion has been entered into, it appears that four alternatives (or combinations of them) confront the institution:

1. The rule could be changed so as to be completely and easily enforceable. This would mean an implied if not explicit statement as to where students may drink and how much they may drink.

2. Students may be more carefully selected in terms of their drinking habits. While this is an alternative open to some extent to a few private institutions, it is not one open to many institutions. Furthermore, it does not present a practical solution, since it would require a kind of investigation that is not usually open to college admissions officers. Admissions officers can do a great deal to assist in this prob-

lem, however, by making the attitude of the college quite clear to prospective students.

3. Police action may be heightened, and an atmosphere developed in which fear is the motivating factor, so that the penalty for drinking is severe, automatic, and immediate. Extreme action is taken in every case. This tends to create an atmosphere in which it becomes a kind of "game" to elude the policing thus established. Furthermore, it carries over to other relationships in the college, creating attitudes which are not characteristic of most intellectual communities where personal responsibility is emphasized, and where a mature level in compliance with the rules and regulations of the community is encouraged.

It must be quickly observed that to some extent "police" action is, of course, entered into in the apprehension of violators, but to create a kind of "gestapo" environment is expensive, ineffective, and conducive to other attitudes which seem out of place in a college atmosphere.

4. As in the case of other college problems, the matter of the use of alcohol can become an educational concern. This involves full information as to the college's attitude, and the creation of an atmosphere of expectancy that students will respond in a mature way, with accompanying assurance that appropriate action will be taken in case of violations. In addition, it involves conscious attempts to engage in education concerning alcohol.

A number of problems in the area of values faces every college administrator as he works with the various aspects of the use of beverage alcohol on the part of college students.

Philip Jacob reports in his study of values that the American student apparently tends "to value self-interest first, then social acceptance, friendship and the moral principles in that order when they are in conflict" (8, p. 25). While this may appear to be a discouraging finding, in many respects it has the possibility of being of positive use in the control of the use of alcoholic beverages, because if enough self-interest can be established through the facts and the truth about alcohol, then as a matter of self-interest some students will not drink and others will exert an intelligent control over their drinking.

Whether this can outweigh or outrun the increasing social acceptance of beverage alcohol is a basic problem.

Student values include a large degree of permissiveness in regard to the conduct of others. This protective attitude leads to a peculiar philosophy in groups who profess character-building standards and who claim to encourage action leading to the development of the most wholesome personalities of their members. When it comes to the matter of alcohol, many organizations refuse to take much of a stand except on the matter of drunkenness, which is usually taboo. Students characterized by leadership potential and integrity in most relationships sometimes seem not to be embarrassed by violations of a drinking regulation. There exists a feeling that "rules are good for most people, but not for me if I choose for purely personal reasons not to follow them." Furthermore, says this attitude, "I'm not going to tell anyone else how to run his life, therefore I'm not saying much if I observe violations in my group—it is up to the individuals concerned."

This results in collegiate irresponsibility and a very critical attitude if "the college" does not apprehend all the violators known to students. After all, it is "their" responsibility, and the student has made a poor gamble if he gets caught. It is a calculated risk, but if one is caught he deserves whatever he gets.

Along with this fact is another which may give some encouragement; namely, that students will respond to positive leadership when they respect this leadership among their own peers. In a fraternity known to have had some drinking problems, a young man successfully ran for the office of president on a "dry" platform. His success in achieving office and his subsequent success in carrying out his determination that the house should be free of drinking is to be accounted for on the basis of the fact that he was highly respected among all the members of his group. This suggests the possibility of more use of the respected leadership on college campuses.

Somehow students expect administrative officers and faculty members to represent official pronouncements, and therefore often tend to discount what they say about such matters as regulations concerning alcohol. If student leaders are personally convinced that it is to the best interest of their fellows to eliminate or control their drinking, they will exert a more important influence than faculty, administrative officers, or parents. Peer leadership is of primary importance in the solution of problems such as this one.

It becomes of paramount importance that we continue to have a staff of persons whose skilled leadership is effective in the area of encouraging the development of values. This is no task for the easy moralist, but requires an understanding of people, the means of their growth and development, and above all a steady personality, healthy motivations, and professional skill as advisors and counselors, not managers of persons.

The most enlightened approach to discipline problems on college campuses today embraces a mental hygiene philosophy. This results in every case being treated in terms of its own peculiar aspects, and with the best interests of the particular persons involved in focus as well as the interest of the college community. When this is done, the results sometimes seem weak to uninformed observers. The charge has often been made that college officials really do not mean to "crack down" on drinking because they have not always taken obviously severe action in cases of known drinking. The fact that *appropriate* action has been taken is often completely overlooked, and there appear to be as many solutions to what constitutes "appropriate" action as there are observers.

Appropriate action in cases involving violations of drinking regulations need not be severe, automatic or without regard to the background of each case. Appropriate action may range from counseling referrals to dismissal from the college. Public relations pressures must be resisted in favor of what is best for the offender.

Much harm may result from the use of routine penalties applied without reference to the psychological reasons for the behavior under consideration. Although a strong division of opinion on this matter is recognized, it is asserted here that successful counseling situations can emerge out of what originally was a disciplinary context. A more effective contact is possible when human personal factors are recognized.

It is the role of education to insist that recovery is more important than punishment, and yet not to be weak or indecisive in declaring a stand on the use of beverage alcohol among college students. To accept persons as individuals of worth can be achieved, even though one may not accept what they have done. Not to confuse these two things becomes the important problem for all who work with young people in this area. We know that persons who use alcohol regularly are often people who have a low sense of self-esteem and a loss of sense of dignity. Being accepted as a person may be the beginning of the rebuilding of some of this sense of dignity and personal worth.

VI

Administrators must consider that there are sociological and psychological aspects of the college drinking problem that surround the existence of a final statement of a campus rule or regulation.

Experience has shown that where students participate in the formulation of the drinking regulation there is more effective student support in enforcing the rule and better understanding of, and hence cooperation on, the problems involved.

In an unpublished survey of 60 returns from Methodist-related colleges and universities in the United States, only 30 per cent reported students as having participated in the formulation of their basic drinking regulations. Students who frequently share in formulating regulatory policies in campus life on other matters are frequently not involved in the formulation of alcoholic beverage rules. Here is one place administrators can (with confidence gleaned from the experience of others) take steps to improve student cooperation on the campus drinking policy by involving them in its formulation.

In the survey mentioned above, 25 per cent of the schools reporting said that in the year before the survey the question had been raised complaining about faculty drinking as being a poor example for students. In the complex life of a college campus, faculty drinking presents a very real problem because a small minority of professors can by their example create an ambiguous situation for the campus community.

Some schools make it clear that faculty and staff members are expected not to drink with students. Others expect consistency with the college policy for students, allowing for drinking in faculty-student groups as long as this behavior is in keeping with the college traditions and regulations.

Dr. Preston Munter, writing about alcohol and values, says, "Values that are relevant to the use of alcohol in the university setting rest on the tradition of the particular school. I don't believe it is possible, except over long periods of time, and surely not within a single college generation, to change tradition. Drinking traditions, especially, have enormous persistence. They come at students through all kinds of literature, and in particular through word of mouth. Traditions can't be disguised or camouflaged, ignored or denied. Rules seem absolutely inadequate against them. What the faculty and administrative officers of the university do, however, does have impact upon traditions. Unless the faculty and administrative officers at the university use alcohol intelligently and reasonably themselves and unless they take a sensible position on its use, I don't think any rules will be effective, nor will the less desirable drinking traditions be eliminated or even made relatively ineffective. Some sort of consistent behavior is necessary on the part of adults. It is simply not acceptable any more for the faculty to say one thing on problems of this sort and to do something else privately. To assume the students don't know is foolish. They do know it. There is no communication system as accurate and sensitive as the scuttlebutt lines in the college. I can tell you from vivid experience that no university president or college student should ever say anything that he thinks is in the privacy of his office or room without knowing that it can be and will be repeated very shortly within the school community. Unfortunately, even what happens in the privacy of our homes becomes currency in the college community. There is no hiding place. Ambivalence on the part of a faculty or school administration, in my view, is the most negative force in the control of the use of alcohol, whereas consistency in adult statements and behavior is a strong positive force in establishing reasonable drinking habits on the campus" (9, p. 26).

"The continued development of a sense of responsibility

regarding beverage alcohol on the college campus will only come about with leadership shared by faculty, staff and students. No one group can do it alone. Faculty and staff must share in this. While student leadership is of critical importance, it must be supported and inspired by consistent and unapologetic help from faculty and staff members" (7, p. 3).

In analyzing data from the survey of Methodist colleges by size of the schools and the size of the communities in which they were situated, the size of the community seems to have an important relationship to reports of problems with drinking regulations. For example, a college reporting a considerable problem with alcoholic beverages was the largest school in the group in a community whose population was under 10,000 persons. There is a subtle indication that a small college located in a large community reports fewer problems with drinking than a large school located in a small community. Likewise, large schools in large communities report fewer problems. The anonymity provided by a large community seems more often to shield the problems that may exist as compared to the problems reported by colleges in small towns where the college may dominate the community.

A factor of importance may be that the larger schools, regardless of size of community, more often apply their restrictions chiefly in terms of the campus and official college functions, whereas colleges in smaller communities often extend the influence of their restriction of drinking by students (even those of age) to any place in the community.

It may be that smaller schools have unrealistically responded to what they consider to be community pressures of the small town, whereas they would have better control of drinking problems if they limited their use of authority to support state law and to those situations affecting the college.

To fully understand any one student body in regard to attitudes about drinking, it needs to be known what the parents of these students think and do about alcohol. There is evidence that parental influence is of great importance in the ultimate formulation of a student's decision about the role of alcohol in his life. Many parents appear to recognize the special nature of the college experience because when asked specifically they express support of the college drinking regulation whatever it may be. These same parents are often the ones who serve alcoholic beverages to their children in their homes and have thus laid the groundwork for their sons or daughters to continue drinking practices while attending colleges where there are restrictions on drinking. Those parents seem to be asking the colleges to say "no" while they have said "yes."

The student coming from such a home is confronted with a genuine dilemma. The college seems to be restricting him in an area his parents have allowed more latitude. This presents another reason for college students understanding the unique nature of the college community and that their social responsibility as members of the college community is often different than their responsibilities at home.

When invited to write expressing opinions on the drinking rule of a particular college, less than 7 per cent of parents of the student body responded in support of the college's position. Two persons expressed mild doubt about the wisdom of the particular rule and the rest remained silent. We must better understand that the parents of our students participate in the midst of a culture that appears at best to be uncertain about a strong stand for the elimination of the use of alcoholic beverages. There is more agreement on controls, but still many differences about the degree and nature of the controls. The best agreement in our culture seems to be on the undesirability of drunkenness and extremes in the use of alcoholic beverages. Our students have their roots in this culture.

These findings throw light on the fact that there are important sociological aspects of the problem. No thorough study of a campus situation can be made properly without taking these factors into account.

VII

The problems surrounding control of alcoholic beverages on the college campus are numerous and complex.

The position of the college must be clearly stated and interpreted in terms of the mission of the college. Action on the part of college officials must be clearly motivated and enforcement efforts must be consistent.

Students must be confronted with maturely presented facts in the hope they will respond constructively for their best personal development and for the common good. These are factors that relate peculiarly and clearly to personal development and group welfare in the campus community with its rather uniquely constituted authority-responsibility constellation. These educational efforts must be a part of the college experience. They must be presented in such a manner as to create an atmosphere in which each individual may find his personal growth, his self-respect, and his concern for others enhanced.

The use of alcoholic beverages is still a personal choice. It appears worth considering how such freedom of choice can be effectively used in preserving human values in individual and group life on the campus. Students will respond to presentations of fundamental values and appeals to reason based on sound information.

College students have an unusual opportunity to be a creative force in society. It is a high privilege to have a part in developing this exciting possibility.

May we be wise enough and patient enough and human enough to rise to our challenge and opportunity in working with college men and women toward understanding the important issues surrounding the use of alcoholic beverages in society as well as on our campuses.

REFERENCES

1. RIGGS, LAWRENCE, in a symposium, "How Can Methodist Colleges Control Drinking on the Campus?" *Together*, Vol. IX, No. 3, March, 1965, p. 27.

2. REGAN, J. ROBERT, Jr. *What About Alcohol*, National Council of the Churches of Christ, New York, New York, 1962, p. 11.

3. BARRINGTON, THOMAS. "The Rights of College Students," *National Association of Student Personnel Administrators Journal*. Vol. IV, No. 1, July, 1966, p. 23.

4. BENDER, RICHARD. *College Drinking—A Moral Problem*, Pamphlet, General Board of Christian Concerns, Methodist Church, Washington, D. C.

5. *Alcohol and College Youth*, Proceedings of a conference

sponsored by the American College Health Association under a grant by the National Institute of Mental Health, June 10-12, 1965.

6. RIGGS, LAWRENCE. "Are College Drinking Rules Effective?" *Bulletin of the Association for the Advancement of Instruction About Alcohol and Narcotics,* Vol. X, No. 1, May, 1964, pp. 32-39.

7. RIGGS, LAWRENCE. "Alcohol on the College Campus," *President's Bulletin Board Supplement,* Division of Educational Institutions, The Board of Education, the Methodist Church, Nashville, Tennessee, November, 1959, pp. 2-3.

8. JACOBS, PHILIP. *Changing Values in College,* The Edward W. Hazen Foundation, New Haven, Connecticut, 1956, p. 25.

9. MUNTER, PRESTON K. "The College Community and Alcohol," AAIAN *Bulletin,* Vol. X, No. 1, May, 1964, p. 26.

Chapter 20

EDUCATION ABOUT ALCOHOL IN THE UNIVERSITY: OBLIGATION AND OPPORTUNITY

ROBERT D. RUSSELL
Southern Illinois University

THE MAJORITY of young Americans who attend colleges and universities drink alcoholic beverages of various sorts, on various occasions, in varying amounts, with various results. The educational implications of this fact are related to two other facts: that consumption of alcoholic beverages for a variety of reasons and motivations is part of man's cultural heritage, and that for some number of drinkers problems develop as a result of drinking experiences. It seems appropriate, then, that young drinkers understand how these beverages have been used by others before them, as well as the nature of the potential harm that may follow drinking. The thesis of this chapter is that this is a proper and legitimate educational responsibility of the college or university, and that there should be some interrelationships between and among the curricular and extracurricular forms of such education.

Health education, the discipline with which I am identified, can be described as a way of studying man in total and man in function, particularly in relation to man's dynamic interaction with substances and other forms of life that affect his well-being for good and for ill. Now I also recognize that health education can be—and often is—seen as "the science and art of proscription—the discipline set up to tell people what they should and should not do, with scarcely a thought as to what they enjoy doing, except, perhaps, to infer that 'if you enjoy doing it, it's probably bad for you.'" In such a context the student in health education is faced with a rather dismal picture of the effects of alcohol use and is nudged to conclude that "Don't Drink" is probably the only "healthy" answer to this problem.

But if we go back to the first description, the student of health is urged, instead, to examine the motivations behind drinking—the nature of man and of society that makes drinking an appealing practice, the variety of effects, social and emotional as well as physical, which follow alcohol use—in order to have some perspective in which to view the potential dangers. Health education had its origin in the drive of the temperance movement of the late nineteenth and early twentieth centuries to "educate" young people about the evils of alcohol (and progressed to educating people about the "evils" of many other things), but hopefully, as a field, it has outgrown the compulsion to indoctrinate people "for their own good."

In 1948 the World Health Organization was formed as an international cooperative agency designed to help nations assist people in achieving health, which the definition-developers told us was "a state of complete physical, mental, and social well-being, and not merely the absence of disease or infirmity." The years that followed found health textbook and curriculum writers giving this definition considerable lip service, but no genuine commitment to it and its implications was evidenced. In 1963, however, the School Health Education Study, a foundation—and, later, an industry-supported national project—began the development of a "structure of knowledge" for the health field, which took those WHO dimensions of well-being and said of them: "Any decision made about health takes into account, in some way and to some extent, the physical dimension (the possible or actual physical and physiological consequences of an action or issue), the mental-emotional dimension (what the individual knows and how he feels about the issue), and the social dimension (how others react, recommend, and what the social consequences are or might be)."

Now as in many cases, the theoretical concept is more

difficult to state with clarity than the concrete applications. Therefore we shall turn to the issue at hand—alcohol. This educational approach encourages health education about alcohol to include the effects of alcohol on the physical body and its physiological processes (immediate and long range); its effects on learning, on various emotions and motivations, and on the development of self-concept; its social uses, effects on human relationships, and the sociological consequences of its use. Here learners begin to see, in the dynamic, how one choice may favor maximum physical well-being, but at the expense of social acceptance; that when another choice is made social well-being may come at the expense of a completely clear conscience, etc. Well-being is not automatically guaranteed by any particular decision. Abstinence is thus not the predestined condition for good total health—but neither is drinking a necessity. "The answer" is not determined before study begins, and hence the possibility of real learning taking place is much increased.

But do these "dimensions" help in pointing to necessary information and understandings that students should have? A sample of some of the pertinent content follows.

Physical. Alcoholic beverages or drinks are a form of food; alcohol is a drug; alcohol affects brain cells, but effects from moderate amounts are reversible; drinking is most often done, in college communities, in ways that would be called "dissipating"; after some time of drinking the drinker experiences diminished coordination and sense of caution and hence becomes more susceptible to physical harm from accidental causes, and is more apt to cause harm to others, intentionally or unintentionally; long term, deteriorative effects on organs and tissues begins with repeated heavy drinking.

Mental-Emotional. Drinking has the general effect of blunting feelings of tension, fatigue, and frustration; drinking has the general effect of reducing the power of certain inhibitions and of blunting developed, learned aspects of self-criticism; how a drinker feels—after drinking—is related to how he felt or wanted to feel before drinking; what a person does under the influence is a function of the motivations he takes into the drinking experience; drinking may be part of the learning-about-self process, particularly in terms of what inhibitions are diminished; drinking may be part of the process of developing a sense of self, as an independent adult rather than a dependent child.

Social. Drinking may be a part of a number of social occasions and may be the *raison d'être* for certain ones; alcoholic beverages have the social reputation of being associated with friendly, less inhibited occasions; drunkenness may result in anti-social behavior by certain individuals (causing harm to persons or property); the general social attitude toward drinking, even to drunkenness, is generally a live-and-let-live tolerance; the laws in regard to drinking are mostly preventive in nature, assuming that some harm may come and therefore making the drinking situation itself illegal; drinking is an activity where getting around or breaking the law is reluctantly acceptable, because there seems to be no possibility of change.

Thus far it has been posited that education about alcohol is a legitimate aspect of the higher education curriculum, and that health education which points to better understanding and achievement of total well-being is an appropriate framework for such instruction. The argument is *not* that this is the only context in which valuable learning can take place, but health education is fairly unique among course offerings in its capacity to include a consideration of *personal* drinking behavior without departing from its normal objectives.

Education Comes in Many Ways

Now that the "what" has been described, albeit briefly, the "how" becomes the next subject of inquiry. Education in the college or university obviously occurs in many settings and under many circumstances. Some learning comes via teaching—or at least is guided in some ways; other learning comes out of independently conceived and directed efforts by students; still others are the result of some combination of teaching and personal involvement by the learner. Each of the following is a means of educating about alcohol, its use, non-use, and misuse.

Lecture. The lecture is a phenomenon characteristic of the university, based on the premise that a professor knowledgeable in his field can organize material from various sources and can present ideas and information in new, uniquely structured, stimulating and communicative ways so that the students learn. Research seems to indicate that the lecture is as good a method as any for learning material that needs to be recalled (and which can be quantifiably compared). Note also that the selective factor working in all pre-college grading results in a college population who basically *can* learn by reading and listening. Lectures on various aspects of alcohol studies, including the phenomenon of alcoholism, in regular classes or in special sessions, with regular university faculty or with visitors, can give a base of information for and stimulate interest in many students on a campus.

Reading. While lectures select, condense, and efficiently present a topic, books amplify and expand. Lectures and readings are, in the ideal, complementary to one another. For a number of years I had the opportunity of teaching a Senior Colloquium at Stanford University, entitled "Beverage Alcohol and Society." The two hours per week I met with the class were spent in discussion of assigned and selected readings. The major text was McCarthy's book of readings, *Alcohol Education for Classroom and Community,* an excellent representative source book of facts, ideas, and approaches to alcohol studies based mostly on references to the published scientific study of the phenomena with which alcohol use is associated. A second reading was Roueché's paperback, *Alcohol,* a collection of three essays originally published in the *New Yorker,* which presents a skillful writer's interpretation of facts and values on man's use of the intoxicating substance. In addition, each student sought out and read a novel, play, or biography wherein drinking was a major part of the life, the action, the plot; a written analysis of this at the course's end focused on the particular role drinking played in the account. Sometimes the aggregate of these readings suggested a consistent point, with material from the factual presentations being represented through accounts of human interaction in the play or story. But probably just as often the readings were contradictory and non-reinforcing, leading students (with some professorial guidance) to the realization that the scientific and predictable aspects of alcohol use must always be mediated by the somewhat unpredictable humanity of those who drink. Reading is something that can continue long beyond the termination of a course and the last echo of a professor's wise words. Some introduction to the range of written materials seems to be an important educational responsibility in the college or university.

Discussion. As used here this is a broad term, encompassing a number of things that occur in classrooms which encourage critical thought, the asking and answering of questions, and the conscientious dealing with problem situations. Discussion may simply arise from lecture presentations, readings, or both—or may be provoked by the professor. In addition, problem discussions may be structured, and I particularly like to use mimeographed case accounts or problem situations, with some questions to be answered or statements with which students must agree or disagree. In most problem discussions involving alcohol use, students must utilize some combination of facts and values. Such discussions often serve admirably in showing how facts and values do interrelate and that values finally tell us how to consider and regard facts.

Another interesting variation of the discussion is the sociodrama, where a selected group of students assume roles and personalities at least partly defined and interact with "each other" in some sort of definitive situation (a meeting, a beach party, a coffeehouse discussion, etc.). Such a presentation is a stimulus to thought and discussion by the total class.

Printed reports on provocative material also can serve as the focus of a discussion. A one-page report on a pre-test, drinking, and post-test demonstration relative to driving skills, where different adult male subjects showed different recorded degrees of impairment with identical amounts of alcohol rarely fails to raise new questions and stimulate new insights. A printed dialogue between a Dean of Students and a junior-level student on the subject of student drinking is often effective in showing how facts are interpreted differently in different value systems.

One must use discussion approaches such as these with a bit of faith at first, for it usually seems as though they are not nearly as efficient as the lecture, where order reigns and students are quiet and docile (and, hopefully, still awake). One has to be willing to be inefficient on the faith that somehow "inefficiency" adds a dimension to the learning process which cannot be done with the more efficient presentation of information. But if one feels that learning is more than just information-storing, then the results of such student involvement are often quite gratifying.

Student Investigation and Inquiry. The basic assumption about how learning should take place in the university could be diagrammed as a fork with two tines: (1) students are to learn what professors and textbooks have to say; and (2) students are to become facile and familiar with the skills and resources necessary for finding answers to questions, both those assigned and those self-conceived. This out-of-class or self education has many forms, each of which can be exemplified in a number of ways; the examples which follow are from my own personal professorial experience.

Library Research. A student was dissatisfied with the explanations of alcoholism given in the assigned readings and was stimulated by the suggestions that different disciplines saw the condition in different ways. So she proceeded to read books and periodical writings of physiologists, psychologists, psychiatrists, sociologists, biochemists, and members of AA in order to understand better the diversity of views. Though one could not argue that she had the complete picture, her research probably put her into the top 1 per cent in the country in terms of answering the question "What is Alcoholism?" Another student studied the generalizations and experimental results regarding alcohol's effects on the liver; unable to complete the picture to his satisfaction he arranged and conducted an interview with a physiologist at a nearby medical school, a man currently doing research on this phenomenon. Another student went through five years of back issues of the *National Voice,* the oldest "dry" newspaper in America, to establish a picture of representative "dry" arguments in this era. Several students read as much as they could find about the fellowship of Alcoholics Anonymous and then attended some open meetings, much better prepared to understand what they observed than if they had gone without any background or preparatory reading.

Surveys. Some students seem always to be dissatisfied with present knowledge and eager to conduct their own surveys of drinking behavior and patterns of their fellow students. One survey focused on freshmen women, another on Jewish students, another on upper class women in three different collegiate institutions (the survey director, a senior male, was going with a woman from each institution simultaneously and had some research problems the typical investigator does not have!), and yet another on the "drink-oriented segment of the student body." In such surveys the techniques are not always the most rigorous and the instruments often are not subjected to enough critical validation, but students often have a unique access to their peers and to information only they have which is simply not "gatherable" by adult—or even graduate student—researchers.

Experiments. On several occasions students devised and carried out experiments that demonstrated, in systematic and often imaginative ways, the after-drinking effects on the performance of various tasks. Some of these showed, in direct ways, an understanding of how experimental research is done. One report, still one of the "gems" of my academic collection, was a magnificent spoof of performance research, showing both a grasp of research technique and a willingness to smile at the hyper-seriousness often communicated from research reports. "Research" such as this has much potential meaning for those doing the experiment, for those participating as subjects, and for those who see or hear of the results. A student may actually learn more from an experiment going on in the upper hall of a fraternity house than from a dozen carefully conceived and statistically reported ventures done in labs in Finland, Toronto, New Brunswick, Boston, or wherever.

Systematic Observation. At one time a senior student of mine worked as a bartender in one of the local beer gardens frequented by students. The paper he finally presented, as an independent study project, was an analysis based on six months of systematic observation of the patrons, their patterns of drinking, and the range of behaviors after drinking. (This is at least akin to anthropological research, locally applied.) A woman student who was a member of Al-Anon while a university senior did a commendable observational report on her group, creatively presented in dialogue form.

Field Trips. A student was particularly interested in researching the beer industry (because he had worked two summers for a brewery and owned three shares of company stock), and, in lieu of a detailed final paper, he arranged for the class to go to the nearby plant of "his" company and take a specially conducted tour of a major brewery in production. He assisted the regular guide throughout the tour in commenting on and explaining the operations we were observing and the nature of the industry in general.

Personal Recall. In my judgment this is a particular, peculiar form of research where the data reside in the student's past experiences and can be sorted and assembled only by the individual student. Examples of this would include a paper tracing the steps in the development of the writer's own drinking style or in the maintenance of abstinence when drinking has become a real possibility; a description of high school drinking patterns as experienced by the writer; and the writer's descriptions of the progressive deterioration of an alcoholic parent. Some of these, as final products, come close to being therapy-type recall, but they often are obviously of value and benefit to the writers and, used carefully to preserve anonymity later, provide valuable insights for subsequent students.

Education beyond the Instructional

All education, even in the college or university setting, does not occur in classrooms or other instructional environments. In fact, about alcohol and its use a student will learn much of what he comes to know in these "extracurricular" ways.

Informal Sessions With Professors, Members of the Helping Professions, and Others. Students seem to feel considerable enthusiasm for chances to sit informally—individually or in small groups—and talk with knowledgeable faculty members, health service or medical school physicians, social workers, deans, members of AA, and others about issues such as drinking or not drinking. The colloquium to which I have referred met at least once each quarter in my home, a change of environment (including beer as one of the beverages served) which obviously increased the total educational experience of the course. When a member of AA visited the class I often noticed that much important education took place during the "break" in the hall outside the classroom. In the hall he spoke more informally with individuals and small groups and apparently was more comfortable than when he was facing a class gathered more formally around tables in a classroom.

Campus Rules and Their Enforcement. Though the rules of an institution relating to drinking by students and the way such are enforced constitute a very informal, unstructured "learning experience," it still can be argued that this whole phenomenon teaches students some very practical things about drinking in our society. On most campuses freshmen learn early that drinking is not allowed on campus (or at least that *they* are not allowed to drink); at the same time, however, they also learn how and where to get a false ID, how and where to get beer, how you can and cannot drink in a dorm, fraternity, or other campus residence hall, which Resident Assistants or other officials acting *in loco parentis* are likely to turn drinkers in and what liberalities others will tolerate—and a host of other such educational nuggets. These learnings are often a significant "boost" to the general perception that American attitudes toward drinking, particularly by those in late adolescence, are more than a bit ambiguous. And because these learnings come from personal experience or from the related personal experiences of contemporaries, they are somewhat difficult to counter with mere lectures and readings.

Bull Sessions and Other Informal Student Gatherings. Bull sessions in dorms, fraternity and sorority houses, discussions in shower and locker rooms, and talk at mealtime illustrate the university as a community in which information, opinion, and "absolute knowledge" is being shared constantly. Some of it is experiential; some of it is faulty, inaccurate, incomplete, or misinterpreted. But also, much of it is a sharing of what has been heard in a lecture, read in a book, discovered in an experiment or survey or observation, and, often enough to mention, the comments of professors and other authorities in non-formal discussion and question-and-answer sessions. In this subject area much of what is learned is learned from peers or is shared with peers in some informal talk session.

"Laboratory Sessions" (or Drinking Parties). Last but not least, the student learns about drinking and its effects on him and on others in actual drinking situations. From varied experiences such as a surreptitious beer while studying, a roaring keg party in the hills, a stag party with dirty movies, an overnight party with dates, a fraternity-sorority exchange, a formal date in the city, a formal dinner in a home with cocktails and wine, he or she learns different things. Yet what the students learn is to an extent what they are conscious of, attuned to, and looking for. Some instruction and some other kinds of education, particularly involving some of the varieties of problem-solving, then, can make the actual "lab" sessions more instructive. As one senior man put it:

. . . one may rightly ask if there is any reason for drinking in college. In other words, should college men drink? The answer is yes, if they so decide. College is a maturing place for many students. We enter college not knowing what we want out of life, or even what it is for. One might say that college is a fenced-in proving ground wherein all of the student's values are questioned and tested by the individual himself. We are more excessive drinkers because we are testing, and the exuberance shown even after one beer comes from this. The basic question to us becomes one of how far society will let us let down our inhibitions given the rationalizing element of alcohol. We can test in this surrounding whereas if we were placed directly in society we would be restricted to follow doggedly what it proclaims. In college we have the friends who will put us to bed if we go too far, whereas if we were in society we would only receive the disdain of our friends and probably a night in jail. College is also a time when there are very few responsibilities placed on us and so we can afford to experiment, as it were, without the risk of hurting family or friends. It is while in college that the most can be accomplished toward gaining an understanding of the outside world without hurting or being hurt.

This is a very moral statement based on the premise that choosing to drink is a legitimate option, for it focuses on the need to drink without hurting self or others. It also strongly implies that drinking can be a personal educational experience— in the sense of self-discovery.

Are There No Problems?

Obviously, the three forms of informal education chronicled last operate for virtually all students in this drinking society, to a greater or lesser extent. But the college or university is not just a social institution where young people educate each other, but an educational institution. One of its aims is the purposeful and systematic expanding and deepening of the student's view of the world and its phenomena in order that the truth might make him freer to live effectively. Since I am no mortarboard Pollyanna claiming that where education is not purposively provided it is just a simple matter of attention and concern, I must present my version of current and inherent problems.

The Stuff Is Too Tough, Except for the Buff. The field of alcohol studies is not only a multi-disciplinary one, as illustrated by the number of university departments involved. Alcohol studies also include insights from both the basic and clinical disciplines, from sociologists and social workers, research and practicing psychiatrists, psychologists and counselors, and many others. This fact makes the current research findings and expository writings voluminous and complex. Consequently, the problems of understanding the field, keeping up to date, and dealing with all of the value problems inherent in the subject tempt many conscientious professors to skip over it or give it a very abbreviated coverage. Generalists in a field who recognize that some of their colleagues devote their whole professional life to the study of alcohol may find it difficult to assume the kind of authority they would like to offer students. Professors doing research in some other sub-field may realize even more sharply how relatively little they know about another research area. Even health education professors, who typically have felt they can handle any and every topic, show signs of wariness particularly

when there are suggestions that "Don't Drink" is not necessarily the preconceived conclusion.

Thus, realistically, most undergraduates never are offered the opportunity for any systematic learning or directed discussion on the subject. At the most they hear a lecture or two, and then probably on alcoholism or some other harmful result of drinking.

The Curry Is Too Thick. The possible, potential subject matter for any course, whether it is Personal Health, Introduction to Sociology or Psychology, Abnormal Psychology, or whatever, increases each day without any commensurate increase in teaching time. Alcohol studies is always in competition with all other areas of interest and frequently receives little attention. Also, the individual professor tends to select those areas for emphasis with which he is most familiar and feels most confident.

Because the available printed materials in all specialized fields also are increasing, because libraries never have funds to purchase all materials requested, and because professors request materials related most specifically to their teaching or their own research, the situation pictured regarding professors is usually reflected in library materials. In all fairness to learners, this should not be so. If not much is going to be taught in classes then at least the information should be available for self-study. But, it rarely works this way.

Learners Can Be Burners. Among the students in any class there is an unknown but predictably ample range in knowledge, experience, attitude and background with regard to alcohol use. For some professors this is no problem—either in the sense that they're willing to deal with possible diversity or that they're not interested in recognizing it. But some instructors still become somewhat apprehensive when they find out or suspect that the father of a particular student is a practicing alcoholic, or a strong-mouthed Baptist preacher; when they know they have some Jews and some Irish in a class; or when they are dealing with a behavior which is illegal. Some instructors are pretty staunchly middle class, with smaller or larger remnants of the conviction that drinking is, finally, bad. Some are "first-generation drinkers," still a bit uncomfortable with themselves as drinkers, particularly on the

occasions when they may stray from moderation. Still others are abstainers, but feel a bit "uneasy" about this continuing choice in a society where the mode is some drinking. With this subject, such underlying feelings may come through or be revealed by responses to student inquiry. For these teachers the task is an uneasy one.

The One Way to Think = Don't Drink! In a recent paper the sociologist Bacon developed, through sociohistorical perspective, the thesis that the dominant way of thinking about this subject developed by the classic temperance movement of the last century still persists today. In essence, it is that alcohol is bad, serves no useful functions, rather inevitably leads to deterioration and disaster, and its use should be curtailed as much as possible. Today there still are those who believe this and there are those who deny it, but the majority of the population, including most faculty, have tried to avoid the whole issue by rejecting both the Drys and the Wets; however, in so doing they have offered no other ways to think about beverage use, and therefore the temperance position remains in force. What we *have* done, as a society, is to declare that it does not apply to adults at certain times, and in certain places, but that prohibition and temperance teaching *does* apply to youth, including most college students.

Therefore because there are, in most states, a variety of illegalities related to the act of drinking, particularly by minors, students in general really don't expect any final summary other than DON'T! Material from scientific studies may be presented—and it may be perversely interesting—but essentially it will paint a negative picture. The drinker always seems to come out weak, stupid, immature, and lacking in self-control, and his behavior under the influence is usually reprehensible; the road to ruin while not inevitable, is clearly well traveled. Another postulate of the Movement was that all drinking is the same and all drinkers the same. So if the student is going to drink he would rather enjoy it than have the experience berated and bedeviled. He might want to learn something about drinking, but he doesn't wish to be told—or led to conclude—that he really shouldn't. If this is the way he perceives alcohol education he probably does well to avoid it. Some students never lose such a threatening

expectation and probably will go on to continue the classic way of thinking, simply by rejecting it, but still believing it. Other students can be encouraged in genuine learning by an openness they did not expect.

The Essentials of a Minimum College Alcohol Education Program

Each of the following items is important as a part of the whole; an effective program of instruction about alcohol occurs only when they all function together, complementing and supplementing one another, each developing the strength and effectiveness of the others. When all function regularly and abundantly, the way is open for excellence in understanding. The necessities are:

1. At least one member of the faculty, administration, or helping profession staff who is interested, knowledgeable, up-to-date, and somewhat active in the alcohol studies field. The larger the institution the less "visible" one person is, obviously, and more than one would increase the educational possibilities, but at least one is essential. To have one or more individuals actually doing research in some facet of the field is an added bonus. To have such a person or persons to teach, to be available as a resource person and available speaker, to direct students to materials, persons and other sources and resources necessary for their investigations, even to do some unique counseling, is a primary requisite for the institution of higher education.

2. A library containing a number of basic references, kept up to date, and relevant current periodicals plus some index to other relevant but not readily available materials. Practically speaking, having the person or persons described above is fundamental to having these library resources, because, as noted earlier, librarians rarely order materials not requested by faculty members or other university personnel. In any specialized field it would be a rare librarian who would know what to order. Nevertheless, a college or university without such source materials is not fulfilling its educational and societal function in relation to an area where under-

standing is one fundamental way of avoiding or alleviating personal and social problems.

3. Encouragement of student inquiry in its many forms. Students have great potential for creative approaches to topics, and to the extent that this inquiry is encouraged, critically appraised, and valued when the performance is one of excellence the atmosphere for learning is a healthy one.

4. Establishment of a repository for student-prepared materials. A portion of the main library or of a specialized library, such as Health Education, might be set aside for such materials. The Student Health Service is another interesting possibility for such an educational collection. The really excellent materials which students can produce should not be lost or simply given back to disappear into the student's basement, closet, or wastebasket. With credit given where credit is appropriate and with respect for anonymity when it seems called for, student-prepared materials can provide information and insight and can stimulate, in some mildly competitive way, additional work by other students.

These are the essentials for formal, curricular, and research-type educational experiences for college students. To complete the picture requires two recommendations relative to the informal, non-curricular "education."

5. Acceptance of drinking as possibly appropriate behavior on the campus, particularly at campus residences and dining facilities. This would involve a "new way of thinking" for most college administrations and would require an important distinction between responsible and irresponsible drinking rather than between drinking and not drinking. This new way of thinking would put abstinence and responsible drinking together and both would be distinguished from irresponsible, destructive drinking. The accent would be on actual behavior rather than this supposed "potential for destruction" view of any drinking.

Education about drinking will always have a sort of "spooky" quality to it as long as societal and college rules are so out of line with social custom and as long as appropriate, genteel or social drinking cannot be recognized and practiced for its positive values. Rules against destruction of property, disorderly conduct, and other overt acts can be maintained, even strengthened. But making drinking automatically an offense is a deterrent to sound education. There are other reasons for such a change in what is defined as legal, appropriate behavior, but I call for it as an aid to better education. On the other hand, it can be argued that the educational institution cannot be too different from the society it serves. Certainly there is marked ambivalence about drinking in the society at large, so perhaps the college actually is educating well for the society as it is. Perhaps the drinking rules on most campuses are really not meant to be strictly enforced. Rather, they are meant to encourage careful conduct and to be available in case of some real infraction of the general welfare. They are prototypes of some common laws of the larger society such as speed laws and jaywalking laws. We live in a society that talks about peace and prepares for and makes war; that supports the United Nations and yet acts unilaterally for its own interests; that seeks a smooth-running, do-something government but encourages each political party to thwart the other; that talks about the need for birth control and still admires the large family. In short, if we condemn alcoholic beverages and yet drink them, we are not unique in the ambivalence we exhibit. It can be argued, then, that there must be some leadership out of this confusion. I would argue that this role belongs to the university community.

6. The education of certain students, possibly selected ones, in order to indirectly affect the informal system of communication. Students talk to each other, share with each other, and seek judgments from one another. This suggests the possibility of educating certain students in a special way. Perhaps fraternity and sorority presidents, resident hall assistants and other selected or self-selected members of the student body are the ones to educate about alcohol exceedingly well and in some depth. Such student leaders could be taught and encouraged to use a number of approaches to informal instruction about alcohol among their peers. This would seem to be an important and somewhat unique way to develop awareness and understanding of alcohol and its use and misuse on a campus. Much education goes on by way of these peer group communications. Making sure that those

who are likely to be influential are knowledgeable may be much more efficient in terms of final learning results than just educating at random those who show up in classes.

A Final Representation of the Educational Problem

Though the difficulties in educating clearly and well in this subject area have been delineated and interpreted, one fundamental dilemma remains. In a lecture which I entitled "Tippling and Togetherness," developed for a course in Marriage and Family, I described ways in which alcoholic beverage use serves to make family life more pleasant and other ways in which they were part of that human devastation that can occur in deteriorating family relationships. I closed the lecture with two quotations, each presenting a view of the fluid in question which represents a facet of reality. Though they sound contradictory—or unrelated—they represent the basic dilemma: what kind of a substance is alcohol? And with these I close.

The first, a quotation from the book *Should Christians Drink?* by the Methodist theologian Everett Tilson, portrays alcohol in this stark fashion:

Drivers under the influence of alcohol annually commit more murders than all the most wanted criminals in the past two decades have committed. Though the courts seldom confront drunken drivers with any more serious charge than that of manslaughter, they are responsible for getting drunk if not for what they do after becoming so. What of its influence on the family? Between one fourth and three fourths of all divorces have it as a primary cause or a major contributing factor. While the degree of its influence on industry, sports, crime, juvenile delinquency and other aspects of our individual and corporate life greatly varies, in each area the nature of its influence falls in the same disruptive and destructive category. In other words, it more often encourages the kind of realism we meet in Erskine Caldwell and Tobacco Road than in Jesus Christ and the Sermon on the Mount.

The second is in the form of a toast, offered by the late author-editor-critic Bernard DeVoto, presenting the beverage in this gentle fashion:

The water of life was given to us to make us see for awhile that we are more nearly men and women, more nearly kind and gentle and generous, pleasanter and stronger than without its vision there is any evidence we are. It is the healer, the weaver of forgiveness and reconciliation, the justifier of us to ourselves and to one another. One more—and then with a spirit made whole again in a cleansed world—to dinner.

ANNOTATED REFERENCES

CHAFETZ, MORRIS E. *Liquor, The Servant of Man.* Boston: Little, Brown, and Co., 1965. 229 pp. A positive look at liquor and its relationship to man's good life, by a psychiatrist who works regularly with alcoholics.

JELLINEK, E. M. *The Disease Concept of Alcoholism.* New Brunswick, N.J.: Hillhouse Press, 1960. 245 pp. A definitive work by the most significant thinker in the field, introducing the concept of several alcoholisms, based on much cross-cultural data and observation.

KELLER, MARK, and JOHN SEELEY. *The Alcohol Language.* Toronto: University of Toronto Press, 1958. 32 pp. A lexicon of selected terms defined in terms of use throughout the world.

LOLLI, GIORGIO. *Social Drinking. The Effects of Alcohol.* New York: Collier Books (paperback), 1960. 278 pp. A discussion of how a substance like ethyl alcohol can be used for social purposes.

MADDOX, GEORGE L., and BEVODE C. McCALL. *Drinking among Teen-Agers.* New Brunswick, N.J.: Rutgers Center of Alcohol Studies, 1964. 124 pp. Based on a study in Michigan, this monograph includes many illuminating sociological insights on the phenomenon of youth drinking.

McCARTHY, RAYMOND G. (ed.). *Alcohol Education for Classroom and Community.* New York: McGraw-Hill Book Co., 1964. 294 pp. A collection of nineteen readings, well organized to cover the alcohol studies field, rather than merely alcohol education.

McCARTHY, RAYMOND G. (ed.). *Drinking and Intoxication.* New Brunswick, N.J.: Rutgers Center of Alcohol Studies (paperback), 1959. 445 pp. Selected readings focused on social attitudes and controls relative to alcohol, with considerable material on non-American cultures.

PITTMAN, DAVID J., and CHARLES R. SNYDER (ed.), *Society, Culture, and Drinking Patterns.* New York: John Wiley and Sons, 1962. 616 pp. A large variety of social and cultural readings on alcohol use.

ROUECHÉ, BERTON. *Alcohol.* New York: Grove Press (Black Cat Books; paperback) 1960. 151 pp. A collection of three essays, originally featured in the *New Yorker,* the happy combination of an excellent writer and the many facts about alcoholic beverage use.

STRAUS, ROBERT, and SELDEN D. BACON. *Drinking in College.* New Haven: Yale University Press, 1953. 221 pp. Description and analysis of the findings of the only major study of the drinking patterns of students in college in the U.S.

Quarterly Journal of Studies on Alcohol. New Brunswick, N.J.: Rutgers Center of Alcohol Studies. Approximately 800 pages per year in four issues. Now in Volume 30. The major professional journal in alcohol studies, including original research reports, reviews, and summaries, and news of the field.

Journal of Alcohol Education. Lansing, Michigan: Association for the Advancement of Instruction about Alcohol and Narcotics (212 S. Grand Avenue). Approximately 140 pages per year in three issues. Now in Volume 13. A useful reference for those planning to be or those furthering their education as teachers.

Chapter 21

COLLEGE DRINKING: SO WHAT AND
WHAT NEXT?

Selden D. Bacon [1]
Rutgers University

THE QUESTION "so what?" is felt to be rather imper-
tinent by some academic researchers, especially if the
question is pointed toward their own research by some
representative of the untutored laity: "Don't people realize
that research is important?" Strangely enough, that question
is often asked with sincerity as deep as it is naive. Many
academic researchers have spent years in graduate training
followed by years in a faculty setting in which there was
consistent and constant acceptance of the inherent truth and
value of disciplined intellectual study and reports thereon.

To others, however, the question of relevance is not only
pertinent, it is crucial. More than 70 years ago William Graham
Sumner, one of the three or four founders of sociology, is
reported to have posed three questions about dissertations
to every Ph.D. candidate: What is it? How do you know?
What of it? In more technical terms, he was perhaps referring (1) to definition, (2) to the method of obtaining and
the substance of the obtained evidence, and (3) relevance.
A generation later Robert Lynd, a sociologist perhaps best
known for *Middletown,* published a book with the title
Knowledge For What? When, 25 years after that, the editor

---

[1] Director, Center of Alcohol Studies, Rutgers, The State University,
New Brunswick, New Jersey. The Center receives its basic support from
the National Institute of Mental Health (USPH-MH-05655).

asked me to write a concluding chapter, to this book on college drinking, entitled "So What," he was adhering to a respectable sociological tradition. That he should ask one of the authors of probably the first sociological publication on this subject to state "what of it?" some 15 years (and at least 15 authors) later would perhaps shock Sumner and Lynd: the question might seem to have arrived a little late.

But the editor also requested that to the question "So What" be added the second question, "What Next?" I hesitate to suggest that the range of possible answers might include "damn little" and "hopefully, nothing" at one extreme. However, the editor knew his man: the answers will be more positive, as well as longer.

There are thousands of human behaviors which could be and are subjected to more or less serious study. Whether weddings or nose-blowing or attending horse races or plying a trade, whether these ways are activated by Presbyterians, city-dwellers, juveniles or the mentally ill, it seems that Alexander Pope's dictum about mankind being the most appropriate subject for our study will be followed. And although it is probable that study of any human behavior will have some value, I shall assume here, first, that some "studies" have greater value than others (in terms of questions, methods, conclusions, applicability for further research or for policy making) and that some subject matters have greater potential than others for eliciting such value; second, that resources for study—such as time, trained personnel and social support—are limited, and that selection would be necessary even if all questions and all subject matters and methods were of identical utility.

Why should the limited resources of time, money, and competent personnel be devoted to the study of drinking alcohol beverages, let alone drinking by boys and girls in college? One answer, perhaps an answer of emotional significance to many, was presented by a nationally syndicated columnist at the time the original college drinking study was announced (1949); it was included in the Straus-Bacon book produced by that research and will be repeated here. Referring to the survey as a "Booze Kinsey," the author wrote:

I can save the researchers a lot of time and trouble. And heaven knows how much wear and tear on the tabulating machines. I can tell you now why college boys drink. They drink because it is fun. Or else they do it because the prexy says they shouldn't. But in any case it is my scientific observation that nobody ever got hurt much by college drinking—unless he was the sort of guy who would have been a drunk in college or out, before or after.

A college student is a puppy. He will chew any shoe, hat or soapbar that is placed before him. If he is a smart puppy he will stop chewing the articles which make him sick. If he is a dumb puppy he will keep on munching, and nobody can ride sufficient herd on him to stop him.

The researchers, for some odd reason (maybe they haven't got enough work to do) . . . would like to amass a flock of statistics. The snoopers would like to know if rich kids drink more than poor kids, or if the sons of teetotallers lush it up more than the scions of soaks.

Every so often I despair of the work that Satan finds for idle professional hands to do. . . .

The college boy or girl is one animal I should like to see protected from too much second guess and explanation. College is a fine, prime, giddy period of coltishness, where the hobble-de-hoys cavort according to their nature. Their youthful troubles and their method of handling same swiftly serve as groundwork for the tough chores of adulthood, and as swiftly split the men from the boys. . . .

This viewpoint is not restricted to the illiterate, is not merely a belief of embattled old-time "Wets" or "Drys" (in this instance, presented in its Wet costume). It represents a more universal and traditionally popular position. Above all, this viewpoint incorporates the fear of new knowledge, expressed by asserting the validity, even sacredness, of old beliefs and practices, by ridiculing the meddling and even "Satanic" efforts of questioners or innovators, by denying either the existence of problems or, if they should be present, the possible applicability of new knowledge to their solution. That the proposed research dealt with human behaviors rather than with planets or microbes or metallurgy evidently enhanced the fear; questioning on that level strikes home deeply and immediately. The popular columnist in that instance retaliated in the classic mold: (1) the answer to the question the innovators propose (a question the columnist created for his own purpose) is already known—that is, kids drink because they want to; (2) there isn't any problem anyway; (3) college students are puppies, "good ones" or "bad ones", and you can't do anything about that; (4) but they're nice puppies, should be protected from academic-scientific meddlers, and college is a nice time and place for "natural" growth to occur.

The Dry version of negativism runs in similar fashion except for a different assertion of the existence or quality of the problem ("it's big and terrible") and a different answer ("take the alcohol away and then 'natural growth' will take place as it ought"). But from the point of view of those concerned with the development of knowledge and understanding, and of those concerned with the education of youth, both versions are utterly nihilistic. They both assert that education is fruitless, although the Drys are strongly for indoctrination of particular (not to be questioned) behavioral rules.

The preceding discussion indicates that the question "should time, money and trained personnel be devoted to studying college drinking" cannot be effectively posed until a previous question has been answered: "Should time, money and trained personnel (especially if in limited supply) be devoted to study?" Moreover, history suggests that study of man and his behavior, despite Pope's lofty assertion, will require particular consideration; many who might grant positive value to studies of air currents or cancer-producing elements or potential food sources in the sea, might draw the line at studies of religion, family life, or property. For them, these things are better left alone and people should be protected from such studies and harebrained plans for extending understanding of these topics. As the columnist put it: if, indeed, certain phenomena seem on occasion to be difficult or painful, this is the proper groundwork from which maturity will [may?] naturally develop.

If the answer to the first general question should be negative, there is no reason to proceed to specific examples of the general; they have already been ruled wasteful if not, indeed, dangerous. If an affirmative answer is given to the question "are disciplined objective studies of man and his behavior worthwhile," then the question of studying drinking behavior, and more specifically, in the collegiate setting, becomes pertinent. There should be no doubt in the reader's mind or emotions about my stand on the value of study, especially relative to man and his behavior: it is affirmative.

But what about drinking behavior? Why not study playing poker or use of slang or styles in clothing or modes of earning a living or the formation or dissolution of marriages? These are all highly patterned forms of behavior differentiated primarily in terms of different societies, forms which persist beyond the life of individual members of a society, forms which are learned or learned about by the members. They are patterns of behavior with distinct labels. They are held to be appropriate at different times and places, are equipped with various notions of worth, serve functions both for satisfying individual desires and also for maintaining the structure and strength of groups. Many such ways are held differentially appropriate for this or that segment of the population—for example, correct for men but not for women, correct for freemen or the aged but not for bondsmen or the young. Individuals often show great differences in their skill or style in activating these ways. Teaching, criticism, and even punishment may accompany faulty or inappropriate activation. Moreover, all the behavioral ways within a society are more or less interactive, influence each other, tend toward some minimal state of consistency, and, singly and *in toto*, manifest change.

Study of any of the ways will lead to some understanding of this order of phenomena. But some customs seem more promising for study than others, especially in terms of specific purposes. Drinking behavior has the values for study characteristic of almost any patterned, repetitive human action. However, it has in addition certain aspects which suggest more than usual potentiality.

(a) *Sharply discrete meaning combined with broad social and psychological scope.* In studying any phenomenon, the more exactly it is defined, both by excluding all other matters and by precisely including every relevant matter, the more useful the resulting knowledge will prove. Unfortunately for those interested in social phenomena, most of the behaviors which can be so defined are things or techniques of only the most specialized interest, forming but small parts of matters of broader concern. Such phenomena as love, war, property, health, achievement, government, employment, money and the like are enormously difficult to define, to separate from other phenomena while including all relevant items in the category. The use of alcoholic beverages forms a striking exception. This is true both of the material, alcohol, whose unique definition is rooted in precise chemistry, and also of its use; both in popular terminology and in the special terminology of students of behavior, there is little serious question (there may be pretenses and mistakes) as to what is included or excluded when the term "drinking," meaning ingestion of alcohol beverages, is utilized. There may be 50 or 100 kinds of "drinks" and even more modes of "drinkings" and types of drinkers, but there is no confusion of this behavior with consumption of soup or soda or with sports or religion or any other activity. There is no "almost drinking" or "half drinking." In this sense, the student is dealing with a unique and definable phenomenon, quite different from housing or art or transportation or aggression or gambling. This specificity of definition presents a major, unusual, incalculably valuable asset for disciplined study of human behavior.

(b) *Multi-disciplinary relevance of drinking behavior.* A major value for students of human behavior lies in relevant convergence of biochemical, neurologic, psychologic, and sociocultural studies. None of the structures and processes covered by these disciplines are absent from social behavior of any sort, but descriptions of behavior are rarely couched in terms of more than two disciplines and usually only one is utilized. The use of alcohol beverages involves direct impact of this specific chemical agent on the central nervous system; that impact produces changes on sensory, learning, feeling-tone, and other psychologic functions. Not only does this occur when, under controlled laboratory conditions, alcohol is introduced into the system in measured fashion; it also happens (or does not happen under similar circumstances with the same people) under natural conditions, in millions of cases every day. It is the outstanding example of a psycho-pharmacological entity of clearly significant impact, both social and psychological, being widely, frequently, and openly used in everyday life. It could well prove to be a Rosetta stone for the useful translation of the different scholarly "tongues" used to explain man and his behavior.

(c) *Human behavior consists of responses to stimuli (originating internally or in the socio-physical environment).* All socially significant behavior is a product of learning, based upon experience, upon imitation, upon the reward of effective and approved practice; actions require individual mobilization of emotional and physical structures and processes; the behaviors of individuals are accompanied by some degree of self-approval or self-disapproval or other self-evaluation. Whether the action be shaking hands, paying a bill, saying a prayer, stealing a purse, laughing at a joke, praising or cursing someone, at least these phases are present: sensing of cues which elicit action; use of learned attitudes and behaviors; mobilization of biological and psychological structures and capacities; the action; and self-evaluation. Although the precise influencing mechanisms of alcohol on the central nervous system are not well understood, it is generally agreed that alcohol directly affects (1) sensing, (2) the use of learned patterns, (3) the mobilization of biological and psychological capacities, (4) the nature of activation, and (5) the process of self-evaluation. Therefore, whether in laboratory or in real life, alcohol can provide a means of measuring the interplay of biological, psychological, and sociological factors in human behavior. Other phenomena, such as marriage, training, employment, social-class status, success, and "personality," frustrate attempts at such measurements because they are *not* single, constant, identical entities but rather diffuse characteristics of many different natures, meaning different things to and for different individuals. Although the emotional status, previous relevant learning, surrounding situation, and organic capacities of individuals consuming alcohol may differ, and differ in the same individual at various times, the alcohol concentration in the nervous system at any given moment can be established with great

exactitude and is a "constant"—not true of other frequently
tried yardsticks for the measurement of human behaviors.
A popular application, rather remote from disciplined analysis, of this potential for explaining human behavior residing in alcohol is seen in the statements exculpating or fault-
ing, praising or blaming behaviors because the actor had
been "drinking." These explanations are found in law, religion,
literature, everyday conversation, and even quasi-professional
studies. The undisciplined character of these popular rationalizations is evident not only in the conflicting conclusions about
the nature of change in behavior which is alleged to emerge,
but also from the common knowledge that most of the time
no noticeable change occurs at all. Even so, of all widespread
and continuing practices and of all widely available substances, drinking and alcohol are perhaps the most common
popular explanations, in all societies which have the custom,
for changes in human behavior. Nevertheless, scientists dealing with human phenomena have largely avoided dealing
with this substance and activity.[2]

(d) The three previous aspects of alcohol and its use, as
they provide an effective subject for disciplined research,
have been more meaningful to the researcher than to the
general public. The third aspect did raise the question of
"behavior itself" which, especially as it includes deviant
behavior, is almost always of popular interest, but the emphasis was on the peculiar value of measurability, not on
the pathological or bizarre occurrences which occasionally
take place. The fourth aspect, however, is directly related
to "social problems" and to "what do people do about them."
It comes much closer to the lay interest in problems and
policy.

The use of alcoholic beverages has been associated with
problems, all sorts of problems, in almost every society of
which there is record. These problems may be presented
under three headings: the occurrence of socially deviant actions in which one or more actors had sufficient alcohol in

[2] See S. D. Bacon, "The Classic Temperance Movement of the U.S.A.:
Impact Today on Attitudes, Action and Research," *British Journal of
Addiction*, Vol. 62, pp. 5-18, 1967.

the system so that this was considered causal, to some significant degree, in bringing about the deviant event; this includes behaviors of those chronically heavy users who, even if at the moment of the deviant action were without alcohol, were supposed to have so behaved because of their "alcohol-determined" careers. Under this heading would come accidents, disease, death, crime, economic or familial disruption, and social shame, when these events are supposed to be connected with someone's consumption of alcohol.

The second class of "problems" concerns the means for dealing with such deviant acts and actors when those means are widely and long-lastingly inefficient, immoral, creative of further problems, or otherwise "bad." For example, jailing, gaining pledges of abstinence, psychoanalysis, failure of authorized agents to act, imposition of fines, or commitment to mental institutions might in a given society come to be widely considered as inefficient, silly, expensive, bad, or otherwise undesirable as means for dealing with drunken persons or with alcoholics. As one or more of these disapproved means persists, as people continue to "get drunk" and irritate or damage others, and as no substitute means for response are developed, social friction increases.

The third classification, also dealing with responses to the problem-causing uses of alcohol, concerns intended preventive actions within a society which in the long run prove inefficient, immoral, creative of new "problems," or otherwise provoking disapproval. Laws, systems of youth training, rules of etiquette or hygiene, fiscal policies, ethical codes, industrial personnel practices, etc., can include specific requirements, prohibitions, limitations, etc., on the use or availability of alcoholic beverages, or even on the expression of attitudes about them. As significant segments of a society over many years consider such attempts at long-range control to be "bad," social friction will ensue.

All three problems are represented in striking fashion in our own and in many other societies in relation to the use of alcoholic beverages. The only other specifically substantive usages which seem to have an equally widespread and continuing history of problems in our society would be weapons, money, modes of mass communication, and means for voting on political matters. For purposes of study, the distinction of these others from the phenomena of alcohol was indicated earlier: none of them possess the combination of assets listed (though they may well have unique assets of other types).

A few examples will indicate the scope and intensity of these problems in our society. The first type of problem is marked by behavioral disorder directly related to ingestion of alcohol or to a career distressed by "excessive" use. The following are usually cited: (1) the existence of about 5,000,000 alcoholics; (2) about half of the roughly 50,000 "accidental" deaths occurring annually on the highways involve significant amounts of alcohol in driver or victim; (3) perhaps a third of all patients in tuberculosis sanatoria have chronic problems with alcohol; (4) aside from minor traffic rule violations (as overtime parking), between half and two-thirds of all arrests made by police are directly related to alcohol.

The second type of problem concerns the continued exercise of responses to the deviation or deviator which are widely held to be at the least ineffective and frequently thought to be harmful or immoral in themselves. Among the more obvious of these commonly criticized means of immediate response are (1) the jailing of "drunks," (2) the avoidance of professional care or the lack of professional facilities for care and treatment of alcoholics, (3) either the use of license withdrawal, imprisonment, and fines to punish "drinker-drivers" or the failure of enforcement agencies so to act (neither course of action being regarded as effective or proper), (4) the social permissiveness frequently exhibited toward blatant drunkenness.

The third type of problem, namely, persistent and widely recognized inefficiency (if not worse) of standard means for long-range control, offers the most dramatic cases to those interested in social rather than individual phenomena: the century-old and continuing religious conflicts; the enormous, possibly unmatched, volume of law on the subject, frequently bizarre, and widely if not generally violated; the inept if not irrelevant educational programs in the schools; the unusual purposes, structure, and functioning of alcoholic beverage taxation; the long history of alleged (and often proved) graft, hypocrisy, avoidance, mislabeling, mass hostility, and futility in attempts at long-range control of problems related to alcohol. All these provide an almost inexhaustible source of case study in social pathology.

Not only for increasing understanding of individual and social behavior in general but also for increasing understanding of individual and social pathologies (including short- and long-range responses thereto), the subject matter comprising beverage alcohol, its use, and the sociocultural phenomena of drinking form an area of high relevance both for research as such and also for the development, implementation, and evaluation of social policy and social action. I do not suggest that this field of study is the "greatest" or comes "first" in some hierarchy of research subject matters in social science. Rather, I emphasize the special and in some ways unique assets of this field of study, and urge that if research and education should be directed toward particular customs (as contrasted to study of process, e.g., social maturation, or of structure, e.g., the family), then the constellation of practices dealing with alcohol and its use possesses a high, extraordinarily high, relevance. This viewpoint may be called an argument. It argues against the widespread influence of nihilists who deprecate or oppose both research and education, especially as they relate to social and human phenomena. It argues also against the failures of some researchers in our society (with recent exception of a score of sociologists), such as neurologists, experimental psychologists, political scientists, economists, etc., and against the structures which support such researchers, e.g., universities, foundations, industrial complexes, philanthropists, and (until some small action since 1965) the federal government, in having avoided this subject matter as if it were the plague.

Granted the relevance of alcohol and drinking as subject matter for research, why study "drinking in college"? What makes this category of drinking more or particularly relevant for development of understanding or for consideration of policy and action? Why not study Skid Row excessive drinkers, alcohol use in preliterate societies, or the bizarre legislation in our own society on alcohol beverages? There is no reason for not studying these and other topics within the wide scope of subject matter available under alcohol studies. It happens that the collegiate scene represents some particular values.

One of these values deals with a crucial age-grade, in our society a seven- or eight-year span, roughly from 15 to 22. This is when (for most of the population) the drinking custom becomes "available" to members of the society, is experimented with, talked about, anticipated, avoided, practiced, adopted, rejected, etc. Whether this starts at age 14 or 15 or doesn't start till 18 or 21, it includes the stage of inception and, thus, is especially relevant for the understanding of any custom. This is not presumed in a psychosocial sense (e.g., "as the twig is bent . . .," which may or may not be significant in a given life history) but in the sociological sense; namely, the places, times, amounts, types of beverage, accompanying acts, associates, attitudes, expectancies, and the like, will be, so to speak, experimented with, will be subjected to positive and negative responses of self and others. Rules, preferences, styles, emphases, avoidances and the like can be seen during the stage of inception in broad scope and in quantity as they emerge into patterns which, a few years later, may become quite narrow and rigid. If there are inconsistencies, difficulties and "friction points" in the structuring of a given social way, description of the stage of "taking on" such a way can provide a particularly effective tool for analysis.

School and college settings form naturally attractive arenas for study of this behavior in the 14–22 age grade. Although drop-outs and non-collegians clearly form necessary additional categories, both for a picture of the American scene as a whole and as essential "control" study populations, it is more difficult, time-consuming, and expensive to gain descriptions of these individuals. The high-school population has special assets in that this age-grade represents the "first trial period" for a majority of the population (whether they become users or abstainers) and because of the particular "social maturation" situation which usually involves the parental, neighborhood, peer group, school, and "adult world" pressures. The collegiate situation usually marks a physical separation from family and neighborhood influences and provides something similar to a fairly persistent total environment of a highly specialized community; the proportion of users, many of them "beginners," is considerably larger than in the high-school category.

In the collegiate setting the pertinent role of the educational institution is far greater than in the high-school which usually is held responsible for the behavior of students for only a few hours a day, five days a week, and can regard parents and other local groupings as the major agencies of modeling, sanctioning, and maintaining the social ways of the student body. At college, however, the situation is more like that of a quasi-sub-society in which "almost-adults" for about four years are in a setting characterized by potential status uncertainty: Are they still "children," are they participants in a viable culture, are they transients, are they frustrated adults? Students, parents, and functionaries of the college try different answers to these questions; real difficulties are encountered. In this situation the custom of abstaining from or using alcohol beverages—and, if using, "how"—can be seen in a multiplicity of phases and orientations. Although "alcoholism" is rare among students, the other problems, whether deviant behaviors, immediate responses, or preventive activities and programs, are all present. Although a microcosm, and a specialized one at that, the collegiate drinking scene represents an effectively available sample for analysis of much of the phenomena of alcoholic beverage use, attitudes, problems, and patterning of response to problems, in our society. And this particular phenomenon allows insight, often in unique fashion, into social and human phenomena in general.

However, what has preceded suggests values for the study of drinking in college only in terms of drinking. What about collegiality? Is this phenomenon worth study? And, if the answer should be affirmative, would the subject matter of drinking or abstinence provide an effective basis for such an analysis? Very much the same procedure that answered the question about drinking will answer this question. The perhaps amusing and certainly frightened nihilism of the newspaper columnist should not be overlooked; it may well represent the view of a major proportion of the population. The particular expression of that view was to the effect that the students were predetermined "good" or "bad" puppies, somewhat playfully going through a "natural" growth process in an environment which, hopefully, would be protected from meddling social analysts and "do-gooders." The style of the expression is relatively unimportant; the substance is to the effect that the collegiate experience (apart from the passage of time) is of no significance to the development of the person, and that studying the person or the collegiate process is pointless. Closely related to this opinion are beliefs that this sort of education is a "good" (or a "bad") thing, but it is not to be questioned or analyzed or altered—merely to be sustained (or eliminated).

A somewhat cynical viewpoint may be adopted about colleges—that the economy does not need these hundreds of thousands of potential jobholders, that families are not socially or emotionally geared to their continued living at home, and that this "holding operation" has come to possess such an enormous economic role in itself that any challenge to its continuation would be economic folly. This view I label as cynical because, despite peripheral relevance, it utterly fails to explain the quality or quantity of investment and clearly is intended to deprecate if not deny any constructive value.

The needs for technical knowledge in our society are obviously sufficient to explain the maintenance of training institutions, but that they would require either the number or type or duration characteristics of our current colleges is surely not manifest, if anything is manifestly ridiculous.

The more serious explanations of college education are usually couched in what may be termed the pre-scientific language of the humanities. I do not mean that the assumptions or logic or style of communication of these explanations are "improper" or "wrong." In fact, they seem more graceful, if not more mature, than the emerging "scientific" rationales. They are, however, inadequate by themselves for explaining social phenomena at this stage of history. For the institution of "higher education" this inadequacy seems peculiarly inappropriate. The use of refined definition, of observation of controlled representative data, of hypothesis formation, of empirical testing, of systematic questioning, need not be the "only" or "best" approach, but the absence of such an orientation in twentieth century American collegiate philosophy is difficult to justify.

Drinking, whether knowledge about it, facility in abstaining or in practice, or effectiveness in responding to personal or social problems related to it, is hardly the focus of any collegiate department. No so-called extracurricular programs of the administration are devoted to this activity. Some of the student organizations and ways involve drinking as a fairly significant activity, but in such instances a quasi-cloak of secrecy or of ridicule is frequently employed by all concerned, though sometimes strong criticism, even sanction by the college, community, or government may be invoked. The overall picture, however, is fairly clear: this is not an area of recognized social concern, leadership, training, education, or other major function of the American college. If anything, avoidance of consideration of the subject, broken only by occasional spurts of disapproval, is as characteristic of the college scene as it has been of American medicine, government, welfare, research, and religion.

We all now know that this network of behaviors and attitudes labeled "drinking" has major impact on and relationship to physiological, psychological, and social phenomena; that it has been directly related to almost every category of personal and social deviation; that it represents major social problems in immediate responses and in long-range programs of control and prevention. Does the college experience, curricular or other, have any impact on personal or social behavior in this sphere? *Could* any part of the college experience have any relevant measurable impact? Could it fail to have?

Just because the subject matter is *not* central to any planned collegiate program, it may be in some ways a more useful yardstick for evaluating those possible purposes or functions of college which are stated to transcend the goals of technical training. Does the curricular training (in physics, language, philosophy, mathematics, history, biology, fine arts, economics, etc.) have any measurable effect on the individual's behavior or attitudes about drinking, about how to deal or set policy for dealing with immediate problems, or for developing long-range controls? Does the relevant policy or does the relevant reality of college administration have any impact? Does the sort of drinking (or non-drinking) experienced at college have any measurable impact on later life?

If the answer could be "no," then two questions would arise: One, *could* the collegiate experience (whether through activation of relevant curricula, through administrative, student-life organization and practice devices) have a planned effect? Two, does the collegiate experience have any impact on any aspect (aside from possible technical abilities) of the graduate's life?

It might be more difficult to gain objective analysis of collegiate functioning in areas felt to be the responsibility or privilege of particular departments or programs than in areas avoided by all. Furthermore, the area of drinking (and abstaining) is felt to be of direct and continuing relevance to almost all American individuals; it has also been a matter of extensive and dramatic social import for more than a century. It seems likely that on this academically neutral yet both individually and socially significant phenomenon a testing of collegiate functioning would be both possible and useful. This would involve questions about the college not only in terms of the impact of formal teaching, but also in terms of administrative functioning and of extracurricular living.

The "so what" and "what next" of research on collegiate drinking may be viewed in the context of drinking in America, in the context of social science research, and in the context of collegiality. Relevant studies of the period 1949-1959 were significant as studies of alcohol and drinking, and should be viewed as fact-finding and exploratory in an area characterized by avoidance, ignorance and the consequent power of stereotypes, myths and special pleading. Merely to report on the extent of drinking in a factual fashion which could be (and was) subjected to validation, formed a contribution. To note further that most of this usage was not accompanied by social misadventure, was usually no secret to parents, but was even similar to their behavior and was reported to occur with their consent—this also contributed to a more mature and objective understanding. Perhaps the most obvious message of the first studies was that "drinking" was a social behavior, in many ways like all other social behaviors (e.g., learned, patterned, closely related to other modes of living); that it was not something unique, fearful, or to be reacted to as if apart from other experience, knowledge and feeling.

Some of the succeeding research remained primarily in the area of alcohol relevance, extending into studies of alcoholism, alcohol control laws, changing drinking patterns, and methods of teaching youth about alcohol; examples of all these are to be found in this volume.

But even in these studies, explicitly as well as by implication, a broader scope of relevance can be seen emerging. That further knowledge, insight, and questioning about alcohol and drinking can be productive both for research and policy purposes in the field itself can hardly be denied. The discrepancies between attitudes and behavior, between legislation and social reality, between educational doctrine (for youth or the public at large) and mass popular practice are dramatic; one of the authors in the present volume has even described the situation in the Old South in terms of "majority deviance." The whole sphere of the use of alcoholic beverages in our society is replete with social discrepancy, with unresolved problems, with personal suffering so extensive and persistent as to merit the term epidemic. Studies of drinking among those aged 14 to 22, perhaps with special emphasis on the collegiate setting, can be of direct value. But wider scope in relevance would seem a natural development.

If one is concerned with the operation of law or social rules, with situations which can be characterized as conflictful, with the process called deviation, with social structures and processes attempting to meet "social problems," then the phenomena of drinking, of alcohol-related problems, and of programs to cope with those problems can serve as effectively as any other subject matter for description, comparison, analysis and the development of verifiable hypotheses. The collegiate setting happens to provide an available and peculiarly

474 SELDEN D. BACON

appropriate model for such study. The relevance here is not alcohol and drinking problems as such. Rather they serve as a vehicle for the study of social pathology.

The other relevance concerns collegiality. It may be true that colleges, whether the administrators, teachers, or changing student bodies, could gain a great deal in dignity and efficiency, and diminish a great deal of pain, awkwardness, and bewilderment, if they learned something about drinking in college—learned about it in academically appropriate fashion. However, it seems possible that a greater relevance may emerge from the study of drinking in college, namely, the development of insight and of verifiable hypotheses about curricular teaching and about collegiate life as educational processes: Can measurable changes in attitude, in style of behavior, in capacities for reacting to personal and social questions and problems—changes significantly related to the factors of educational life—be identified? If so, can the limitations and potentialities of students, faculty, administration and situation be labeled, tested, and evaluated? As a vehicle for developing greater understanding of the collegiate process, the constellation of ideas and practices called "drinking" might well prove to be of extraordinary value. So far, the studies of drinking in college have been valuable chiefly in terms of knowledge and insight and policy development within the field of drinking itself. In the years to follow, such studies may well have even greater values for analysis of the whole gamut of social problems as well as for the emergence of more rational understanding and development of the American college.

Index

INDEX

Abstinence, 135ff; (Negro sample), 146ff, 163, 170ff

Abstinence, patterns of, 101-02

Abstinence and church affiliation, 268ff

Administration of regulations, 408ff

Administrators' drinking, 218ff

Adolescent drinking, 107ff, 177ff, 287ff

Age, legal, for drinking, 43, 388

Age and education factor, 86, 90-91

"Alcohol and College Youth" conference, 1965, 386ff

Alcohol as a drug, 165

Alcoholism, 16-17, 35, 224ff, 343ff

Alcoholism, adolescent risk of, 118-19

Alcoholism and education, 91ff

Alumni drinking, 218ff

Ambivalence, 147ff

American college drinking, 361ff

Anomie and permissiveness, 248ff

Anxiety and depression, 356

Armed forces experience, 35-36

Attitudes, church members', 268ff

Attitudes, students', 176ff

Attitudes toward drinking, 15ff, 20ff, 36ff, 107ff; toward society, 40ff

Automobiles and drinking, 42ff

Background, Negro sample's, 157ff

Behavioral effects, 33-34

Beverages drunk, 32

Bull sessions and other gatherings, 446ff

Carry-over drinking, 220ff

Change in drinking patterns, 194ff

Church affiliations and drinking, 268ff

Conference on "Alcohol and College Youth," 1965, 386ff

Conformity, norms of, 121ff

Courses about alcohol, 437ff, 451ff

Cultural norms and drinking pathology, 239ff

Data bases, 29

Dependency in alcoholism, 351ff

Depression and anxiety, 356

Deviant drinking behavior, 234ff

Double standards, 37-38, 193ff

Drinking, attitudes toward, 15ff, 20ff, 36ff, 107ff

Drinking, college, history of, 45ff

Drinking age, see Age, legal, for drinking

Drinking motivations, 17ff

Drinking prescribed, 234ff

Drinking problems for research, 457ff

Drinking profiles, 372ff

Drinking proscribed, 234ff

Drugs (other than alcohol), 41ff

Drunken driving, see Automobiles and drinking

Education about alcohol, 437ff, 451ff

Education and alcoholism, 91ff

Education and amount of alcohol consumed, 87ff; and heavy drinking, 91ff

Educational level and drinking, 81ff

Eighteenth Amendment, 56ff; repeal, 66-70

Enforcement of drinking rules, 425ff, 446

"Epidemic drinking," 70ff

"Escapist drinking," 388ff

Ethnic drinking, 34

Executives' drinking, 103, 218ff

Expectation and drinking, 326ff

"Facilitative drinking," 388ff

Faculty-Student drinking, 205ff

Finland, drinking in, 248-49, 361ff

Fraternity drinking, 142ff, 293ff, 314ff

Frequency patterns, 32-33, 292ff

477

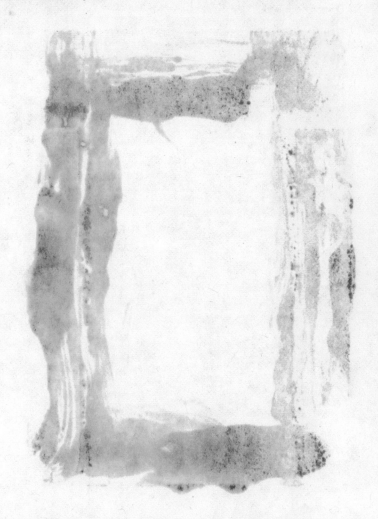